Meningococcal Disease

Meningococcal Disease

edited by
KEITH CARTWRIGHT
Public Health Laboratory, Gloucester, UK

JOHN WILEY & SONS
Chichester · New York · Brisbane · Toronto · Singapore

Other Wiley Editorial Offices

John Wiley & Sons, Inc., 605 Third Avenue,
New York, NY 10158-0012, USA

Jacaranda Wiley Ltd, 33 Park Road, Milton,
Queensland 4064, Australia

John Wiley & Sons (Canada) Ltd, 22 Worcester Road,
Rexdale, Ontario M9W 1L1, Canada

John Wiley & Sons (SEA) Pte Ltd, 37 Jalan Pemimpin #05-04,
Block B, Union Industrial Building, Singapore 2057

Library of Congress Cataloging-in-Publication Data

Meningococcal disease / edited by Keith Cartwright.
    p.   cm.
    Includes bibliographical references and index.
    ISBN 0–471–95259–1
    1. Meningitis, Cerebrospinal.   I. Cartwright, Keith.
    [DNLM: 1. Meningitis, Meningococcal.   WC 245 M545 1995]
    RC124.M46   1995
    616.8'2–dc20
    DNLM/DLC
    for Library of Congress   94–32088
                                                                  CIP

British Library Cataloguing in Publication Data

A catalogue record for this book is available from the British Library

ISBN 0 471 95259 1

Typeset in 11/12pt Palatino by Vision Typesetting, Manchester
Printed and bound in Great Britain by Biddles Ltd, Guildford

Contents

Contributors

Mark Achtman DSc, PhD
Senior Lecturer, Max-Planck Institut für molekulare Genetik, Ihnestrasse 73, 14195 Berlin, Germany

Norman Begg MFPHM
Deputy Director, PHLS Communicable Disease Surveillance Centre, 61 Colindale Avenue, London NW9 5EQ, UK

Petter Brandtzaeg MD, PhD
Consultant Paediatrician, Department of Pediatrics, Ullevål University Hospital, N-0407 Oslo, Norway

Keith Cartwright MA, FRCPath
Director, Public Health Laboratory, Gloucestershire Royal Hospital, Great Western Road, Gloucester GL1 3NN, UK

Carl E. Frasch PhD
Chief, Bacterial Polysaccharides Laboratory, Division of Bacterial Products, HFM-428, Center for Biologics Evaluation and Research, 8800 Rockville Pike, Bethesda, Maryland, USA 20892

J. McLeod Griffiss MD
Professor, Centre for Immunochemistry and Department of Laboratory Medicine, University of California San Francisco, San Francisco, California, USA

Parviz Habibi PhD, MRCP
Senior Lecturer, Department of Paediatrics, St Mary's Hospital Medical School, London W2 1NY, UK

Dennis M. Jones MD, FRCPath, Dip Bact
Director, Meningococcal Reference Unit, Public Health Laboratory, Withington Hospital, Manchester M20 8LR, UK

Michael Levin PhD, FRCP
Professor of Paediatrics, St Mary's Hospital Medical School, London W2 1NY, UK

Peter A. van der Ley PhD
Head, Department of Molecular Biology, Laboratory of Vaccine Development and Immune Mechanisms, National Institute of Public Health and Environmental Protection, Bilthoven, The Netherlands

Simon Nadel MRCP
Meningitis Research Appeal Lecturer, Department of Paediatrics, St Mary's Hospital Medical School, London W2 1NY, UK

Jan T. Poolman PhD
Head, Laboratory of Vaccine Development and Immune Mechanisms, National Institute of Public Health and Environmental Protection, Bilthoven, The Netherlands

Neil Steven MRCP
Senior Registrar, Department of Infection and Tropical Medicine, Birmingham Heartlands Hospital, Birmingham B9 5ST, UK

J. Tommassen PhD
Associate Professor, Department of Molecular Cell Biology, University of Utrecht, The Netherlands

Martin Wood FRCP
Consultant Physician, Department of Infection and Tropical Medicine, Birmingham Heartlands Hospital, Birmingham B9 5ST, UK

1
Introduction and Historical Aspects

KEITH CARTWRIGHT
Public Health Laboratory, Gloucester, UK

INTRODUCTION

Why does meningococcal disease excite such interest in health professionals and in the general public? A number of factors may contribute. *Neisseria meningitidis* is the commonest cause of bacterial meningitis in the Western world, markedly so in those countries which have introduced national immunisation programmes against *Haemophilus influenzae* type b (Hib) disease. Mortality in meningococcal disease as a whole (both meningitis and septicaemia) is considerably higher than in Hib disease (though there is probably little difference in mortality in *meningitis* caused by the two organisms). Unlike Hib infections, which are essentially sporadic, outbreaks and epidemics of meningococcal disease occur throughout the world, providing visible evidence of bacterial transmissibility from person to person. It is a source of considerable frustration that, though we can treat individual cases with antibiotics, usually with great success, we cannot as yet influence the epidemiology of the disease.

For doctors and epidemiologists, it is a paradoxical and mystifying infection. After almost two hundred years of observation and research we know much about the transmission of the organism from person to person, about the different types of outcome which may result and their underlying pathophysiology. We know a little about immunity to systemic infection and about variations in meningococcal virulence. Yet we are unable to explain why one particular individual, on acquiring a meningococcus, develops invasive disease whereas several hundred others acquiring the same strain do not. We do not understand why sub-Saharan Africa

Meningococcal Disease. Edited by Keith Cartwright © 1995 John Wiley & Sons Ltd

experiences epidemic waves every 5–10 years[1], nor why serogroup A infections predominate in this part of the world, yet when introduced into Europe and the United States, fail to spread[2]. We do not know why serogroup A disease, once common in Europe and the United States, is now very rare. We do not know why outbreaks start, nor how to bring them to an end. Following an upsurge of serogroup C disease in eastern Canada in the winter of 1991–2, some provinces adopted a policy of mass vaccination in target population groups, whereas others did not. The incidence of serogroup C disease declined in both the vaccinating and the non-vaccinating provinces!

Meningitis or septicaemia in a young child is a terrifying experience for the whole family. When septicaemia occurs, the rapid onset makes this a medical emergency; the sense of urgency in the medical and nursing attendants transmits itself easily to the anxious parents of a sick child. Fulminant infection leading to the death of a child can be devastating for the parents, who may be overwhelmed with guilt as well as with sorrow. The need to give treatment to the close family in an attempt to prevent further cases only adds to the pressures on the family. Chemoprophylaxis and vaccination of family contacts needs to be handled with great sensitivity to avoid parents feeling that they have been responsible for passing on infection to their child. Parents remain worried that other children in the family will fall ill.

Sometimes school friends and neighbours who do not understand the ubiquitous distribution of meningococci amongst children and young adults may shun a family where there has been a case, for fear of infection. Many doctors and nurses are also concerned about the risk of becoming infected, or of passing on infection to their own families when they are involved in the management of a case in hospital. Most UK hospitals operate a policy of isolation of cases for at least the first 24 hours, but as 20% or more of the attending nurses and hospital doctors are likely to be colonised with meningococci, the only logic in this precaution is to guard against the possibility that the index case may be infected with a more than usually virulent strain.

Though communication between health professionals and affected families has improved greatly, it still has far to go. Meningitis charities, such as the UK National Meningitis Trust* have an important role to play in supporting affected families, providing additional information, counselling and encouraging contact with other affected parents.

Communication between public health medicine specialists and the communities they serve has also improved with the realisation that widespread public alarm after one or more cases of meningococcal disease

---

*National Meningitis Trust, Fern House, Bath Road, Stroud, Glos. GL5 3TJ, UK.

(sometimes fuelled by inaccurate or sensationalist journalism) is best allayed by dissemination of as much information as possible about the disease. Alarm rises quite disproportionately if deaths occur, particularly in teenagers who have wider circles of friends than very young children. A death in a teenager attending a large school will be communicated informally to all pupils and teachers within a few hours.

Information issued by public health authorities must be accurate. When cases of meningococcal disease are occurring within a community there is an added advantage in raising awareness. Widespread familiarity with the early symptoms and in particular, an explanation of the significance of a haemorrhagic rash accompanied by fever, may save lives by permitting early recognition and early treatment of incipient disease[3]. A woman recently admitted to my hospital with fatal meningococcal septicaemia had not sought medical assistance for four days after the onset of her severe haemorrhagic meningococcal rash, thinking that she was experiencing an allergic reaction to a garden plant. Early treatment might well have saved her life.

EARLY HISTORICAL ASPECTS—EPIDEMIC MENINGITIS AND 'SPOTTED FEVER'

'Spotted fevers' were relatively common in times past. Typhoid, typhus, other rickettsial infections, perhaps streptococcal infections and even syphilis would have been difficult at times to differentiate from meningococcal infection. The most easily identifiable features of meningococcal disease are its haemorrhagic rash and the propensity for cases to occur in clusters or as large-scale outbreaks. It is most unlikely that the disease is a new one; Hippocrates described headache and tinnitus in association with inflammation of the brain, noting the high mortality of the condition. Other early physicians such as Galen and Rhazes also apparently recognised meningitis.

Thomas Willis (1621–75), an English physician, was probably the first to report an outbreak of cerebrospinal fever[4], though Vieusseux, a skilled Swiss physician, is usually credited with the first clear account of the disease in modern times. He described an outbreak of epidemic meningitis in Geneva and its environs in March 1805[5]. The outbreak began on the left bank of Lake Geneva in the suburb of Eaux-Vives and later became more widespread throughout the city. There were 33 recorded deaths. Viesseux noted symptoms of violent headache, vomiting, stiffness of the spine, and livid patches on the skin in some cases. The pathological findings in some of the fatal cases were described clearly by Matthey, a local pathologist, who found pus at the base of the brain, congestion of the meningeal vessels and a bloodstained gelatinous exudate over the surface of the brain.

In the following year came the first formal description of an outbreak in the New World, at Medfield, Massachusetts, USA[6]. Meningococcal disease spread throughout New England and elsewhere in the eastern United States and Canada over the next ten years. In describing the early part of this prolonged outbreak, North wrote the first treatise on cerebrospinal meningitis[7]. In it, he recommended the use of the thermometer, not widely employed at the time, and he popularised 'spotted fever' as a descriptive term for cerebrospinal fever.

MENINGOCOCCAL DISEASE IN THE 19TH CENTURY

Outbreaks and early clinical descriptions

Once recognised as a disease entity on both sides of the Atlantic, descriptions of outbreaks came thick and fast from both Europe and the United States. Amongst the more notable were outbreaks in Lippisch, near Danzig, where an astonishing attack rate of 1 250 per 10 000 was recorded, and large-scale outbreaks in both the civil and military populations of Dublin in 1866–7 and again in 1885–6. August Hirsch compiled comprehensive and detailed descriptions of those outbreaks published in the medical literature from 1805 to 1882[8]. Subsequently, Netter and Debré supplemented Hirsch's work and updated the record of outbreaks to 1911[9].

The clinical characteristics of the disease came to be clearly recognised during the first half of the 19th century, as well as its contagious nature, though the cause was at that time unknown. The predilection of the disease for the military was an early observation; for example, an epidemic in France during the 1840s began in the south west of the country and spread northwards, apparently in association with the movements of one particular regiment (the 18th).

The sudden onset of meningococcal disease, the extremely high mortality, the capacity to infect most members of a family within a few days, and the lack of any specific treatment combined to make it a dreaded affliction. There are few, if any, practising clinicians today who worked in the pre-antibiotic era, and it is therefore hard for us to grasp the impact which the disease must have had on small communities at this time. Several accounts of family outbreaks in which most members died within the course of a few days attest to the severity of the disease and the thrall in which it must have been held.

Stillé, Professor of Medicine at the University of Pennsylvania, wrote a monograph on meningitis following his experiences during an epidemic in Philadelphia[10]. He attributed the lack of clear-cut clinical descriptions of the disease to a failure to distinguish it from typhus, the other prevalent 'spotted fever' of the 18th and earlier centuries. (In this context it is interesting to note that both diseases have a predilection for the military, and that both can occur as outbreaks.) The frustrations of not being able to offer specific treatment are apparent. Remedies of the time included emetics (also recommended earlier by Vieusseux), cold to the head, blistering of head, neck and spinal column, alcohol, opiates, quinine, mercurials, potassium iodide, belladonna and ergot. Clearly, most compounds known to possess any pharmacological activity were tried. Mortality remained very high.

First isolation of the meningococcus

With the rapid progression of laboratory methods and the evolution of bacteriology from an art into a science in the last quarter of the 19th century, pathologists made repeated attempts to isolate an organism from patients who had died of meningitis. A plethora of reports in the medical literature describe the varied microscopical findings, but the fastidious meningococcus eluded attempts at culture for several years. Some workers found no organisms in cerebrospinal fluid; others described organisms resembling pneumococci. Marchiafava and Celli saw and described oval micrococci within the cytoplasm of leucocytes—almost certainly meningococci; cultures were, however, negative[11].

The breakthrough came in 1887 when Anton Weichselbaum, working in Vienna, isolated an organism (which he called *diplococcus intracellularis meningitidis*) from the meningeal exudate of six out of eight cases of primary, sporadic meningitis. He isolated a pneumococcus from the other two cases and was therefore cautious in his interpretation of these findings[12].

The waters were immediately muddied by Jaeger who, on investigating a small epidemic of meningitis in a military garrison in Stuttgart, reported an intracellular bacterium which resembled Weichselbaum's oval micrococcus on microscopy. Cultures, however, yielded a gram-positive chaining coccus (presumably a streptococcus)[13]. In retrospect, Jaeger's microscopic findings were probably correct, but the organism he isolated was likely to have been a culture contaminant, a common laboratory problem at that time. There were supporters of both men and confusion reigned for some time, but eventually a series of further reports were published confirming Weichselbaum's findings and establishing firmly the association between the meningococcus and cerebrospinal fever.

Lumbar puncture

Eight years after Weichselbaum's report came the first account of lumbar puncture in the living patient[14]. Shortly after, meningococci were isolated for the first time from the cerebrospinal fluid of patients acutely ill with meningitis[15]. Isolation of the causative organism and the introduction of lumbar puncture as a routine clinical procedure paved the way for intraspinal immunotherapy in the early years of the new century. At about the same time the epidemiology of meningococcal disease was advanced crucially by the first demonstration that patients with meningococcal meningitis could also carry the germ in the oropharynx[16].

MENINGOCOCCAL DISEASE IN THE 20TH CENTURY

Immunotherapy—the first effective treatment

That there was an urgent need for further work on the meningococcus was driven home forcibly by the large epidemics of disease which broke out in the early years of the new century—in New York in 1904–5 and in eastern Germany in 1905–7. At this time, bacteriologists in Germany and in the United States were working almost simultaneously on the development of anti-meningococcal sera. The German workers first showed that rabbits and horses immunised with meningococci developed agglutinating antibodies. They then developed a crude animal model of infection in the guinea pig, in which they were able to demonstrate protection by the prior injection of their immune horse serum[17]. This led to the first human trials of the new serum in meningococcal meningitis. The first injections were given subcutaneously, with subsequent doses administered by intraspinal instillation[18]. Twelve of seventeen treated cases survived—excellent results when compared with the mortality of 70–80% which was common at that time.

Simon Flexner and James Jobling, of the Rockefeller Institute, New York, were working in parallel with the German team. As well as developing their own immune serum, they were responsible for demonstrating clearly the value of immunotherapy and in particular, the benefit of the intraspinal route. By 1908 they were able to report a series of 400 cases from Europe and the USA who had been treated with the Flexner anti-meningitis serum and in whom the overall mortality was 25%[19]. There were complications of this novel and highly effective form of treatment[20]—up to half the patients developed 'serum disease' with fever, skin eruptions, arthritis and digestive disturbances. Secondary (fatal) bacterial meningitis caused by introduction of extraneous bacteria into the subarachnoid space was recorded occasionally. However, intraspinal immunotherapy remained in use until the 1930s, when it was superseded by the introduction of the sulphonamides.

Supra-renal apoplexy—the Waterhouse–Friderichsen syndrome

Rupert Waterhouse, a physician working in Bath, UK, was the first to report (in 1911) a case of 'supra-renal apoplexy'(haemorrhage into the adrenals) on post-mortem examination of a fatal case of fulminant meningococcal septicaemia[21]. This was followed by the report of a series of similar cases by

Friderichsen in Copenhagen in 1918[22]. The existence and importance of the syndrome have since been called into question, but the Waterhouse–Friderichsen syndrome was a term widely used to describe fulminant meningococcal sepsis until the recent past.

Notification of infections

Compulsory notification of infectious diseases was introduced in a piecemeal fashion in the UK in the early years of the century. Its value was soon recognised, and a formal notification system was in place in many cities by 1906, in time to assist in the more accurate documentation of substantial outbreaks of cerebrospinal fever in Glasgow in 1906–7 and in Belfast in 1907–8. Meningococcal disease in the UK at this time appeared to be a particular problem in large cities, perhaps associated with poverty and overcrowding.

Nationwide compulsory notification of many infectious diseases, including cerebrospinal fever, was introduced in Britain in September 1912. During the following three years (1912–14) there was little meningococcal disease activity; annual numbers of notified cases in England and Wales varied from 87 to 315, whereas in the first full year of World War I (1915) there were 3496 notified cases. Though the annual numbers of notified cases then declined, they remained high for the remainder of the war.

The Great War 1914–18

Meningococcal disease at the start of the war

The predilection of meningococcal disease for the military had been noted on many occasions throughout the 19th century in France[8]. It had also been recognised that when outbreaks occurred, for example, amongst garrison troops, the disease often appeared to spill over into the adjacent civilian population[9].

There is always a tendency for outbreaks of infection to be blamed on others. In the past, the French have referred to syphilis as the 'English disease', whereas the English used to describe it as the 'French disease'! (With increasing scientific sophistication one might have expected less xenophobia, but more recently influenza has been commonly described as 'Asian flu', and Haitians were held responsible, at least in part, for the introduction of AIDS into the USA in the early 1980s.)

When cases of cerebrospinal fever began to occur in British and colonial army recruits in the winter of 1914–15, the Medical Research Committee's Special Advisory Committee suggested that the causative organism was a new strain of meningococcus introduced into the UK by Canadian troops.

There had been cases of cerebrospinal fever amongst the Canadian recruits in their camp at Valcartier prior to embarkation, and during the Atlantic crossing[23]. However, there had also been cases of the disease in British troops[23,24]. The causative strains appeared similar and there is no good evidence to suggest that Canadian troops introduced disease into the UK. (Not surprisingly, the accusation is refuted vigorously by Adami, the Canadian war historian.)

Britain and Canada were not the only combatant nations to experience outbreaks of cerebrospinal fever. There were cases in Australian and New Zealand troops[23], both in recruit mustering camps in the Antipodes and on board ship in transit to England. There were also increased disease rates in Germany in 1915[25], and numerous outbreaks in US recruit training camps in 1917[26]. It was known at the time that high disease rates occurred amongst new recruits, and that once training had been completed, the disease rate in seasoned troops declined to a more normal level, so that meningococcal disease was much less of a problem in troops in the field. Cerebrospinal fever in naval recruits followed the same pattern. Three cases out of four occurred in personnel at shore-based establishments and there were few cases amongst sailors on board sea-going ships.

In Britain, the winter of 1914 was unusually wet—unhappily so for the massive influx of new recruits who spent the winter under canvas owing to shortages of barracks and accommodation. Cases of cerebrospinal fever began to occur increasingly frequently with outbreaks at Portsmouth, Winchester, and in particular, amongst troops stationed on Salisbury Plain for final training[27]. (The impact of the disease, and the added misery caused by quarantining of contacts, were sufficient for cerebrospinal fever to be included in fictional accounts of the period[28] as well as in the official records.)

Investigations at the Guards Depot, Caterham, London

As the war progressed, troop losses, particularly on the Western Front, mounted inexorably. To make good the enormous manpower requirements of the New Armies the numbers of new recruits at training depots increased to many times the normal peacetime levels. Against this background, a substantial programme of investigation into cerebrospinal fever was carried out at the Guards Depot, Caterham, in South London, led by Captain JA Glover of the Royal Army Medical Corps (RAMC)[29].

Recruits for the five regiments of Foot Guards were trained at the Caterham Depot. From a peacetime establishment of 800 the total number of troops stationed within the Depot rose to over 13 000 at times of maximum overcrowding; the extra recruits were accommodated in huts and in tents in addition to the permanent barracks.

Peacetime accommodation standards for the British Army had been established in 1861, at the time of the Crimean War. It was decreed then that each soldier should have 60 square feet of floor space, 600 cubic feet of air space, and that beds should be separated by a minimum distance of 3 feet. At times of extreme pressure at Caterham, the distances between beds were less than 6 inches. (In later years the British military authorities decided that when severe overcrowding became necessary, troops should sleep alternately head to foot.) Glover found a close correlation between the periods of severe overcrowding and the meningococcal carrier rate (Figure 1.1). He also showed that in this environment, higher carriage rates were associated with the development of cases of disease. Small outbreaks associated with periods of extreme overcrowding occurred at the Depot in each of the first three winters of the War but were controlled by the end of 1918.

Preventive measures

A number of practical measures were implemented in an attempt to reduce carriage rates (and thereby, it was hoped, cases of cerebrospinal fever); these included spacing out of sleeping accommodation, fixing open of windows in huts, shortening of parades and deferral of typhoid inoculation (enteric fever was another scourge of the Army at war) until the second month of training. Meningococcal carriers were treated by inhalation of 1% zinc sulphate solution. A final small outbreak of disease, again heralded by a sudden rise in the carrier rate, occurred in May 1917, but was managed by the deployment of emergency tentage to create more sleeping space.

After the implementation of these various measures the winter of

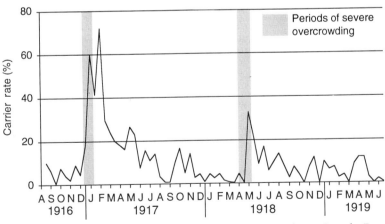

Figure 1.1 *Meningococcal carrier rate in recruits, Caterham Guards Depot, August 1916 to June 1919. After Glover[29] (reproduced with permission)*

1917–18 was the first in which the Depot was free of meningococcal disease. The policy of enforcing adequate sleeping space was so successful that when the first wave of influenza passed through the Depot in July 1918 (4000 cases and 15 deaths) there were only two cases of cerebrospinal fever. Meningococcal disease had been controlled by the application of simple epidemiological principles.

The sceptic will read Glover's lucid and compelling account and will note the lack of controls, of multivariate analysis and of meningococcal strain discrimination. The epidemiologist may acknowledge these deficiencies but will recognise the dedication and skill which went into this long and detailed study. Though the conclusions have since been called into question, the study stands as an early classic of meningococcal epidemiology. It may well be that Glover's findings, of an association between rapid rises in rates of meningococcal acquisition (as well as high rates of carriage) and subsequent development of cases of disease, may be perfectly valid. The circumstances under which he carried out his study are so unusual that they are unlikely ever to be repeated.

The first meningococcal classification systems

Glover's epidemiological investigations were supported by parallel developments in the laboratory. In 1915 MH Gordon and EG Murray, RAMC microbiologists, published a system of meningococcal classification based on antisera raised in rabbits[30]. Their scheme, which divided meningococci into four groups (I, II, III and IV), was adopted widely in English-speaking countries* only falling into disuse in 1950 (see below). Other systems were devised elsewhere, the French scheme[31] becoming popular in continental Europe. Most cases of meningococcal disease in the Great War were due to strains of groups I and III (now known as serogroup A). Group IV has remained a rarity since the time it was first defined.

In 1950, a new meningococcal nomenclature based on the French system was agreed by a committee of the International Association of Microbiologists; the new classification has been used ever since. The relationships between the classification schemes are set out in Table 1.1. All the major outbreaks described between 1914 and 1945 were due to strains which we would now designate as serogroup A.

---

* In researching this historical section in the Wellcome Institute for the History of Medicine, I encountered a copy of *Meningococcus Meningitis* written in 1913 by Heiman and Feldstein, two New York paediatricians. The book had been purchased in 1915 by Mervyn (MH) Gordon and contained his marginal notes. To read his (sometimes trenchant) comments created an unexpected and pleasurable link with a meningococcal enthusiast of the past!

Table 1.1   Relationships between historical and present-day classifications of meningococcal serogroups

Gordon and Murray[30]	1915	I	II	III	IV		
Nicolle, Debains, Jouan[31]	1918	A	B	—	—	C	D
Common use since	1940	I	II	I	IV	II	
Recommended by Committee	1950	A	B	A	D	C	

The inter-war period (1919–39)

With the end of the Great War interest in meningococcal disease subsided, only to be re-awakened by the advent of large epidemics affecting both the USA and Canada in the late 1920s. These outbreaks, peaking in 1929, once more predominantly affected city-dwellers[32,33]. Most infections were again due to group I (serogroup A) organisms, though as the epidemic settled, group II (serogroup B) strains began to be isolated more frequently. Soon after the decline of the 1928–29 epidemic, Geoffrey Rake, in a series of detailed experiments, demonstrated the presence of capsules on freshly isolated meningococci[34] and established the significance of 'smooth' and 'rough' colonies. This led to the use of fresh, capsulated meningococci in the preparation of therapeutic antisera, leading to an improvement in efficacy. Two years later Rake and Scherp reported that the group I capsule was composed of polysaccharide[35]. Rake also carried out studies to determine the duration of meningococcal carriage, and showed that though very variable, oropharyngeal carriage could be prolonged over many months.

In her excellent historical review[36], Branham noted that the intensity of work on many aspects of meningococcal infection increased substantially during the decade of the 1930s, reflecting the rapid advances in biology, bacteriology and immunology which were being made at the time. It was recognised that Gordon and Murray's group I and group III strains were so closely related that it was impractical to distinguish them. Laybourn[33], and subsequently others, showed that high meningococcal carriage rates were not necessarily related to the incidence of meningococcal disease. The development of a reproducible animal model of infection[37] allowed confirmation of the long-suspected variability of meningococcal virulence, effectively removing the logic for swabbing surveys as a means of predicting meningococcal disease activity.

First use of sulphonamides

The development of an animal model also occurred at exactly the right time to permit the evaluation of the first group of specific antimicrobial agents—the sulphonamides. The successful result of the first tests of sulphonamides in preventing meningococcal infections in mice were reported in *The Lancet* in 1936[38] and in the following year Schwentker published his account of successful treatment of human infections with sulphanilamide (Prontosil)[39,40]. In 1939 Long reported still better results with sulphapyridine, also known as M & B 693[41].

World War II

Large outbreaks in combatant countries

The new antimicrobials, which were active against many bacterial pathogens, fortunately became widely available in time to be used in the large outbreaks of meningococcal meningitis which occurred in combatant countries during mobilisation at the outset of World War II. These outbreaks were by far the largest to be recorded in recent times. In 1940 there were more than 12 000 notified cases in Britain (as opposed to a peak of 3500 notified cases in the Great War), over 6000 cases in Germany and comparable or larger increases in disease rates in other involved countries, including Norway, Denmark, France, the Benelux countries, Austria[42] and Australia and New Zealand[42,43]. Interestingly, Sweden, a neutral country, did not experience a major epidemic in 1940[25], though Switzerland did.

The USA, which did not enter the war until December 1941, experienced an epidemic of comparable size to the European outbreaks, but peaking later, at 18 000 cases, in 1943. In most of the affected countries the epidemic died away only slowly. In Britain there were 11 000 notified cases of meningococcal meningitis in 1941 and more than 2000 cases in each subsequent year up to 1945.

Spread of the disease within communities

As in the Great War, meningitis selectively picked out recruit camps, particularly affecting new drafts[44] (Figure 1.2) and was uncommon in troops who had completed their basic training. However, whereas in the Great War the military were relatively more severely affected, the World War II epidemic was primarily a civilian one, both in the USA[44] and in the UK[45]. At the start of the 1940 outbreak in Britain, there was some evidence that the disease flared up first in recruit camps, later spilling over into the civilian population; several cases occurred in the families of soldiers home on leave (the same phenomenon had been observed in the Great War[46]). Early in 1940, attack rates were highest in areas where troops and evacuees made up substantial proportions of the population[45], but this pattern disappeared later in the year as infection became widespread, as it then remained for the rest of the war.

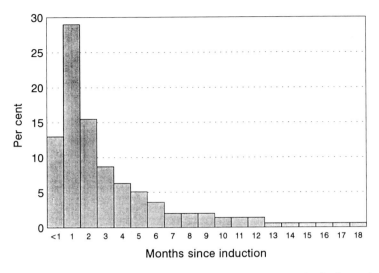

Figure 1.2   *Meningococcal infections in US military recruits. The high attack rate in new recruits is probably due to the continuous influx of new susceptibles, and to a high acquisition rate. After Phair[44] (reproduced with permission)*

Effective treatment—sulphonamides

Sulphonamides provided the mainstay of specific treatment during the war years. When sulpha drugs were first introduced, combination treatment with immune serum was regarded as optimal, but by 1939 Stanley Banks had demonstrated the superiority of sulphonamide treatment alone[47]. Meningococcal meningitis was so prevalent in the early war years that large series of successfully treated cases could be accrued and published[48]. The introduction of sulphonamides had a dramatic effect on mortality in meningococcal meningitis (Figure 1.3). Sulphonamides were also used for the first time during the war to treat successfully meningococcal nasopharyngeal carriage[49]. Then as now, no prospective placebo-controlled trials were undertaken to establish whether such treatment actually reduces the incidence of meningococcal disease in contacts, or whether it merely reduces nasopharyngeal colonisation for a period.

Penicillin

Later in World War II, penicillin became available following Fleming's 1929 discovery[50] and the subsequent purification of the active agent by Florey and Chain. Though penicillin is the antibiotic of choice today, sulphonamides remained in widespread use for the treatment of meningococcal meningitis

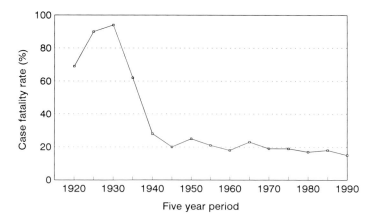

Figure 1.3   Case fatality rate in meningococcal disease in England and Wales, 1916–90. Five year average mortality. Sulphonamides for treatment of meningococcal disease were introduced in 1939, following during World War II by the introduction of penicillin. Data derived from UK Office of Population Census and Surveys figures

for many years. Disappointingly, there has been little further improvement in mortality rates since the end of World War II (Figure 1.3).

Case fatality rates

Though Figure 1.3 gives a fair representation of trends in meningococcal disease case fatality rates over time, the absolute rates in each five year period should be treated with some caution. Many clinical cases of meningococcal disease are not confirmed and may not be reported; it is known that there is substantial under-notification of meningococcal disease, even when the diagnosis has been confirmed in the laboratory. Over the time period covered by Figure 1.3 the precise disease condition to be notified has changed several times—in the 1970s, meningococcal meningitis alone (and not meningococcal septicaemia) was notifiable. Though hard to prove formally, most epidemiologists believe that deaths from meningococcal disease are notified more efficiently than surviving cases. Therefore, in recent years at least, the case fatality rate has probably been much lower than the level shown.

THE POST-WAR YEARS

Whether because of the introduction of polysaccharide vaccination for US military recruits (and, much later, for the UK armed forces as well), or for other less obvious reasons, meningococcal disease has been rather less of a problem for the military since the end of World War II. In the Korean war, for example, there were only seven cases of meningitis in US combatant troops in the war zone[51]. However, meningococcal disease in US army recruits did become a problem again in the Vietnam war. The responsible strains were frequently sulphonamide resistant, obviating the use of this agent for widespread prophylaxis.

The pace of work on the meningococcus has not slowed since 1945, but the great majority of the important advances occurring during this final period are described in the individual chapters. It is perhaps invidious to single out three such developments which have increased our understanding of, or have altered the way in which we manage, meningococcal disease. If one were to do so, one might pick out the series of classical immunological studies of Emil Gotschlich and his colleagues in the late 1960s[52-56], in which the inverse relationship between the presence of bactericidal antibodies and the risk of subsequent meningococcal disease was so elegantly demonstrated, and which were associated with the development of the first purified polysaccharide vaccines; the phenomenally rapid development of molecular biology, permitting a start to be made on the unravelling of meningococcal genetics, and the equally rapid progress in both immunology and in protein and polysaccharide chemistry. These advances underpinned the development of the first conjugated meningococcal vaccines—vaccines which may give lifelong protection against meningococcal disease.

MENINGOCOCCAL DISEASE TODAY

Outbreaks continue to occur throughout the world. At the time of writing, a large epidemic in Burundi, in east central Africa, has just been reported with peak attack rates of 612 per 100,000 population in the worst affected province[57], Canada has just experienced a (much smaller) wave of hyperendemic disease, as has the UK. Though we can now treat the majority of individual cases successfully, we remain unable to control the disease itself. We cannot even agree on the best way to use vaccines and chemoprophylactic antibiotics!

There are further causes for concern. Though meningococci, unlike gonococci, remain almost uniformly sensitive to penicillin, the slight but progressive decrease in penicillin susceptibility observed in British clinical isolates over the last 4–5 years is a trend that needs careful monitoring. More worrying still is the demonstration that genes encoding β-lactamases can be inserted into meningococci *in vitro*, and the (thus far unconfirmed) reports from South Africa[58] and Spain[59] of β-lactamase producing clinical isolates.

Improved understanding of the pathological processes in meningococcal disease has confirmed the prime importance of endotoxin and the inflammatory cascade which it provokes, in determining the outcome in meningococcal disease. However, despite rapid advances in immunology and indeed across the broad front of biological sciences, a new generation of sophisticated immunomodulating agents has yet to be shown to have any effect on mortality in meningococcal disease.

Vaccines

Interest in vaccines, as in all other aspects of meningococcal disease, has waxed and waned over the years. In Chapter 10, Carl Frasch presents a detailed account of the history of the development of meningococcal vaccines up to the present day. He puts into accurate perspective the prospects for effective control of meningococcal disease by vaccination.

The outstanding success of conjugated protein–polysaccharide vaccines in preventing Hib disease in Finland, the USA and the UK offers hope that conjugated meningococcal serogroup A and C vaccines which are now entering clinical trials will be as effective, protecting even young infants and giving long-term immunity without the need for booster doses. Though recent trials of serogroup B outer membrane vesicle vaccines in Norway and Brazil have been somewhat disappointing, this is but one of several different approaches to the development of vaccines for serogroup B disease. One hundred years after the first isolation of the meningococcus, it is hard to escape a sense of optimism that its demise as a human pathogen may now, at last, be imminent.

ACKNOWLEDGEMENTS

Literature reviews are so much a part of today's medical practice that any work of significance is certain to be scrutinised and evaluated, often repeatedly. This was not the case in the last century, when the reviewer was faced with a formidable organisational and linguistic task in bringing together the accrued knowledge about a particular specialist area. The 19th century literature on meningococcal disease is distributed about equally between French, German and English language publications, and some articles are now difficult or impossible to obtain. Any new account of meningococcal disease must therefore depend heavily on the work of previous historians. In compiling this chapter, I am indebted to those who have reviewed the historical aspects of this fascinating disease in past years. Without their detailed research, early references would undoubtedly have been lost forever.

I also owe my thanks to staff at the library of the Wellcome Institute, London, and to Margaret Clennett and her colleagues at the PHLS Library,

Colindale, London, who located (usually almost immediately) many references over 100 years old. Dr Dennis Jones, Manchester Public Health Laboratory, very kindly made available to me his collection of historical references. The comprehensive review of meningococcal disease by Neylan Vedros and his expert contributors in the two-volume *Evolution of Meningococcal Disease*[60] has made the preparation of this book far easier, but at the same time, has set a standard that is hard to equal. I hope readers will find as much to interest and enthuse them in this book as I have found in Vedros' work.

REFERENCES

1. Moore PS. Meningococcal meningitis in sub-Saharan Africa: a model for the epidemic process. Clin Infect Dis 1992; *14*: 515–25.
2. Moore, PS, Harrison LH, Telzak EE, Ajello GW, Broome CV. Group A meningococcal carriage in travelers returning from Saudi Arabia. JAMA 1988; *260*: 2686–9.
3. Thompson APJ, Hayhurst GK. Press publicity in meningococcal disease. Arch Dis Child 1993; *69*: 166–9.
4. Willis T. A description of an epidemical feaver in 1661. In: *Practice of physick*. London: T Dring, 1684, Treatise VIII; 46–54.
5. Vieusseux M. Memoire sur la maladie qui a régné à Genève au printemps de 1805. J Méd Chir Pharmacol 1806; *11*: 163–82.
6. Danielson L, Mann E. The history of a singular and very mortal disease, which lately made its appearance in Medfield. Med Agric Reg 1806; *1*: 65.
7. North E. *A Treatise on a Malignant Epidemic, Commonly Called Spotted Fever.* New York: T & J Swords, 1811.
8. Hirsch A. Epidemic cerebro-spinal meningitis. In: *Handbook of Geographical and Historical Pathology. Vol III – Diseases of Organs and Parts* (translated from the German by Creighton C.) London: New Sydenham Society, 1886; 547–94.
9. Netter A, Debré R. *La Méningite Cérébrospinale*. Paris: Masson et Cie, 1911.
10. Stillé A. *Epidemic Meningitis or Cerebro-spinal Meningitis*. Philadelphia: Lindsay & Blakiston, 1867.
11. Marchiafava E, Celli A. Spra i micrococchi della meningite cerebrospinale epidemica. Gazz degli Ospedali 1884; *5*: 59.
12. Weichselbaum A. Ueber die Aetiologie der akuten Meningitis cerebro-spinalis. Fortschr Med 1887; *5*: 573–83, 620–6.
13. Jaeger H. Zur Aetiologie der Meningitis cerebospinalis epidemica. Zeitschr fur Hyg und Infect 1895; *19*: 351–70.
14. Quincke HI. Ueber Meningitis serosa. Samml Klin Vort (Leipzig) 1893; *67*: 655–94.
15. Heubner JOL. Beobachtungen und Versuche über den Meningokokkus intracellularis (Weichselbaum-Jaeger). Jb Kinderheilk 1896; *43*: 1–22.
16. Kiefer F. Zur Differentialdiagnose des Erregers der epidemischen Cerebrospinal-meningitis und der Gonorrhoe. Berl Klin Woch 1896; *33*: 628–30.
17. Kolle W, Wasserman A. Versuche zur Gewinnung und Wertbestimmung eines Meningokokkenserums. Dtsch Med Wschr 1906; *32*: 609–12.
18. Jochmann G. Versuche zur Serodiagnostik und Serotherapie der epidemischen Genickstarre. Dtsch Med Wschr 1906; *32*: 788–93.

19. Flexner S, Jobling JW. An analysis of four hundred cases of epidemic meningitis treated with the anti-meningitis serum. J. Exp Med 1908; 10: 690–733.

20. Flexner S. *Mode of Infection, Means of Prevention and Specific Treatment of Epidemic Meningitis.* New York: Rockefeller Institute for Medical Research, 1917.

21. Waterhouse R. A case of supra-renal apoplexy. Lancet 1911; i: 577–8.

22. Friderichsen C. Nebennierenapoplexie bei kleinen Kindern. Jb Kinderheilk 1918; 87: 109–25.

23. Rolleston H. Lumleian lectures on cerebro-spinal fever. Lecture 1. Lancet 1919; i: 541–9.

24. Reece RJ. Notes on the prevalence of cerebrospinal fever among the civil population of England and Wales during the last four months of the year 1914 and the first six months of the year 1915; together with a short account of the appearance of the disease and of its distribution among troops in the British Isles during the same period, and of the military administrative measures adopted to deal with the prevalence of the disease. JR Army Med Corps 1915; 24: 555–68.

25. Peltola H. Meningococcal disease: still with us. Rev Infect Dis 1983; 5: 71–91.

26. Brundage JF, Zollinger WD. Evolution of meningococcal disease epidemiology in the US Army. In: Vedros NA, ed. *Evolution of Meningococcal Disease. Volume I.* Boca Raton, Florida: CRC Press Inc, 1987; 5–25.

27. Treadgold CH. Cerebrospinal meningitis in the Salisbury Plain area during the early part of 1915: a laboratory study. J R Army Med Corps 1915; 25: 221–30.

28. Forester CS. *The General.* London: Michael Joseph, 1958; 86–7.

29. Glover JA. Observations of the meningococcus carrier rate and their application to the prevention of cerebro-spinal fever. Special Report series of the Medical Research Council (London) 1920; 50: 133–65.

30. Gordon MH, Murray EG. Identification of the meningococcus. J R Army Med Corps 1915; 25: 411–23.

31. Nicolle M, Debains E, Jouan C. Etudes sur les méningococciques et les serums anti-méningococciques. Ann Inst Pasteur 1918; 32: 150–69.

32. Norton JF, Gordon JE. Meningococcus meningitis in Detroit in 1928–1929. J Prev Med 1930; 4: 207–14.

33. Laybourn RL. A study of epidemic meningitis in Missouri: epidemiological and administrative considerations. Southern Med J 1931; 24: 678–86.

34. Rake G. Biological properties of 'fresh' and 'stock' strains of the meningococcus. Proc Soc Exp Biol Med 1931; 29: 287–9.

35. Rake G, Scherp HW. Studies on meningococcus infection. III. The antigenic complex of the meningococcus—a type specific substance. J Exp Med 1933; 58: 341–60.

36. Branham SE. Milestones in the history of the meningococcus. Can J Microbiol 1956; 2: 175–88.

37. Miller CP. Experimental meningococcal infection in mice. Science 1933; 78: 340–1.

38. Buttle GAH, Gray WH, Stephenson D. Protection of mice against streptococcal and other infections by p-aminobenzene sulphonamide and related substances. Lancet 1936; i: 1286–90.

39. Schwentker FF. Treatment of meningococcic meningitis with sulfanilamide. J Pediatr 1937; 11: 874–80.

40. Schwentker FF, Gelman S, Long PH. The treatment of meningococcic meningitis with sulfanilamide. Preliminary report. JAMA 1937; 108: 1407–8.

41. Long PH. Sulphapyridine. JAMA 1939; 112: 538–9.

42. Gover M, Jackson G. Cerebrospinal meningitis. A chronological record of reported cases and deaths. Pub Hlth Rep 1946; 61: 433–50.

43. Holmes MJ. Report on cerebro-spinal meningitis. Med J Aust 1941; *1*: 541–8.
44. Phair JJ. Meningococcal meningitis. In: Coates JB, Hoff EC, Hoff PM, eds. *Preventive Medicine In World War II. Vol IV – Communicable Diseases Transmitted Chiefly Through Respiratory And Alimentary Tracts.* Washington DC: Office of the Surgeon General, Department of the Army, 1958; 191–209.
45. Banks HS. Cerebro-spinal fever. In: Cope VZ, ed. *History of the Second World War: Medicine and Pathology.* London: HMSO, 1952; 170–94.
46. Flack M. Report on cerebrospinal fever in the London District, December 1915, to July 1916. J R Army Med Corps 1917; *28*: 113–45.
47. Banks HS. Chemotherapy of meningococcal meningitis. A review of 147 consecutive cases. Lancet 1939; *2*: 921–7.
48. Beeson PB, Westerman E. Cerebrospinal fever. Analysis of 3,575 case reports, with special reference to sulphonamide therapy. Br Med J 1943; *1*: 497–500.
49. Fairbrother RW. Cerebrospinal meningitis. The use of sulphonamide derivatives in prophylaxis. Br Med J 1940; *2*: 859–62.
50. Fleming A. On the antibacterial action of cultures of a penicillium with special reference to their use in the isolation of *B. influenzae.* Br J Exp Pathol 1929; *10*: 226–36.
51. Cowdrey AE. *The Medics' War.* Washington DC: Center of Military History, United States Army, 1987: 147.
52. Goldschneider I, Gotschlich EC, Artenstein MS. Human immunity to the meningococcus. I. The role of humoral antibodies. J Exp Med 1969; *129*: 1307–26.
53. Goldschneider I, Gotschlich EC, Artenstein MS. Human immunity to the meningococcus. II. Development of natural immunity. J Exp Med 1969; *129*: 1327–48.
54. Gotschlich EC, Teh Yung Liu, Artenstein MS. Human immunity to the meningococcus. III. Preparation and immunochemical properties of the group A, group B and group C meningococcal polysaccharides. J Exp Med 1969; *129*: 1349–65.
55. Gotschlich EC, Goldschneider I, Artenstein MS. Human immunity to the meningococcus. IV. Immunogenicity of group A and group C meningococcal polysaccharides in human volunteers. J Exp Med 1969; *129*: 1367–84.
56. Goldschneider I, Gotschlich EC, Artenstein MS. Human immunity to the meningococcus. V. The effect of immunization with meningococcal group C polysaccharide on the carrier state. J Exp Med 1969; *129*: 1385–95.
57. Control of a cerebrospinal meningitis epidemic. Weekly Epidemiol Rec 1993; *68*: 237–8.
58. Botha P. Penicillin-resistant *Neisseria meningitidis* in southern Africa. Lancet 1988; *i*: 54.
59. Fontanals D, Pineda V, Pons I, Rojo JC. Penicillin-resistant beta-lactamase producing *Neisseria meningitidis* in Spain. Eur J Clin Microbiol Infect Dis 1989; *8*: 90–1.
60. Vedros, NA ed. *Evolution of Meningococcal Disease, Vols I and II.* Boca Raton: CRC Press, 1987.

2
Surface Structures and Secreted Products of Meningococci

J.T. POOLMAN[1], P.A. VAN DER LEY[1] and
J. TOMMASSEN[2]
[1] National Institute of Public Health and Environmental Protection,
Bilthoven, The Netherlands and [2] Department of Molecular Cell
Biology, University of Utrecht, The Netherlands

INTRODUCTION

Neisseria meningitidis is a gram-negative diplococcus very closely related to the gonococcus. The only known host for both species is man. Meningococci are normally carried in the nasopharynx, occasionally invading to cause systemic disease. The meningococcal cell surface constitutes that part of the organism which interacts most intimately with the host, and meningococcal cell surface structures are known to be critical in colonisation, invasion and disease pathogenesis. Perhaps to facilitate host colonisation by allowing evasion of host immune responses, exposed epitopes of many meningococcal cell surface structures are found to vary. This variation has been exploited in the development of classification systems.

A characteristic of meningococci is the high level of 'blebbing' i.e. the shedding of outer membrane vesicles (Figure 2.1). Such blebs contain outer membrane proteins (OMPs) and lipopolysaccharides (LPS) and are important in the pathogenesis of meningococcal disease. Blebs bind antibodies that would otherwise attach to whole bacteria and they play a crucial role in the induction of LPS (endotoxin)-mediated septic shock. 'Blebbing' is observed in other gram-negative organisms (e.g. *Escherichia coli* mutants that are devoid of OmpA and the major outer membrane lipoprotein[1]) but usually to

Meningococcal Disease. Edited by Keith Cartwright © 1995 John Wiley & Sons Ltd

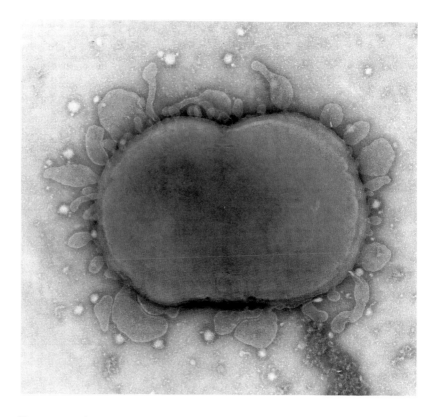

Figure 2.1 *Electron micrograph of a meningococcus showing shedding of outer membrane blebs. The photograph was kindly provided by the Public Health Laboratory Service Centre for Applied Microbiology and Research, Porton, UK*

a lesser extent than in the meningococcus. The major components of the meningococcal cell surface are discussed below.

CELL ENVELOPE

Meningococci typically display a double membrane structure characteristic of gram-negative bacteria, with a peptidoglycan layer sandwiched between the two membranes (Figure 2.2). The cytoplasmic membrane contains a terminally branched electron transport chain[2] allowing the organism to use different electron acceptors. The components of meningococcal peptidoglycan are unknown, in contrast to gonococcal peptidoglycan which appears to be composed of the common N-acetylglucosamine and N-acetylmuramyl-peptide structures[3].

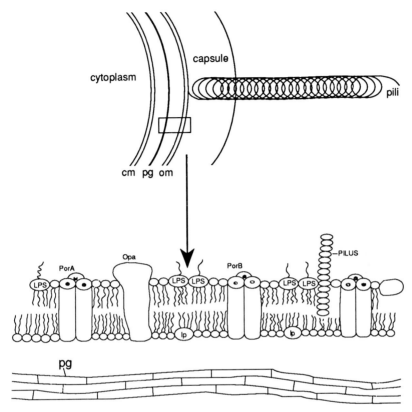

Figure 2.2   *Surface structure of the meningococcus with emphasis on the non-capsular antigens. cm, cytoplasmic membrane; pg, peptidogylcan; om, outer membrane; lp, lipoprotein; LPS, lipopolysaccharide*

Most research has been focused on the outer membrane since this is the site where the pathogenic meningococcus interacts with the human host. Table 2.1 lists meningococcal outer membrane proteins (OMPs) that have been identified to date. In addition to OMPs the outer membrane contains lipopolysaccharide (LPS) and phospholipid. The meningococcal phospholipid composition has not been studied, but gonococcal phospholipids include phosphatidylglycerol, phosphatidylethanolamine and diphosphatidylglycerol[4].

LIPOPOLYSACCHARIDE (LPS)

Meningococcal LPS (endotoxin) has been investigated in relation to the pathogenesis of meningococcal disease[5]. The saccharide and lipid A structures have been determined[6,7]. The terminal glc-gal-glcNAc-gal

Table 2.1 Meningococcal outer membrane proteins (OMPs)

Protein	Molecular mass	Function/characteristics
AniA (Pan 1)	54 kDa	anaerobically induced protein
CtrA		polysaccharide biosynthesis, capsule transport
FrpB	70 kDa	unknown; Fe restriction protein
IroA	~ 100 kDa	induced by iron limitation, maybe Lbp
Laz	17 kDa	lipoprotein, lipid-modified azurin
Lip (H8)	18 kDa	lipoprotein
Lbp	~ 100 kDa	lactoferrin binding protein
Omc	~ 200 kDa	outer membrane macromolecular complex protein, secretion?
Opa (class 5 OMP)	26–30 kDa	adhesion, opacity protein
Opc	25 kDa	invasion, opacity protein
PorA (class 1 OMP)	44–47 kDa	porin
PorB (class 2/3 OMP)	37–42 kDa	porin
Rmp (class 4 OMP)		reduction modifiable protein, unknown; OmpA related
Tbp-1	~ 100 kDa	transferrin binding protein
Tbp-2	64–85 kDa	transferrin binding protein

(lacto-*N*-neotetraose) structure is endogenously sialylated, rendering meningococci serum-resistant[8]. The same structure is also present on glycosphingolipids made by human cells, an example of molecular mimicry by the meningococcus. This structure is present within the L2 and L3 immunotypes that predominate amongst case isolates of serogroup B meningococci[9]. Immunotyping is described briefly at the end of this chapter. Carrier isolates are more heterogeneous and include a greater proportion of strains expressing the L1 and L8 immunotypes, which are associated with serum sensitivity. Gonococci expressing non-sialylated LPS are able to invade epithelial cells[10].

There is no evidence for the existence of O-side chains in meningococcal LPS. The genes involved in the biosynthesis of LPS are being investigated. Mutants lacking the lacto-*N*-neotetraose structure have been constructed by inactivating the *galE* gene[11].

CAPSULAR POLYSACCHARIDES

Meningococci can be divided into a number of serogroups (A, B, C, 29-E, H, I, K, L, W-135, X, Y, Z) on the basis of structural differences in the capsular polysaccharides[12]. Serogroup H strains are very closely related to serogroup B strains. The disease-associated serogroups B, C, Y and W-135 all have sialic acid in their capsular polysaccharide. Sialic acid containing polysaccharides confer resistance to host complement-mediated attack mechanisms[13]. The disease-associated serogroup A capsule is composed of mannosaminephosphate. Serogroup B strains are a predominant cause of meningococcal disease in the developed world. The B polysaccharide is poorly immunogenic, probably because of immunotolerance resulting from cross-reactivity between this polysaccharide and polysialic acid expressed on host neural cell adhesion molecules (NCAMs)[14]. The synthesis of B capsular polysaccharide has been studied intensively and the biochemistry is now well understood[15]. The gene complex involved has been cloned and is designated cps[16]. It contains genes encoding enzymes required for capsular polysaccharide biosynthesis in the cytoplasm, for phospholipid substitution and for the production of proteins whose function is the translocation of polysaccharide across the inner and outer bacterial cell membranes. A number of inner and outer membrane proteins play a role in these processes.

PILI

Pili are filamentous projections from the meningococcal cell surface; analogous structures are found in gonococci. Meningococci express two different classes of pili—class I and class II, which are antigenically and structurally distinct[17,18]. Pili are involved in adhesion and play a role in transformation (acquisition of heterologous DNA from the environment); they show a very high degree of antigenic variability. The biosynthetic mechanisms of pilin formation and the translocation of pilin protein across the cell envelope are currently being analysed.

SURFACE-EXPRESSED PROTEINS

Major outer membrane proteins

The OMPs which are expressed at high levels, the so-called major outer membrane proteins, were recognised early on[19]. Five different classes (1 to 5) of OMP exist, based on differences in molecular weight. Black lipid film experiments have shown that the meningococcal class 1 (PorA) and class 2 and 3 proteins (PorB) are porins, permitting the passage of ions across the cell membrane; they show cation- and anion-selectivity, respectively[20]. The subsequent sequencing of the encoding genes has confirmed the porin nature of these proteins, in that some homology with well-characterised *E. coli* porins was observed[21].

Gene sequencing also permitted the construction of topology models[22,23]. Whereas the transmembrane parts of these proteins are highly conserved, the strain-variable domains, which play a crucial role in the host immune response, are located at the tips of various surface loops in these models. The surface-exposed loops are the longest (and therefore the most exposed) in the class 1 protein which might explain why antibodies against this protein are particularly effective in bactericidal assays and in conferring protection in an animal model[24]. An example is shown in Figure 2.3, which depicts the P1.7,16 serosubtype variant of meningococcal class 1 OMP, showing variable regions at loops 1 and 4. In contrast to class 2 and class 3 OMPs, expression of class 1 protein is variable. Variants with different levels of class 1 expression can be isolated from a single strain *in vitro* and similar variation has been observed *in vivo*[25]. This variation can arise as a result of mutations in the promoter region of the *porA* gene (van der Ley, unpublished results).

The class 4 OMP (Rmp) reveals homology with *E. coli* OmpA[26]. For a long time the exact function of this intensively studied *E. coli* protein

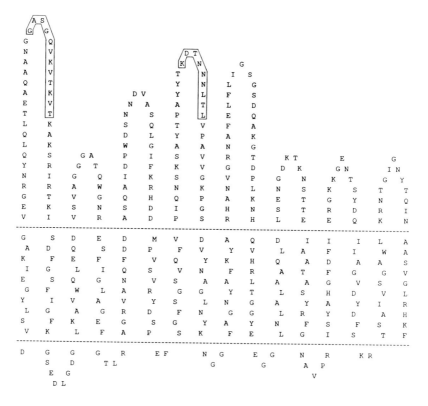

Figure 2.3 Two-dimensional model of the meningococcal porin PorA which is based on the criteria that amphipathic β-sheets form the membrane-spanning regions, the hydrophilic areas are surface-exposed and the protein has the structure of a cylinder

remained an enigma, but recently some evidence for pore-forming properties has been obtained[27,28]. OmpA protein consists of two domains separated by a hinge region[29,30]; the N-terminal half is embedded in the outer membrane whereas the C-terminal half extends into the periplasm. Meningococcal class 4 OMP shows structural homology with *E. coli* OmpA in the periplasmic extension, but its N-terminal half is much smaller. Therefore, the homology with OmpA does not immediately indicate similar pore properties. The class 4 protein can be reduced with mercaptoethanol and it binds with specific antibodies that can block the bactericidal activity of class 1 and class 2 and 3 OMP-specific antibodies[31]. It has therefore been suggested that class 4 OMP might adversely affect the immunogenicity of meningococcal vaccines based on, or containing outer membrane proteins. However, the concentrations of class 4-OMP antibodies required to demonstrate this effect are higher than those found *in vivo*.

Class 5 OMPs, Opa and Opc are so-called heat-modifiable proteins that demonstrate a change in apparent molecular weight on SDS PAGE (sodium dodecyl sulphate polyacrylamide gel electrophoresis) when treated at 37 or 100 °C[32]. Opa and Opc proteins are thought to be important in bacterial adhesion to, and invasion of host cells[33]. Meningococci contain four copies of *opa* genes, each of which can be switched on or off independently by changing the number of CTCTT repeats in the signal sequence-encoding part of the gene[22]. Control of Opc protein production lacks this feature. However, meningococci are capable of switching expression of Opc protein between different levels[34]. Thus these genetic features result in variability of Opa (level and nature of protein) and Opc (level of protein) expression by meningococci.

A model has been proposed for the topology of the Opa proteins in the membrane[35]. In this model, the polypeptide spans the membrane eight times in a β-sheet structure with four cell-surface-exposed regions. Although the membrane-spanning segments are well conserved, the exposed regions appear to be hypervariable when the sequences of different Opa proteins are compared. Hence, a large repertoire of different Opa proteins might be produced, allowing meningococci to evade the host immune system. Opa proteins may be related to the members of a recently discovered family of enterobacterial OMPs, consisting up to now of five members' i.e. Ail (*attachment invasion locus*) of *Yersinia enterocolitica*[36], PagC[37] and Rck[38] of *Salmonella typhimurium*, OmpX of *Enterobacter cloacae*[39] and Lom, encoded by coliphage lambda[40]. A model has been proposed for the topology of OmpX[39], which is very similar to the proposed topology model of the Opa proteins[35]. Again, the cell-surface-exposed regions are hypervariable. In addition, there is some sequence similarity between the Opa proteins and the members of this enterobacterial OMP family, especially in the C-terminal halves of these proteins (unpublished observation). Furthermore, as has been suggested for the Opa proteins, the product of the *Y. enterocolitica ail* gene seems to be involved in adhesion to, and invasion of, eukaryotic cells[41].

Iron limitation induced OMPs

Most gram-negative bacteria including *E. coli* produce and secrete small iron-chelating compounds called siderophores during iron starvation. Under these conditions additional outer membrane proteins are produced which function as specific receptors for ferric–siderophore complexes. These complexes are subsequently transported across the outer membrane by a process that requires cytoplasmic membrane energy. This energy is coupled to the transport process via a mechanism in which TonB protein plays a key role[42,43]. Meningococci do not produce siderophores when grown under conditions of iron limitation[44,45]. Nevertheless, the efficient acquisition of iron is essential for an obligate host-dependent bacterium like the meningococcus, since in the host, iron is only available bound to proteins like lactoferrin and transferrin.

When starved of iron, the meningococcus expresses a number of OMPs that serve to capture these iron-binding proteins and to release and internalise iron into the bacterium. Some of these OMPs are expressed at a level comparable with the major OMPs. In particular, a 70 kDa OMP (FrpB), whose function is still unknown, is abundantly expressed. Antibodies against this 70 kDa OMP showed a level of bactericidal activity comparable with class 1 OMP-specific antibodies[46]. Meningococci appear to express two different transferrin-binding OMPs, transferrin-binding proteins 1 and 2 (Tbp-1 and Tbp-2). Tbp-1 and Tbp-2 (as well as FrpB) are antigenically heterogeneous[47]. Meningococci also express lactoferrin binding-OMPs (Lbps) which appear fairly homogeneous amongst different strains.

The structural genes for Tbp-1 and for another iron-limitation inducible OMP, tentatively designated IroA, have recently been cloned and sequenced[48,49]. Interestingly, the encoded proteins displayed homology with the TonB-dependent siderophore receptors of *E. coli* and other gram-negative bacteria, suggesting some structural and/or functional relationships. There are some indications that IroA is in fact Lbp (Pettersson A. *et al.*, unpublished results).

The 37 kDa Fbp (Fe-binding protein) plays a key role in the internalisation of Fe; it binds one mole of Fe^{3+} per mole of protein. Fbp is homogeneous amongst meningococcal isolates, probably reflecting its periplasmic (i.e. non-exposed) localisation. Fbp seems to function as a substrate-binding protein[50], probably in conjunction with a transport system of the ABC family in the inner membrane[51,52]. The existence of a common system for iron transport across the inner membrane makes it probable that FrpB functions as an intermediate between the receptors in the outer membrane and Fbp, possibly by releasing iron bound to the different host proteins or by forming the actual channel through which the released iron is transferred across the outer membrane. Consistent with such a central role for FrpB was the observation that a mutant lacking the FrpB protein was capable of utilising neither lactoferrin nor transferrin as a source of iron[53]. However, the mutant was ill-defined and recent results with better defined FrpB mutants show that these strains can still use lactoferrin and transferrin (Sparling, P.F. personal communication).

Secreted proteins

There are several indications that neisseriae are capable of secreting proteins into the extracellular environment. The first exoprotein described was IgA-protease[54]. This protein is produced in precursor form with an N-terminal signal sequence and a C-terminal helper domain. The signal sequence is required for transport across the cytoplasmic membrane, and the C-terminal helper domain probably forms a pore in the outer membrane through which the IgA protease is secreted. After translocation, the helper domain is cleaved off by autolytic processing.

Recently it was discovered that *N. meningitidis* produces a protein under iron limitation, designated FrpA, that is structurally related to members of the RTX family of cytotoxins[55]. Southern blot analysis showed the presence of an additional gene, *frpC*, that cross-reacted with a *frpA* probe. The RTX family of cytotoxins[56] is a group of related proteins, secreted by many gram-negative bacteria in a similar way. The best characterised member of this family is α-haemolysin of *E. coli*. α-haemolysin is produced without an N-terminal signal sequence and is secreted in a one-step process across both membranes, thereby bypassing the periplasm[57]. Its secretion requires three proteins, HlyB, which is a member of the ABC (ATP-binding cassette) family of transporters, HlyD and TolC. No genes related to *hlyB*, *hlyD* or *tolC* have been discovered up to now in *N. meningitidis*.

However, in *N. gonorrhoeae* the *omc* gene, encoding the outer membrane protein-macromolecular complex, has been characterised[58]. The Omc protein appears to be homologous with an outer membrane protein, YscC, of *Yersinia enterocolitica*, involved in the secretion of Yops. Yops are exoproteins that are involved in pathogenesis. Like the members of the RTX family of cytotoxins, Yops are produced without a signal sequence. For their secretion, a large number of proteins encoded by the *virC* region of the virulence plasmid pYV, and including YscC, are required[59]. Furthermore, Omc protein is homologous with the members of a family of outer membrane proteins which are involved in the secretion of proteins via a two-step pathway in many gram-negative bacteria. Proteins secreted via this pathway are produced with a signal sequence that is required for transport across the inner membrane. Transport across the outer membrane is accomplished in a separate step and requires a large set of proteins, encoded in *Klebsiella pneumoniae* by the *pul* genes and in *Pseudomonas aeruginosa* by the *xcp* genes[60]. The Omc protein of *N. gonorrhoeae* is homologous to PulD of *K. pneumoniae* and XcpQ of *P. aeruginosa*. The existence of Omc protein in *N. gonorrhoeae* suggests that this organism is capable of secreting additional, thus far uncharacterised proteins, into the extracellular medium via the Yop pathway of *Y. enterocolitica* or the Xcp pathway of *P. aeruginosa*. In addition, the possibility cannot be excluded that the RTX cytotoxins are secreted via a Yop-like pathway in *Neisseria*, rather than via a pathway requiring proteins related to HlyB, HlyD and TolC of *E. coli*.

Other proteins

In addition to the major OMPs and the Fe-limitation inducible OMPs, meningococci express other OMPs, such as the lipoproteins Lip and Laz whose functions are unknown[61], AniA, the synthesis of which is anaerobically induced[62], and CtrA, which is involved in the excretion of capsular polysaccharide[16].

MENINGOCOCCAL CLASSIFICATION

Traditionally, differentiation of meningococci was achieved by serological means using antisera raised by immunising laboratory animals. With the progressive characterisation of the various meningococcal cell surface structures the biochemical basis for this classification became apparent.

Meningococcal *serogrouping* makes use of variations in the capsular polysaccharide: thus A, B, C etc. *Serotyping* is based on differences in the class 2 and class 3 OMPs (Por B): 1, 2a, 2b etc. *Serosubtyping* exploits variations in the class 1 OMP (Por A): P1.1, P1.2, P1.3 etc. Since class 1 OMPs have two separate variable regions (VR1 and VR2), two separate serosubtyping epitopes can be recognised on one Por A protein, resulting in designations such as P1.5, 2 or P1.16, 7. The first variable region is situated on the first surface-exposed loop of the protein and the second variable region on the fourth surface-exposed loop (see Figure 2.3). This nomenclature system has been formally described[19].

The classification system has been shown to be of great value for epidemiological surveillance. An important point to be recognised is that serogrouping and serotyping antigens are targets for bactericidal antibodies. Changing patterns of serogroup and serotype are therefore linked to changing patterns of herd immunity.

Lipopolysaccharides can also be used as typing antigens, giving rise to so-called *immunotypes*: L1, L2, L3 etc. Double and triple epitopes can be recognised, depending on variability (phase-variation) or the presence of partial, incomplete epitopes on the same bacterium. Characterisation of immunotype is relevant for pathogenesis studies and quality control purposes. It is less useful for epidemiological surveillance[9]. Other OMPs such as FrpB may also be useful for classification purposes[46].

In addition to serological classification methods, meningococci can be divided into clonal types using varying techniques to characterise the bacterial genome. Descriptions of the roles of the traditional, serological classification systems and the newer, clonal typing methods are given in Chapters 6 and 7.

REFERENCES

1. Sonntag I, Schwarz H, Hirota Y, Henning U. Cell envelope and shape of *Escherichia coli*: multiple mutants missing the outer membrane lipoprotein and other major outer membrane proteins. J Bacteriol 1978; *136*: 280–5.
2. Yu EKC, DeVoe IW. Terminal branching of the respiratory electron transport chain in *Neisseria meningitidis*. J Bacteriol 1980; *142*: 879–87.
3. Rosenthal RS, Krueger JM. Promotion of sleep by gonococcal peptidoglycan fragments. Structural requirements for the somnogenic activity. Antonie van Leeuwenhoek 1987; *53*: 523–32.
4. Wolf-Watz H, Elmros T, Normark S, Bloom GD. Cell envelope of *Neisseria gonorrhoeae*: outer membrane and peptidoglycan composition of penicillin-sensitive and -resistant strains. Infect Immun 1975; *11*: 1332–41.
5. Verheul AFM, Snippe H, Poolman JT. Meningococcal lipopolysaccharides. Virulence factor and potential vaccine component. Microbiol Rev 1993; *57*: 34–49.
6. Gamian A, Beurret M, Michon F, Brisson J-B, Jennings HJ. Structure of the L2 lipopolysaccharide core oligosaccharides of *Neisseria meningitidis*. J Biol Chem 1992; *267*: 922–5.
7. Kulshin VA, Zähringer U, Lindner B, Frasch CE, Tsai C-M, Dmitriev BA *et al.* Structural characterization of the lipid A component of pathogenic *Neisseria meningitidisi*. J Bacteriol 1992; *174*: 1793–1800.
8. Mandrell RE, Kim JJ, John CM, Gibson BW, Sugai JV, Apicella MA *et al.* Endogenous sialylation of the lipooligosaccharides of *Neisseria meningitidis*. J Bacteriol 1991; *173*: 2823–32.
9. Jones DM, Borrow R, Fox AJ, Gray S, Cartwright KA, Poolman JT. The lipooligosaccharide immunotype as a virulence determinant in *Neisseria meningitidis*. Microb Path 1992; *13*: 219–24.
10. Putten JPM. Phase variation of lipopolysaccharide directs interconversion of invasive and immuno-resistant phenotypes of *Neisseria gonorrhoeae*. EMBO J 1993; *12*: 4043–51.
11. Jennings MP, van der Ley P, Wilks KE, Maskell DE, Poolman JT, Moxon ER. Cloning and molecular analysis of the *galE* gene of *Neisseria meningitidis* and its role in lipopolysaccharide biosynthesis. Mol Microbiol 1993; *10*: 361–9.
12. Davis BD, Dulbecco R, Eisen HN, Ginsberg HS. The Neisseriae. In: Gotschlich EC, ed. *Microbiology* (3rd edition). Harper, 1980; 635–44.

13. Jarvis GA, Vedros NA. Sialic acid of group B *Neisseria meningitidis* regulates alternative complement pathway activation. Infect Immun 1987; 55: 174–80.
14. Finne J, Bitter-Suermann D, Goridis C, Finne U. An IgG monoclonal antibody to group B meningococci cross-reacts with developmentally regulated polysialic acid units of glycoproteins in neural and extraneural tissues. J Immunol 1987; *138*: 4402–7.
15. Masson, L, Holbein BE. Physiology of sialic acid capsular polysaccharide synthesis in serogroup B *Neisseria meningitidis*. J Bacteriol 1983; *154*: 728–36.
16. Frosch M, Weisberger C, Meyer TF. Molecular characterization and expression in *Escherichia coli* of the gene complex encoding the polysaccharide capsule of *Neisseria meningitidis* group B. Proc Natl Acad Sci USA 1989; *86*: 1669–73.
17. Heckels JE. Structure and function of pili of pathogenic *Neisseria* species. Clin Microbiol Rev 1989; *2*: S66–73.
18. Gotschlich EC, Cornelissen C, Hill SA, Koomey JM, Marchal C, Meyer TF *et al.* The mechanisms of genetic variation of gonococcal pili. Iron-inducible proteins of *Neisseria*. In: Achtman M, Kohl P, Marchal C, Morelli G, Seiler A, Thiesen B, eds: *Neisseriae 1990*. Berlin: Walter de Gruyter, 1991; 405–14.
19. Frasch CE, Zollinger WD, Poolman JT. Serotype antigens of *Neisseria meningitidis* and a proposed scheme for designation of serotypes. Rev Infect Dis 1985; *7*: 504–10.
20. Tommassen J, Vermey P, Struyvé M, Benz R, Poolman JT. Isolation of mutants of *Neisseria meningitidis* deficient in class 1 (por A) and class 3 (por B). Infect Immun 1990; *58*: 1355–59.
21. Jenteur D, Lakey JH, Pattus F. The bacterial porin superfamily; sequence alignment and structure prediction. Mol Microbiol 1991; *5*: 2153–64.
22. van der Ley PA, Heckels JE, Virji M, Hoogerhout P, Poolman JT. Topology of outer membrane porins in pathogenic *Neisseria* spp. Infect Immun 1990; *59*: 2963–71.
23. Feavers IM, Suker J, McKenna AJ, Heath AB, Maiden MCJ. Molecular analysis of the serotyping antigen of *Neisseria meningitidis*. Infect Immun 1992; *60*: 3620–9.
24. Saukkonen K, Leinonen M, Abdillahi H, Poolman JT. Comparative evaluation of potential components for group B meningococcal vaccine by passive protection in the infant rat and in vitro bactericidal assay. Vaccine 1989; *7*: 325–8.
25. Poolman JT, de Marie S, Zanen HC. Variability of low-molecular-weight, heat-modifiable outer membrane proteins of *Neisseria meningitidis*. Infect Immun 1980; *30*: 642–8.
26. Klugman KP, Gotschlich EC, Blake MS. Sequence of the structural gene (*rmp* M) for the class 4 outer membrane protein of *Neisseria meningitidis*, homology of the protein to gonococcal protein III and *Escherichia coli* OmpA and construction of meningococcal strains that lack class 4 protein. Infect Immun 1989; *57*: 2066–71.
27. Saint N, De E, Julien S, Orange N, Molle G. Ionophore properties of OmpA of *Escherichia coli*. Biochim Biophys Acta 1993; *1145*: 119–23.
28. Sugawara E, Nikaido H. Pore-forming activity of OmpA protein of *Escherichia coli*. J Biol Chem 1992; *267*: 2507–11.
29. Morona R, Klose M, Henning U. *Escherichia coli* K-12 outer membrane protein (OmpA) as a bacteriophage receptor: analysis of mutant genes expressing altered proteins. J Bacteriol 1984; *159*: 570–8.
30. Vogel H, Jähnig F. Models for the structure of outer membrane proteins of *Escherichia coli* derived from raman spectroscopy and prediction methods. J Mol Biol 1986; *190*: 191–9.
31. Munkley A, Tinsley CR, Virji M, Heckels JE. Blocking of bactericidal killing of

Neisseria meningitidis by antibodies directed against class 4 outer membrane proteins. Microb Path 1991; *11*: 447–52.

32. Aho EL, Dempsey JA, Hobbs MM, Klapper DG, Cannon JG. Characterization of the *opa* (class 5) gene family of *Neisseria meningitidis*. Mol Microbiol 1991; *5*: 1429–37.

33. Virji M, Makepeace K, Ferguson DJP, Achtman M, Sarkari J, Moxon ER. Expression of the Opc protein correlates with invasion of epithelial and endothelial cells by *Neisseria meningitidis*. Mol. Microbiology 1992; *6*: 2785–95.

34. Olyhoek AJM, Sarkari J, Bopp M, Morelli G, Achtman M. Cloning and expression in *Escherichia coli* of *opc*, the gene for an unusual class 5 outer membrane protein from *Neisseria meningitidis*. Microb Path 1991; *11*: 249–57.

35. van der Ley PA. Three copies of a single protein II encoding sequence in the genome of *Neisseria gonorrhoeae* JS3: evidence for gene conversion and gene duplication. Mol Microbiol 1988; *2*: 797–806.

36. Miller VL, Bliska JB, Falkow S. Nucleotide sequence of the *Yersinia enterocolitica ail* gene and characterization of the Ail protein product. J Bacteriol 1990; *172*: 1062–9.

37. Pulkkinen WS, Miller SI. A *Salmonella typhimurium* virulence protein is similar to a *Yersinia enterocolitica* invasion protein and a bacteriophage lambda outer membrane protein. J Bacteriol 1991; *173*: 86–93.

38. Heffernan EJ, Harwood J, Fierer J, Guiney D. The *Salmonella typhimurium* virulence plasmid complement resistance gene *rck* is homologous to a family of virulence-related outer membrane protein genes, including *pag* C and *ail*. J Bacteriol 1992; *174*: 84–91.

39. Stoorvogel J, van Bussel MJAWM, Tommassen J, van de Klundert JAM. Molecular characterization of an *Enterobacter cloacae* outer membrane protein (OmpX). J Bacteriol 1991; *173*: 156–60.

40. Barondess JJ, Beckwith J. A bacteriophage virulence determinant encoded by lysogenic coliphage. Nature 1990; *346*: 871–4.

41. Miller VL, Falkow S. Evidence for two genetic loci in *Yersinia enterocolitica* that can promote invasion of epithelial cells. Infect Immun 1988; *56*: 1242–8.

42. Postle K. TonB and the gram-negative dilemma. Mol Microbiol 1990; *4*: 2019–25.

43. Bitter W, Tommassen J, Weisbeek P. Identification and characterization of the *exb*B, *exb*D and *ton*B genes of *Pseudomonas putida* WCS358: their involvement in ferric-pseudobactin transport. Mol Microbiol 1993; *7*: 117–30.

44. Archibald FS, DeVoe IW. Iron acquisition by meningococci. Infect Immun 1980; *27*: 322–34.

45. West SEH, Sparling PF. Response of *Neisseria gonorrhoeae* to iron limitation: alterations in expression of membrane proteins without apparent siderophore production. Infect Immun 1985; *47*: 388–94.

46. Pettersson A, Kuipers B, Pelzer M, Verhagen EPM, Tiesjema RH, Tommassen J *et al.* Monoclonal antibodies against the 70-kilodalton iron-regulated protein of *Neisseria meningitidis* are bactericidal and strain-specific. Infect Immun 1990; *58*: 3036–41.

47. Danve B, Mignon M, Dumas P, Maitre G, Colombani S, Lissolo L *et al.* Evaluation of the potential of transferrin binding proteins as meningococcal vaccine candidates. In: Conde-Glez CJ, Calderon E, Morse SA, eds. *Eighth International Pathogenic Neisseria Conference* (Abstracts). Cuernavaca: National Institute of Public Health, Mexico, 1992; 32.

48. Cornelissen CN, Biswas GD, Tsai J, Paruchuri DK, Thompson SA, Sparling PF. Gonococcal transferrin-binding protein 1 is required for transferrin utilization

and is homologous to TonB-dependent outer membrane receptors. J Bacteriol 1992; *174*: 5788–97.

49. Petterson A, van der Ley P, Poolman JT, Tommassen JPM. Molecular characterisation of the 98-kilodalton iron-regulated outer membrane protein of *Neisseria meningitidis*. Infect Immun 1993; *61*: 4724–33.

50. Berish SA, Chen C-Y, Mietzner TA, Morse SA. Expression of a functional *fbp* gene in *Escherichia coli*. Mol Microbiol 1992; *6*: 2607–15.

51. Hyde SC, Emsley P, Hartshorn MJ, Mimmack MM, Gileadi U, Pearce SR *et al*. Structural model of ATP-binding proteins associated with cystic fibrosis, multidrug resistance and bacterial transport. Nature 1990; *346*: 362–5.

52. Ames GF-L, Joshi AK. Energy coupling in bacterial periplasmic permeases. J Bacteriol 1990; *172*: 4133–7.

53. Dyer DW, West EP, McKenna W, Thompson SA, Sparling PF. A pleiotropic iron-uptake mutant of *Neisseria meningitidis* lacks a 70-kilodalton iron-regulated protein. Infect Immun 1988; *56*: 977–83.

54. Pohlner J, Halter R, Beyreuther K, Meyer TF. Gene structure and extracellular secretion of *Neisseria gonorrhoeae* IgA protease. Nature 1987; *325*: 458–62.

55. Thompson SA, Wang LL, West A, Sparling PF. *Neisseria meningitidis* produces iron-regulated proteins related to the RTX family of exoproteins. J Bacteriol 1993; *175*: 811–18.

56. Coote JG. Structural and functional relationships among the RTX toxin determinants of gram-negative bacteria. FEMS Microbiol Rev 1992; *88*: 137–62.

57. Holland IB, Kenny B, Blight M. Haemolysin secretion from *Escherichia coli*. Biochimie 1990; *72*: 131–41.

58. Tsai W-M, Larsen SH, Wilde III CE. Cloning and DNA sequence of the *omc* gene encoding the outer membrane protein–macromolecular complex from *Neisseria gonorrhoeae*. Infect Immun 1989; *57*: 2653–9.

59. Michiels T, Vanooteghem J-C, Lambert de Rouvroit C, China B, Gustin A, Boudry P *et al*. Analysis of *virC*, an operon involved in the secretion of Yop proteins by *Yersinia enterocolitica*. J Bacteriol 1991; *73*: 4994–5009.

60. Tommassen J, Filloux A, Bally M, Murgier M, Lazdunski A. Protein secretion in *Pseudomonas aeruginosa*. FEMS Microbiol Rev 1992; *103*: 73–90.

61. Cannon J. Conserved lipoproteins of pathogenic *Neisseria* species bearing the H.8 epitopes: lipid-modified azurin and H.8 outer membrane protein. Clin Microbiol Rev 1989; *2*: S1–4.

62. Hoehn GT, Clark VL. The major anaerobically induced outer membrane protein of *Neisseria gonorrhoeae*, Pan 1, is a lipoprotein. Infect Immun 1992; *60*: 4704–8.

3
Mechanisms of Host Immunity

J. McLEOD GRIFFISS
Centre for Immunochemistry and Department of Laboratory Medicine, University of California San Francisco, San Francisco, USA

INTRODUCTION. NATURAL IMMUNITY IS REQUIRED TO MAINTAIN THE COMMENSAL STATE

Neisseria meningitidis is a commensal of the human upper respiratory tract[1]. Colonisation of the nasopharynx follows inhalation of infected aerosols from a previously colonised individual. However, as meningococci are susceptible to drying, they do not survive for long in aerosol droplets, and person-to-person transmission requires frequent or close contact.

Meningococcal colonisation is not, itself, dangerous, as it is the expression of the successful commensal relationship. Between 25% and 40% of young adults in temperate climes carry meningococci on their throats in the absence of disease. However, certain *N. meningitidis* do possess a variable, low, but definite pathogenic potential that is expressed as the ability to survive and multiply after entering the bloodstream of certain individuals. It is the non-carrier who is potentially at risk, since her or his ability to establish a commensal relationship with a newly acquired strain is not known.

The pathogenic potential of a meningococcal strain is a function of certain of its surface organelles. Immunological response to these organelles strengthens the commensal relationship by enabling the host to restrict bacteria to mucosal sites of colonisation. The more such immunogenic organelles a strain makes, the greater the likelihood that it will successfully

Meningococcal Disease. Edited by Keith Cartwright © 1995 John Wiley & Sons Ltd

colonise the mucosa without invading and killing its host. Thus, bacteria and host act together to maintain the commensal relationship.

MUCOSAL IMMUNITY

Despite its obvious potential importance, knowledge of mucosal immunity against meningococcal disease remains largely theoretical. Perhaps this is because colonisation so rarely leads to dissemination and disease. To cause disease *N. meningitidis* must not only attach to (colonise), but also *invade* epithelial cells. To be effective, mucosal immunity need not prevent colonisation, just invasion—yet it is colonisation that we record when assessing mucosal immunity. At present we have no ways of measuring mucosal immunity to epithelial cell invasion other than by noting the absence of disseminated disease.

The first step in the highly complex processes by which bacteria invade epithelial cells is adherence to the host-cell membrane. Adherence is mediated by specific ligand:receptor interactions, often of the lectin:carbohydrate sort, and is followed by sequential bi-directional signalling that causes up-regulation of additional pro- and eukaryotic proteins that are needed for active endocytosis[2-6].

Pili

The attachment of *Neisseria* to human mucosal surfaces is initiated by the binding of filamentous bacterial lectins called pili to tissue-specific glycoconjugate structures in the eukaryotic membrane[6,7]. Most, if not all, gram-negative bacteria make pili that adhere to the epithelial cells of the particular mammalian surface that they routinely colonise[8-11]. Pili are found on meningococci and gonococci isolated from human mucosal surfaces[12] and on meningococci isolated from blood and cerebrospinal fluid[6,13,14]. Piliation of meningococci is associated with increased adherence to human nasopharyngeal cells[6].

Structural variations in pili dramatically affect the adherence of *N. meningitidis* and *Neisseria gonorrhoeae* to respiratory and genital epithelial surfaces respectively[10,11]. Neisserial pili are composed of repeating polypeptide subunits termed pilin[15]. More than one pilin may be synthesised by a single strain[15], and neisserial pili undergo rapid phase shifts during infection[16]. Adhesive pilus variants mediate *initial* attachment of meningococci to human nasopharyngeal tissue in organ culture[6,10], but pilus-mediated attachment is later replaced by a tighter adherence mediated by non-pilus adhesins[17,18].

Many pilin epitopes that are common to gonococci and meningococci and among different meningococcal isolates have been described[15,19,20]. Surprisingly, conserved epitopes appear not to be exposed on pili that have been assembled on the surface of meningococci[20], and antibodies against conserved pilin epitopes are rarely found in sera from patients convalescent from bacteraemic meningococcal infections[20]. Furthermore, antisera raised against common pilin epitopes are not able to keep piliated meningococci from attaching to human buccal epithelial cells[20]. These findings raise questions as to whether pilus antibodies could prevent meningococcal colonisation, should they be present on the mucosa[20].

Outer membrane proteins

Meningococcal outer membrane proteins (OMPs) are divided into five classes based on their electrophoretic mobility in polyacrylamide gels (PAGE) after disaggregation in sodium dodecyl sulphate (SDS)[21]. Class 5 proteins are homologous with the opacity-associated proteins (Opas) that have been implicated in the signalling of cervical epithelial cells to engulf *N. gonorrhoeae*[11,17,22,23].

Opas are surface-exposed lectins. By binding to an oligosaccharide motif within the organism's lipo-oligosaccharides (LOS), Opas increase intercellular adhesion between cocci[24]. Human cell-membrane glycosphingolipids (GSL) have the same oligosaccharide motifs as neisserial LOS[25,26], and some studies have implicated Opas in the tight adherence of gonococci to epithelial cells and polymorphonuclear leucocytes (PMNs)—presumably through their binding to GSL sugar sequences[22,27−29]. As yet no studies of the potential effects of class 5 OMP antibodies on either colonisation or invasion have been reported[19].

One meningococcal class 5 protein, Opc, is less closely related to the true Opas (22% amino acid homology)[30,31]. It is over-expressed during colonisation[32] and has been implicated in invasion of cultured epithelial and endothelial cells—but only by organisms that are poorly encapsulated[33]. Abundant circulating Opc antibodies are induced by meningococcal colonisation, disseminated disease, or vaccination with OMP preparations[31]; it is not known whether these same immunising events induce mucosal Opc antibodies. Serum Opc antibodies can initiate lysis of minimally encapsulated organisms that express large amounts of the protein at the cell surface, but not those that express smaller amounts. Whether either mucosal or circulating Opc antibodies can block attachment or invasion is not known.

Capsular polysaccharides

The polysaccharide capsule is the outermost organelle on the meningococcal surface and therefore the prime target for mucosal immunity. Meningococcal capsular polysaccharide vaccines induce serum, and presumably secretory, IgA. Early studies found that vaccination with purified serogroup C polysaccharide reduced colonisation by *circa* 50%[34], but such an effect has not been found consistently, or for the other polysaccharides (Griffiss JMclo, unpublished observations). Polysaccharide vaccines could induce mucosal immunity to invasion even if they did not prevent colonisation, but their failure to prevent disease in those with deficiencies in one or another of the terminal complement components (see below) suggests that they do not do so for any length of time[35].

IgA_1 proteases

All *N. meningitidis*, regardless of serogroup, make a protease that can cleave IgA_1 at the hinge region. This characteristic, which is shared by *N. gonorrhoeae* and other mucosal pathogens, has often been invoked to explain the apparent absence of mucosal immunity, but there are sound reasons for believing that this enzyme plays little, if any, role in mitigating mucosal immunity.

Firstly, meningococci of serogroups that are essentially avirulent make the same IgA_1 protease, in the same amounts, as those of fully virulent serogroups. Secondly, the protease does not affect IgA_2, the more abundant IgA isotype on mucosal surfaces. IgA_2 is a deletion mutation of IgA_1 in which the hinge region cleavage sites for IgA_1 proteases are lost. Thus, man appears to have countered any possible deleterious effects of IgA_1 proteases by a simple deletion mutation. Lastly, IgA_1 proteases are ubiquitous and quite immunogenic; everyone has an abundance of antibodies that inactivate the enzymes.

HUMORAL IMMUNITY

The exact effector mechanism of immunity to meningococcal dissemination remained in doubt until the late 1960s, when Goldschneider, Gotschlich and Artenstein published a set of classic immuno-epidemiological investigations[34,36,37]. Shortly after World War I, Heist had observed that the serum of most humans lysed most meningococcal strains[38]. Through their exquisitely conceived studies that led to the development of meningococcal capsular polysaccharide vaccines, Goldschneider, Gotschlich and Artenstein demonstrated conclusively that it was this bactericidal activity of serum (immune lysis) that effected the host's contribution to a commensal relationship with a colonising meningococcus.

Immune lysis is the effector mechanism of natural immunity

Goldschneider and his colleagues found an inverse correlation between the age-related incidence of disease and the age-specific prevalence of serum bactericidal activity[36]. Then in a prospective study among army recruits during an epidemic, they showed that serum bactericidal activity against the epidemic strain was present in 82.2% of controls, but in only 5.6% of cases. Finally, using a prospective, longitudinal study that took into account the transmission within cohorts of the epidemic strain (serogroup C, type II)[39] as well as non-epidemic strains of the same and other serogroups, they correlated susceptibility with the absence of serotype-specific bactericidal activity[1].

Three subsequent observations provide additional evidence of the primacy of immune lysis as the immunological barrier that restricts the meningococcus to mucosal sites of colonisation[1,35,40–44]. The most compelling evidence is the unique susceptibility to disseminated neisserial infections of individuals who have inherited a deficiency of one or another of the terminal complement components that are required for immune lysis[35,41,43]. Such individuals develop disseminated neisserial infections recurrently, despite having adequate serum levels of meningococcal antibodies[35] and intact C3-dependent opsonophagocytic killing[43].

Secondly, the protective efficacy of meningococcal vaccines seems to be dependent upon the induction and persistence of antibody that is capable of initiating and sustaining immune lysis (bactericidal antibody)[45]. Mammals other than humans, including the other Great Apes, are not colonised by *N. meningitidis* and are not susceptible to meningococcal dissemination. The meningococcal polysaccharide vaccines that have been used successfully worldwide for over 20 years are uniformly non-immunogenic in experimental animals, including apes[46] but reliably induce bactericidal antibodies in humans[45,46]. In contrast, lower mammals make antibodies to different non-capsular antigens upon inoculation than does man during disseminated disease[31,47], and vaccines that were developed on the basis of the antibody response in experimental animals have failed to prevent disease in humans.

Thirdly, susceptibility to disseminated meningococcal disease can be induced by circulating meningococcal IgA which blocks complement-mediated immune effector mechanisms, including immune lysis[40,42,48,49]. Of greater importance is the observation that epidemics of meningococcal disease are associated with elevated levels of serum meningococcal IgA in the at-risk population (see below)[1,50–52].

Glycose structures of the meningococcal surface

The immunochemistry of immune lysis is quite complex, as we shall see, and 'bactericidal activity' in serum is not wholly synonymous with 'bactericidal antibodies' in serum. Before considering immune lysis in greater detail and assessing what is known about bactericidal antibodies, we need to review the structures of meningococcal capsular polysaccharides and cell membrane

LOS, as it is these glycose structures that regulate lytic activity in the absence of antibodies and that bind many of those antibodies that can initiate lysis.

Capsular polysaccharides

Most meningococcal cells are encapsulated within acidic and hydrophilic polysaccharides which provide the surface charge and humid environment that are critical for survival of the bacteria in aerosol droplets. Structural differences among these capsules provide serogroup specificity.

Sialic acid is an N-acetylated nine-carbon acidic ketose (N-acetyl neuraminic acid; NeuNAc or NANA) that results from the condensation of pyruvic acid and N-acetyl mannosamine (ManNAc). Serogroup A meningococci have a polymer of ManNAc-P for a capsule; meningococci of the other four pathogenic serogroups, B, C, Y and W, make capsules that are polymers of sialic acid. The serogroup B and C capsules are homopolymers of sialic acid, linked α2→8 and α2→9, respectively. The α2→9 polysialyl capsule (serogroup C) is variously O-acetylated; the α2→8 polymer (serogroup B) is not. Interestingly, those E. coli strains that most commonly cause sepsis and meningitis (K1) also have an α2→9 polysialyl capsule that is, however, O-acetylated. The serogroup Y and W capsules are co-polymers of NeuNAc linked α2→6 to glucose (serogroup Y) or galactose (serogroup W)[53]. Both are variously O-acetylated.

Lipo-oligosaccharides (LOS)

Lipo-oligasaccharides are short triantennary integral glycolipids of neisserial membranes bearing a structural resemblance to human glycosphingolipids (GSL)[25,54,55]. They have a lipoidal moiety that is inserted into the membrane, a proximal polar and highly variable basal oligosaccharide (Table 3.1), and three short oligosaccharide chains, termed α, β and γ[54]. Their α oligosaccharides share sequence and linkage with oligosaccharides of several human GSL series (Table 3.2)[26,54,56-58].

Neisserial LOS share a conserved basal segment that consists of two heptoses (Hep-1 and Hep-2) and a 2-keto, 3-deOxy, octulosonic acid (Kdo) residue that is attached to the lipoidal moiety[54,56-62]. A second Kdo residue is branched from the first; both heptoses may be substituted with phosphoethanolamine (PEA) residues[63].

Wild strains add a lactose (Lac; Galβ1→4Glc) disaccharide to Hep-1 to begin the α-chain[54]. Glucosamine (GlcNAc) is added α to Hep-2 to create the γ-chain; this GlcNAc residue is usually O-acetylated[54,56,57,64]. Meningococci, but perhaps not gonococci, usually also add either Glc, Gal or β-GlcNAc to Hep-2—thereby creating the β-chain and making a triantennary structure[54,56,59,63].

Table 3.1 *Meningococcal LOS basal region substitutions*

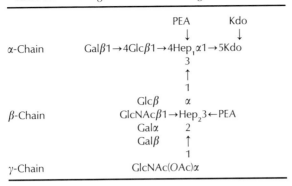

There is not enough variation in meningococcal α oligosaccharides (Table 3.2) to account for either serotypic diversity[65], physical diversity[61] or the conformation of structures that bind different bactericidal antibodies[66]. It is thought that the various LOS basal region substitutions shown in Table 3.1 account for much of the seryptypic diversity among meningococci and that most of the LOS structures that bind bactericidal antibodies to the meningococcal surface are conformationally determined by basal segment substitutents. Available evidence suggests that meningococcal LOS basal regions are more diverse than those made by gonococci, although this may reflect only the different emphases of structural studies of the two species' LOS.

Each LOS molecule has a 'selection' of basal region adornments; one set of substituents predominates, whereas others are at lower abundances. Each basal region, regardless of its abundance, is adorned with the same series of structurally related α-chains. The four known β-chains are probably mutually exclusive. The γ-chain is not elongated, and it is not certain that the β-chain is ever elongated beyond a single glycose substituent.

GSL-like α oligosaccharides

Table 3.2 shows the relationships of known LOS α-chain structures to one another and to GSL structures. Reference to their analogous GSL series provides a way to distinguish LOS structures—a convention that also serves to emphasise the pathogenetic importance of their molecular mimicry[26].

The addition of lactose to Hep-1 creates an α-chain that mimics lactosyl-ceramide GSLs. Such LOS run as 3.6 kDa molecules in SDS PAGE. They bear the L8 and L11 meningococcal LOS serotype determinants[63,67,68] as well as the monoclonal antibody (MAb) D6A epitope, which is a surrogate for an epitope that binds an important population of human IgG molecules that are bactericidal for serogroup B and C meningococci[68,69,70].

Table 3.2 *LOS and equivalent GSL structures, structure-specific MAbs and meningococcal L types*

GSL series	MAb	L type	Structure
Muco-	3G9	? Gc Only	Galβ1→4Galβ1→4Glcβ1→4Hep-1→Kdo
Globo-	Pᵏ	L1	Galα1→4Galβ1→4Glcβ1→4Hep-1→Kdo
Sialoglobo-	None	None	NeuNAc→Galα1→4Galβ1→4Glcβ1→4Hep-1→Kdo
Lactosyl	2.1.L8	L8	Galβ1→4Glcβ1→4Hep-1→Kdo
Lacto-	L6	L6	GlcNAcβ1→3Galβ1→4Glcβ1→4Hep-1→Kdo
Paraglobo-	1B2	L9	Galβ1→4GlcNAcβ1→3Galβ1→4Glcβ1→4Hep-1→Kdo
Sialoparaglobo-	None	L3,7	NeuNAcα2→3Galβ1→4GlcNAcβ1→3Galβ1→4Glcβ1→4Hep-1→Kdo
Ganglio-	1-1-M	Gc Only	GalNAcβ1→3Galβ1→4GlcNAcβ1→3Galβ1→4Glcβ1→4Hep-1→Kdo
Globo-	P₁	? Gc Only	Galα1→4Galβ1→3Galβ1→4Glcβ1→4Hep-1→Kdo

L8 and L11 are commonly made by the same strain[68]. The structural difference between them has not been determined, but probably results from different basal substitutions of LOS that bear lactoside α chains. Many of the other LOS serotypes result from alternative substitutions of the lactosyldiheptaside 3.6 kDa LOS[66]. Addition of glactose (Gal) $\alpha 1 \rightarrow 4$ to lactosyl LOS creates globotriaose, the glycose of human P^k GSL[26,58,63]. All L1 strains of *N. meningitidis* and many *N. gonorrhoeae* and *Neisseria lactamica* strains make LOS with this structure[26]. It bears the L1 antigen[63,71] and is commonly co-expressed with L8. *N. gonorrhoeae* can also add Gal $\beta 1 \rightarrow 4$ to lactosyl LOS to create the mucotriaose structure that is shared with mucoside GSL, but this structure is probably not made by *N. meningitidis*.

The best understood α oligosaccharide is that which mimics paragloboside-series GSL[25,26]. *N. gonorrhoeae*, *N. lactamica*, L9 strains of serogroup A *N. meningitidis* and most serogroup B and C meningococci can add a lactosamine (LacNAc; Gal$\beta 1 \rightarrow 4$GlcNAc) disaccharide $\beta 1 \rightarrow 3$ to the now internal Lac of lactosyl LOS α-chains[26,59,65]. The resulting LacNAc$\beta 1 \rightarrow 3$Lac tetrasaccharide is the lacto-*N*-neotetraose substituent of paragloboside series GSL and the H precursor of human ABO blood group antigens[25,26,54]. The lacto-*N*-neotetraose structure is made so commonly by *Neisseria* that it may be considered the 'mature' neisserial LOS[25,26,54–59,65,72].

The L3, L7 and L9 determinants are all found on LOS molecules whose α-chains terminate with lacto-*N*-neotetraose; they are usually co-expressed. L3 and L7 are made exclusively by serogroup B and C strains that endogenously sialylate lacto-*N*-neotetraose, whereas L9, which is seldom found on serogroup B and C strains, is made by serogroup A strains that cannot endogenously sialylate LOS. This is the basis for assigning L3,7 epitopes to sialylated lacto-*N*-neotetraose moieties and L9 to unsubstituted ones. Tsai and Civin reported that most meningococci, regardless of L-type, make lacto-*N*-neotetraose, but this must await confirmation[65].

$\beta 1 \rightarrow 3$ substitution of lactosyl LOS with glucosamine (GlcNAc) alone, creates a lactoside-like LOS that is reported to bear the L6 antigen[65,71]. Truncated lactoside-like LOS made by *N. gonorrhoeae*, however, do not bind Poolman's L6 MAb. Perhaps L6 requires basal region adornments that are only made by *N. meningitidis*.

Gonococci, but not meningococci, can add a terminal GalNAc $\beta 1 \rightarrow 3$ to lacto-*N*-neotetraose moieties[26,57,58,73] to create V³-(β-*N*-acetylgalactosaminyl) lactoneotetraose[57], a pentaose of X_2 and asialo-G_3 ganglioside GSL[74,75]. A few *N. gonorrhoeae* can also link Gal; $\alpha 1–4$ to the terminal Gal of lacto-*N*-neotetraose[26]. This creates the P_1 GSL; it has not yet been found for LOS made by *N. meningitidis* or *N. lactamica*.

Alternative and/or incomplete substitution of precursor LOS results in expression of more than one L-type by most meningococcal strains.

Sialylation of LOS

Meningococci that can make sialic acid (serogroups B, C, W and Y) usually sialylate their lacto-N-neotetraose LOS substituents (endogenous sialylation) when grown on laboratory media[72,76]. The L1/Pk globotriaose structure is also endogenously sialylated by L1 meningococcal strains[63]. Serogroup A N. meningitidis, N. gonorrhoeae and N. lactamica cannot make sialic acid[77] and do not endogenously sialylate LOS, but nearly all strains of all three species make at least one sialyl transferase (STase) that can transfer sialic acid from the human sugar nucleotide, CMP-NANA, to their LOS (exogenous sialylation)[25,72,76,78].

LOS sialylation is a strain-specific attribute[76] and is also dependent on growth conditions, including medium[65] and growth phase (log versus stationary)[79]. Only 2 of 25 serogroup C isolates from children that we have examined failed to endogenously sialylate their LOS[76]. It is not known whether meningococcal LOS are sialylated during dissemination from the oropharynx.

The endogenous STases made by N. meningitidis strains are probably not the same as the exogenous STases made by them and by other Neisseria. Exogenous STase is anchored in the cell membrane and active on the cell surface[80], whereas endogenous STase is a cytoplasmic or periplasmic enzyme. Meningococci that have endogenously sialylated their LOS can be sialylated further by the exogenous STase[76].

The acceptor-specificity of one meningococcal endogenous STase is C_3 of the lacto-N-neotetraose terminal Gal[81]. It is this carbon that N. gonorrhoeae galactosaminylates to create ganglioside-like α-oligosaccharides. If the acceptor-specificity of the gonococcal exogenous STase is the same as that of this meningococcal endogenous STase, then the former must compete with the gonococcal endogenous galactosaminyl transferase[26,55,57,73,81]. It has been observed empirically that gonococcal paragloboside-like LOS are either galactosaminylated or sialylated in the presence of CMP-NANA; the proportions of molecules that remain unsubstituted, sialylated or galac-tosaminylated in vivo vary.

Complement activation and its regulation

Intravascular defence against invasion by gram-negative bacteria is thought to depend upon recognition of the bacterial surface by either antibody or complement. Intravascular clearance is mediated through the deposition of complement components: C3b for phagocytic clearance; the membrane attack complex (MAC) or C5b–C9 for lysis. C3 is the molecule of convergence of the two pathways of complement activation and the source of opsonically active fragments[82]. C3 binds covalently to primary OH and

NH_2 groups through a reactive thiolester in the C3d domain of its C3b fragment[83]. The quantity of deposited C3 and the extent of its degradation determines the interaction of complement-opsonised bacteria with peripheral blood cells that express receptors for C3 fragments.

The alternative complement pathway (ACP) is activated by the spontaneous low-rate hydrolysis of the C3 thiolester to form C3 (H_2O)[83]. C3(H_2O) then forms a complex with factor B in which factor B can be cleaved by factor D to yield C3(H_2O)Bb, the fluid-phase C3 convertase. C3(H_2O)Bb cleaves the C3a fragment from the amino terminus of the α-chain of C3 resulting in the formation of a metastable C3b which binds covalently via ester or amide linkages to membrane surfaces. Bound C3b binds additional factor B, which in turn is cleaved by factor D to produce C3bBb. C3bBb is the surface-phase C3 convertase of the ACP; by cleaving additional C3 molecules, it increases the number of C3b molecules that are membrane-bound. Properdin (P) binds between residues 1402 and 1435 of the C-terminal region of the α-chain of C3b and stabilises the C3bBb complex. P-binding increases the half-life of C3bBb nearly tenfold[84].

Immune lysis is a complement-mediated function that is effected by the assembly of the fifth to the ninth complement components on the bacterial surface. This assembly results in the rapid conversion of the hydrophilic circulating proteins into an amphiphilic macromolecular aggregate, the MAC. Integration of the MAC into the bacterial outer membrane causes extensive detergent-like disassembly of the outer membrane, formation of transmembrane channels and loss of the membrane barrier to peptidoglycan degradation by serum lysozymes. The simultaneous disruption of the cytoplasmic membrane by the MAC results in irreversible loss of cell viability.

Antibody-independent activation of complement

In the absence of antibodies, bacterial surfaces variously activate the two complement pathways through their binding of different initiating components. The activation process involves cell surface glycoses that provide receptors for the initiator glycoproteins[85,86]. C1q binds to basal LOS and lipopolysaccharide (LPS) structures, and metastable C3b binds covalently to a variety of carbohydrate residues[87]. Other cell surface glycoses interfere with or 'down-regulate' complement activation[88]. Masking of receptors by polysaccharides, either as LPS or capsules, prevents binding of C1q, and sialylation prevents ACP activation (see below). Gradations in efficiency of complement activation are a function of the number and specificity of receptors, both activating and down-regulating, and the affinity with which they bind complement glycoproteins. Bacteria capable of surviving in the bloodstream invariably resist antibody-independent activation of complement by one or another mechanism.

People who have inherited isolated deficiencies of the terminal components of complement are at increased risk only of neisserial infections. Other mucosal bacteria that also routinely cause disseminated disease in the absence of immune lysis[89,90] do not disseminate in the sera of complement-deficient people. Therefore there must be something unique in the way the neisserial surface interacts with complement.

Sialic acid, complement and immune lysis

Sialylation of cell membrane glycoconjugates aborts the assembly of the MAC[91], and sialylation of the meningococcal surface aborts complement-mediated lysis[44,92]. A relative deficiency of sialic acid on red blood cells favours the binding of factor B to particle-bound C3b, whereas an abundance of sialic acid favours the attachment of factor H to C3b. Binding of H to C3b, or displacement of Bi from C3bBb by H, facilitates cleavage inactivation of C3b by factor I. Meri and Pangburn reported that factor H contains a binding site for terminal sialic acid residues but not for polysialyl structures[93]. Occupation of this site caused an increase in the affinity of H for C3b that resulted in down-regulation of ACP activation.

Polysialyl capsules

The $\alpha2\rightarrow8$ polysialyl capsule of serogroup B N. meningitidis is an important virulence factor[94,95]. It confers virulence by stoichiometrically interfering with complement activation. Individual strains vary in their ability to activate the ACP as a function of the amount of capsule that they make[96]. Jarvis and Vedros found that the amount of ACP-initiated C3 bound by a serogroup B N. meningitidis strain in the absence of antibodies was proportional to the amount of sialic acid that had been enzymatically removed from the bacteria[44]. Enhanced C3 binding was accompanied by an increase in factor B deposition. The sialylated capsules of K1 E. coli and serogroup B streptococci have also been shown to render those cells non-activators of the ACP in the absence of specific antibody[97,98].

The interactions between anionic polysaccharides and complement have a stoichiometry that is independent of bacterial origin and distinct from antigenic specificities[44,49-101]. The $\alpha2\rightarrow8$ serogroup B and $\alpha2\rightarrow9$ serogroup C meningococcal polysialyl capsules, the $(NeuNAc\alpha2\rightarrow6Gal)$-R capsule of type III, group B streptococci and the ManNAc-P polymer of serogroup A meningococci can all inhibit immune lysis of meningococci and opsonophagocytosis of streptococci[98] when in the fluid phase—as would occur during *in vivo* bacteraemia—and in the absence of antibody[99]. The $\alpha2\rightarrow8$ and $\alpha2\rightarrow9$ polysialyl structures in the fluid-phase can inhibit lysis even when it is initiated by antibodies that bind other surface organelles[101].

The $\alpha2\rightarrow9$ sialyl polymer, the ManNAc-P polymer and the streptococcal capsule are equimolar inhibitors in native serum in which both complement pathways are available; the $\alpha2\rightarrow8$ sialyl polymer is twice as inhibitory as the other three. This 2:1 molar ratio holds for both opsonophagocytosis of streptococci and immune lysis of meningococci. That is, ManNAc-P inhibits opsonophagocytic killing of B/III streptococci just as well as the streptococcal capsule; $\alpha2\rightarrow8$ polysialyl inhibits killing of both streptococci and meningococci twice as effectively as do their respective capsules[99].

All four polymers, when in the fluid phase, can also inhibit lysis and phagocytosis that is mediated through the ACP alone. The inhibitory capacities of meningococcal capsules for ACP-mediated clearance mechanisms are equimolar and more than twice that of the streptococcal capsule. When expressed as moles of N-acetate, the inhibitory capacities of the four polysaccharides are equal[99]. Varki and Kornfield found that down-regulation of the ACP by red blood cells was also a function of the acetylation of their surface NeuNAc residues[100].

It has been assumed that polysialyl capsules bind factor H directly and increase its affinity for C3b, but the O-acetylated $\alpha2\rightarrow8$ polysialyl capsule of K1 *E. coli* does not interact directly with factor H[93]. Whether the O-non-acetylated meningococcal $\alpha2\rightarrow8$ polysialyl capsule (serogroup B) or the variously O-acetylated $\alpha2\rightarrow9$ polysialyl capsule (serogroup C) directly binds H has not been investigated. Sialylation could also change the density distribution of C3b such that high affinity binding sites for factor H are formed in areas in which C3b is clustered[102].

Sialylated LOS

Sialylated LOS, which have the same sugar structures as erythrocyte glycoconjugates, could also bind H directly, but this has not been studied. Exogenous sialylation of their LOS makes gonococci resist immune lysis[103], but exogenous sialylation of meningococcal LOS has been reported not to have this effect[104]. The effect of endogenous LOS sialylation on lysis of meningococci has not been adequately studied.

Properdin

Men who have inherited an X-linked deficiency of properdin (P) have no ACP activity in their serum and are at high risk of disseminated meningococcal disease with an unusually rapid, fatal course[105]. Curiously, they are not at increased risk of disseminated gonococcal infections, nor of other bacterial infections. P is thought to stabilise the association of factor B with C3b and thereby increase the half-life of this ACP C3 convertase[84]. The unique susceptibility to disseminated meningococcal disease of men who have no circulating P shows that the initiation of complement activation on the surface is just as important as its termination with deposition of an effective attack complex, and that P is absolutely necessary for lysis of meningococci, at least for those who do not possess circulating capsular antibodies[105]. There must be something unique about the meningococcal surface that destabilises C3b and the lytic pathway and that can be overcome by P.

Properdin, which binds a 34 amino acid sequence in the α-chain of C3, serves as a 'recognition' molecule for the ACP. The binding of P to the surface of a cell is independent of that of C3b. P that is bound to the surface provides a site for stable and effective C3b-binding through the latter's α-chain recognition sequence[106].

Serum resistant (ser[r]) N. gonorrhoeae that resist immune lysis do so because their surfaces fail to activate complement stably in the absence of bound antibody[67,107–109]. The proportion of serum sensitive (ser[s]) gonococci that can be lysed through the ACP alone varies among strains and among different populations of a given strain. This variation is a function of the amount of P that each bacterium can bind to a 39 kDa outer membrane protein[110]. We must assume that P also binds directly to the surface of encapsulated meningococci and thereby stabilises nascent C3b and the lytic pathway.

The structures of meningococcal capsules suggest a hypothesis. Serogroup Y capsular antibodies induced in a P-deficient patient by vaccination[105] were lytic in the absence of P; serogroup W antibodies were not. The two capsules are co-polymers of NeuNAc linked $\alpha2\rightarrow6$ to glucose (Y) or galactose (W)[53]. This suggests that the interposition of Gal, but not Glc residues, between sialic acid residues causes C3b to bind to sites where it can be inactivated readily even in the presence of antibody, and that the coincidental binding of P is necessary to prevent C3b inactivation[111,112]. The disaccharide antennae of B/III streptococcal capsules have the same NeuNAc$\alpha2\rightarrow6$Gal structure as the meningococcal W capsule[113].

Antibody-dependent activation of complement

Complement activation is an aggregate phenomenon[102]; i.e. initiator molecules that bind to the cell surface in clusters bind with greater affinity, are less readily disassociated or inactivated, and are more likely to promote effective MAC deposition. IgM and IgG immunoglobulins have various C3b and C1q binding sites in their Fc regions. When they bind in close proximity, their aggregated Fc regions provide a nidus for continuous complement activation[114]. Thus antibody molecules direct complement activation onto the bacterial surface and concentrate it into foci of activation. Antibody molecules that activate complement in such a way that the MAC inserts stably into the bacterial membrane are 'bactericidal'.

LOS antibodies, sialylation and immune lysis

The addition of GalNAc to lacto-*N*-neotetraose LOS moieties creates gangliosyl-like LOS that bear an epitope for IgM molecules that are ubiquitous in human sera and that initiate classical pathway (CP)-mediated lysis of *N. gonorrhoeae*[110]. Sialylation of the same LOS moieties prevents them from being galactosaminylated (see above)[55,65,76,79,115], so that fully sialylated gonococci have no GalNAc-dependent epitopes with which to bind lytic IgM. Sialylation also occludes lacto-*N*-neotetraose epitopes, so that lysis of fully sialylated gonococci must proceed through the ACP, without any contribution from the CP. Since sialylation down-regulates the ACP, fully sialylated gonococci are ser[r].

Meningococci, on the other hand, do not galactosaminylate lacto-*N*-neotetraose LOS structures and do not bind the LOS IgM that initiates lysis of gonococci. Meningococci are lysed by IgG molecules that bind epitopes on basal LOS structures that are not made by gonococci and that are not occluded by sialylation (see below)[63,116,117]. Thus, LOS sialylation has different effects on the sensitivity of the two pathogenic *Neisseria* to immune lysis[103,104].

Lactosyl-like LOS lack the lacto-*N*-neotetraose acceptor for GalNAc, cannot be galactosaminylated and do not bind lytic IgM. Increased expression of these molecules by gonococci decreases the density with which IgM can bind and initiate CP-dependent C3b deposition. Enhanced or sole expression of lactosyl-like LOS also make *N. gonorrhoeae* ser[r67,118]. If such strains bind enough P, they can be lysed through the ACP.

Augmentation of the alternative complement pathway

Cell-bound C3b provides a binding site for factor B regardless of the pathway of its activation[119]. C3bBb continuously activates more C3, thereby generating a positive feedback amplification loop. ACP augmentation can increase the aggregate density on the cell surface of any CP-deposited C3b and thus the efficiency with which the MAC is assembled. Ser[s] strains of *N. gonorrhoeae* that equivalently bind IgM to LOS GalNAc residues are, nonetheless, lysed at different titres by the same human sera, as their surfaces variously bind P and support ACP augmentation of the density of C3b that is deposited through IgM activation of the CP[110].

Capsular antibodies up-regulate the alternative complement pathway

When an antibody molecule binds its epitope it may mask surface components on or adjacent to the epitope that would otherwise down-regulate complement activation. The $\alpha2\rightarrow8$ polysialyl capsule of serogroup B *N. meningitidis* prevents ACP augmentation of C3b molecules that are derived from CP activation by IgG antibodies that bind subcapsular determinants[44,96]. Since man is tolerant to this polysialyl capsule, antibody against it is virtually absent from human serum[101,120]. However, during convalescence from disseminated disease or following vaccination with an appropriate protein/polysaccharide complex, tolerance is partially broken, and IgM that is of quite low avidity[121] and poorly bactericidal[101,122] is produced briefly[120,123]. When this otherwise poorly lytic IgM binds to the capsule it masks the chemical moiety responsible for ACP down-regulation, perhaps N-acetate adducts, thereby sustaining the lytic process[44]. Interestingly, the binding of capsular IgM does not result in an increase in bound C3b, even as it sustains lysis[44].

Antibody binding to bacterial surfaces also increases ACP activation in the absence of CP activity. It remains unclear, however, whether this results from direct activation of other initiator components, masking of surface components, or through decreases in the affinity with which H and I bind to C3 convertases.

Immunoglobulin isotypes

The three major circulating isotypes of immunoglobulins (Igs) vary in their ability to initiate immune lysis[48]. IgM normally circulates as a pentameric aggregate and is the most efficient initiator. IgG normally circulates as a monomer; in order for it to activate the CP at least two molecules must be bound sufficiently closely that a single C1q molecule can bridge their Fc receptors. Because of this requirement for at least doublet formation, the bactericidal power of IgG is, at best, only one half that of IgM[48]. Moreover, IgG_2 and IgG_4 activate complement poorly.

IgA blocks immune lysis

Under most biological conditions of aggregate binding, including those on the surface of bacteria, IgA does not initiate immune lysis[40]. Rather, IgA blocks lysis initiated by IgM or IgG through either pathway of complement activation[49]. IgA blockade is a widespread phenomenon. It was described originally with Salmonella typhimurium as the target cell[124] and has been described subsequently in relation to many additional bacterial species[40,125–127]. It has been shown to occur with polymeric secretory IgA[124,126] and monomeric serum IgA[40,48,125,127], and for both pathways of C activation[44]. IgA binding can also suppress chemotaxis and block opsonophagocytosis by polymorphonuclear leucocytes[126,128,129].

Serum IgA has competitive advantages over IgG and IgM[48]. IgA may displace IgG from antigen binding sites, and the binding of IgG to at least one antigen, the meningococcal $\alpha2\rightarrow9$ polysialyl capsule, causes the exposure of IgA binding sites that were previously not available—a form of positive binding co-operativity between the two immunoglobulins[130]. Since blockage of lysis is an IgA-weighted function of the IgA:IgG ratio, and this remains constant at all inocula, IgA blockade of IgG-initiated lysis is not inoculum-sensitive. IgA blockade of IgM-initiated lysis is a non-competive function of the ratio of IgA to antigen (inoculum) and independent of the concentration of IgM[49]. As a result, a given amount of IgA more effectively blocks IgM-initiated lysis of a small inoculum than a large one. The competitive advantages that IgA has over IgM and IgG led us to hypothesise that blockade of complement activation and its inflammatory sequelae is an important homeostatic regulatory function of circulating IgA that operates most efficiently during entry into the bloodstream of the normally trivial showers of organisms that accompany such biological functions as chewing and defecation[49].

Opsonophagocytosis and sialylation

The observation that people who have inherited deficiencies in one or another of the terminal components of complement have intact complement-dependent opsonophagocytic killing of *N. meningitidis* in the face of a significantly increased risk of disseminated infection[35,43] has been taken to mean that opsonophagocytosis provides little, if any, protection from dissemination[35,43]. However, the discovery that LOS are sialylated has sparked a renewed interest in opsonophagocytosis of *Neisseria*[76,131,132].

In a study of serogroup C *N. meningitidis* consecutively isolated over 4 years in Houston, Texas, USA[101,133], we found that the serotypically diverse strains isolated during the period of endemic disease were variously sialylated. The amount of polysialyl capsule made by each strain and the extent of its LOS sialylation were associated with each other and with resistance to killing by neutrophils[76]. Three strains that were isolated from carriers were among the most easily killed and among the least sialylated.

Toward the end of the 4 years, a C2b:P1.2:L3,7 strain caused a focal outbreak in a school[134]. During the next 4 months this epidemic strain was isolated from nasopharyngeal carriers at the school and from patients outside the school. The several copies of the epidemic strain survived significantly better in the presence of neutrophils than did the endemic strains; eight of 14 epidemic strains completely resisted killing by neutrophils. Endogenous LOS sialylation was fairly homogenous among the different isolates of the epidemic strain and was not associated with polysialyl capsule production. Neither endogenous LOS sialylation nor capsule production affected resistance to neutrophil killing, which was, in any event, higher than among the endemic strains[76].

Exogenous LOS sialylation had little effect on the susceptibility of endemic isolates to complement-dependent neutrophil killing, but it did make resistant two of three otherwise sensitive epidemic isolates. Exogenous LOS sialylation also has relatively little effect on PMN uptake and killing of gonococci[131,132], even as it makes them resistant to immune lysis[103].

These observations suggest that opsonophagocytosis may play a more prominent role in humoral immunity than previously thought. Strains that caused endemic disease resisted neutrophil killing because of enhanced endogenous LOS sialylation and polysialyl capsule production. The epidemic potential of the school-outbreak strain may have been related to its ability to survive in the presence of neutrophils independently of sialylation.

INDUCTION OF ANTIBODY

Antibody to the meningococcus that is present at birth is acquired from the maternal circulation. As this passive immunity wanes, it is replaced throughout life by autonomously induced antibodies.

Maternally derived

That portion of the mother's immunity that is contained in her IgG is passed to the fetus transplacentally[36,135]. Infants who suckle their mothers also receive large quantities of IgA and lesser amounts of IgG and IgM from colostrum. The breast is a part of the mucosal immune system, and colostral IgA reflects the mucosal antigenic experience of the mother. This includes antigens of the meningococcus that were presented to mucosa-associated lymphoid tissue by other organisms[1,136]. The effect of colostrum-derived antibody on immune processing of maternally derived flora during the nursing period is unknown.

Autonomously induced

The sequential colonisation of the child's pharynx by non-pathogenic *Neisseria* induces immunity that then allows commensal colonisation by potentially pathogenic meningococci.

N. lactamica

N. lactamica (a species that can use lactose, the principal disaccharide in milk) and not *N. meningitidis*, is the *Neisseria* that most commonly colonises the pharynges of infants and young children[137-140]. *N. lactamica* colonisation induces antibodies that are bactericidal for meningococcal strains of different serogroups and serotypes[137]. Children previously colonised with *N. lactamica* seldom sicken during epidemics of meningococcal disease. The protective effect of lactamica colonisation on the risk of developing meningococcal disease can be quite striking, as shown in Table 3.3. Lactamica carriage was significantly lower in an area of Qingfeng County in the People's Republic of China that was experiencing hyperendemic serogroup A meningococcal disease (the Meningitis Area) than in an area that had no disease (the Control Area). Meningococcal carriage was higher in the Meningitis Area, but not significantly so. Observations in Connecticut[137], provinces of China[139,140], and Africa[138] show similar associations between *N. lactamica* colonisation and an absence of both endemic and epidemic meningococcal disease.

N. lactamica are not encapsulated[141] and do not cause disease. They do share LOS structures and epitopes, but not serotype proteins, with strains of *N. meningitidis*[141]. *N. lactamica* strains from South China, where meningococcal disease is rare, often make LOS that have infant-immunising epitopes[69,70]; those from areas of epidemic disease do not[141]. Surface expression of conserved LOS epitopes by lactamica strains would account for the induction of protective meningococcal antibody during the early years of life.

Human LOS antibodies

It has been difficult to establish the structural specificities of LOS antibodies in humans[67,101,142–145]. Sialylated glycoses are poorly immunogenic in mammals, and antibodies that bind lacto-*N*-neotetraose are rarely found in human sera, even after neisserial infection[146]—presumably because of their similarity to human GSL structures. Circulating antibodies that bind conserved epitopes on non-sialylated, low molecular weight meningococcal LOS are acquired by most people by adulthood. These antibodies are

Table 3.3 *Prevalence of meningococcal and lactamical colonisation among children in two areas of Qingfeng County, PRC*

	Culture negative	Culture positive with	
		N. meningitidis	*N. lactamica*
Meningitis Area	294	9	4
Control Area	299	3	38
Δ Between areas	$\chi^2 = 30$	$p = 5 \times 10^{-7}$	
For *N. meningitidis*	$\chi^2 = 2.68$	$p = 0.10$	
For *N. lactamica*	$\chi^2 = 24.4$	$p = 8 \times 10^{-4}$	

Data provided by Dr Hu Xujing of the Institute of Epidemiology and Microbiology, Beijing, People's Republic of China.

bactericidal and are responsible for some portion of protective immunity against meningococcal dissemination. Their epitopes are expressed by *N. lactamica*, but not by *N. gonorrhoeae*, and they are probably induced during lactamical and meningococcal colonisation. We have recently identified two such populations of human LOS IgG antibodies that are bactericidal for, respectively, serogroups B and C, and A and Y meningococci[116,117].

Bactericidal antibodies induced in infants and children who do not respond to the capsular polysaccharide of their infecting strain during disseminated serogroup B and C disease can be inhibited by a conserved, non-sialylated LOS molecule that is separate from the various serotype-specific LOS molecules[101]. To find out which LOS bear this epitope, we developed an assay that tests the ability of polyclonal antibodies in human sera to compete for LOS binding sites with monoclonal antibodies (MAbs) that define epitopes of interest[69]. Two epitopes, defined by MAbs D6A and 6B7, induced antibody in 17 children who were convalescing from disseminated disease (14 due to serogroup B)[70,101]. Eleven of these children were ≤ 2 years of age; the youngest was aged 3 weeks. Both epitopes are found on non-sialylated 3.6 kDa LOS; D6A also binds non-sialylated 3.2 and 4.0 kDa LOS. The latter LOS bears the P^k/L1 epitope[147].

By six years most children have MAb D6A-like antibody. The levels of MAb D6A-like antibody in the acute-phase sera of children who sicken are less than those in the sera of healthy children of the same age. Healthy children who are colonised with serogroup B or C meningococci have the highest levels, regardless of age[70]. Their levels were almost as high as those in convalescent sera[69,70]. The population of IgGs in human sera that inhibits MAb D6A initiates lysis of serogroup B and C meningococci[116].

Some years ago we found that naturally acquired bactericidal antibodies against serogroup Y *N. meningitidis* cross-react with, and can be absorbed by agarose, a galactan made by red seaweeds[144,145]. We found that α-lactose (α-Lac; Galα1→4G1c), but not β-lactose (Gal β1→4 Glc) nor mellobiose (Galα1→6Glc), can elute human IgG that is bactericidal for serogroup A meningococci of LOS types L10 and L11 from agarose[117]. Lytic antibody can be completely absorbed from whole human sera by homologous LOS, mostly absorbed by heterologous LOS, and eluted from LOS with α-Lac. *N. lactamica* LOS of molecular weight < 4500 can also absorb antibody that is lytic for serogroup A meningococci. Absorption of capsular polysaccharide antibodies from human sera has little effect on their lytic titre.

Neither serogroup A meningococci, nor *N. lactamica* sialylate their LOS; L10 and L11 LOS are borne on 4.0 and 3.6 kDa LOS, respectively, but the structure of neither type is known with certainty. The presence of α-Lac structures has not been reported in meningococcal LOS, but structural work has concentrated on defining the serotypes, and the α-Lac structure that binds lytic IgG is independent of LOS serotype structures.

N. meningitidis

After age 4, the pharynx of the child is regularly, if intermittently, colonised by strains of *N. meningitidis*. Many of these are either unencapsulated (multiagglutinable) or they elaborate capsular polysaccharides that do not confer pathogenic potential. As with colonisation by *N. lactamica*, these strains induce bactericidal antibody against subcapsular (LOS and protein) or serotypic determinants[148]. Commensal colonisation by encapsulated meningococci induces or augments antibody against capsular polysaccharides (serogroup immunity). Thus, serotype and serogroup immunity 'leap-frog' through the early years of life. Serogroup immunity takes precedence over serotype immunity, regardless of the antigenic specificity of the latter[145].

The prevalence of capsular polysaccharide antibody in a population is not uniformly distributed over time or space[149]. Rather, the prevalence of antibody to each serogroup rises and falls independently. Levels of serogroup A antibody in sequential cohorts of young American adults declined steadily from 1975 to 1983 (the last year for which I have data)[149]. Levels of antibody to serogroups C, Y, and W initially declined, then increased. The distribution of antibody was always biphasic for each serogroup, with some proportion of each cohort remaining unimmunised into adulthood. The changes in antibody prevalence to serogroups A and Y did not reflect contemporaneous changes in the prevalence of colonisation by meningococci of these serogroups and occurred in the absence of nationally appreciable serogroup A or Y disease during the periods over which the individuals were studied. Assays of the prevalence of serotypic immunity have not been attempted because of technical difficulties, but would also be expected to fluctuate over time.

It would be unlikely for meningococcal disease to spread in populations with high levels of immunity. As serogroup (or serotype) immunity declines in a population, the incidence of inapparent colonisation by meningococci of that serogroup (or serotype) should increase, with disease occurring only in that portion of the population that has neither serogroup nor serotype immunity. Increased colonisation would then increase population immunity and abate the wave of colonisation and disease.

If the acquisition of antibody during childhood provided uninterrupted immunity, susceptibility should be clustered in the very young and be independent of serogroup and serotype. During endemic periods, however, age-related susceptibility varies for the different serogroups, and the age-specific attack rate invariably shifts to older individuals during epidemics, regardless of serogroup.

N. gonorrhoeae

N. gonorrhoeae may be encountered in the birth canal or some years later with the advent of sexual activity. The effects of these encounters are controversial. It has been suggested that they could transiently reduce meningococcal immunity[150].

Enteric immunisation by 'cross-reacting' organisms

Enteric colonisation with organisms that have surface antigens that are the same as those on the meningococcus provides an additional route by which individuals may acquire immunity[120,151]. Such organisms are widespread in human populations; when ingested they initially stimulate both secretory and serum IgA[49]. The IgA response is a generalised one that leads to the secretion of the secretory IgA at distal mucosal sites. IgA production wanes several days after colonisation[49], and the response 'matures' with a modest increase in cirulating IgM and/or IgG that contributes 'natural' immunity to meningococcal antigens, particularly capsular polysaccharides. If the same, or a related, organism is encountered during the IgA response, it is opsonised by IgA and either maintained within the stool column or killed by macrophages and monocytes[49,152], depending on the anatomic site of the encounter.

THE IgA RESPONSE TO ENTERIC COLONISATION CAUSES SUSCEPTIBILITY TO MENINGOCOCCAL DISSEMINATION

Epidemics of meningococcal disease occur in populations with elevated levels of circulating meningococcal IgA that can block immune lysis of the epidemic strain when it enters the circulation[1,50–52,153]. That levels of circulating IgA sufficient to abrogate completely immune lysis of *N. meningitidis* can occur *in vivo* was demonstrated by removing IgA from the sera of military recruits susceptible during an epidemic and restoring bactericidal activity for each of their infecting strains[42]. This observation has been extended to a serogroup A epidemic in Finland[50], a serogroup A outbreak among 'skid road' habitués in the Pacific Northwest[154], a serogroup C outbreak among school children in Houston, Texas, and a serogroup A epidemic in The Gambia[153]. During the last, Greenwood *et al.* found elevated total serum IgA in cases, when compared with contemporaneous, age-matched controls, in a village with a 10% attack rate[153]. Levels of meningococcal IgA were so high they raised levels of total IgA.

The time/space characteristics of meningococcal outbreaks demonstrate that risk is environmentally acquired[1,136,149,154,155], i.e. risk is centred within an ecological unit defined by socioeconomic and geographic constraints and delimited by time. Individuals within this environment lose immunity gained from prior antigenic experience, and individuals entering the environment acquire susceptibility[1,42,154]. Thus, both immunity and susceptibility are acquired and lost independently during life. The loss of immunity may be serogroup- or serotype-specific, depending on the specificity of the acquired IgA; disease occurs in those who lose either in the absence of the other.

I proposed in 1977 that enteric colonisation by organisms elaborating meningococcal antigens is the immunising event(s) that causes elevated population levels of IgA within the epidemic focus. Since then, organisms with serogroup A meningococcal surface antigens have been recovered in three outbreaks caused by serogroup A *N. meningitidis*[136,156]. One, a strain of *Streptococcus faecalis*, made surface antigens in common with both the serogroup A capsule *and* the conserved LOS antigen that stimulates antibodies that are bactericidal for serogroup A meningococci (see above)[136,154]. The prevalence in the epidemic focus of enteric colonisation by this streptococcus exceeded that of pharyngeal colonisation by serogroup A *N. meningitidis*[1,136,154].

An unpublished study of an outbreak of serogroup A meningococcal disease among black children in Johannesburg, South Africa provided striking proof that colonisation with organisms that share surface antigens with a meningococcus is associated with elevated levels of serum meningococcal IgA and susceptibility to infection by that meningococcus[157] (Table 3.4). Rates of colonisation with bacteria that reacted with meningococcal serogroup A capsular antiserum, primarily of the genera, *Bacillus* and *Micrococcus*, were lower (3.6%) among healthy white school children in Hillbrow, a middle class suburb that was not experiencing disease, than among healthy black school children living in Soweto (8.1%), where disease was occurring. Colonisation was slightly higher among close contacts of the patients (10.3%) than among the healthy Sowetan children. In contrast, 35.3% of the meningococcal disease patients were colonised!

As detected by whole cell enzyme-linked immunosorbent assay (ELISA),

Table 3.4 *Carriage of bacteria cross-reactive with serogroup A meningococci and serogroup A capsular antibodies in South Africans at different risks of meningococcal disease*

Population	Race	Carriage			Percentage with capsular antibodies			
		N	Carrier	(%)	N	IgA	IgG	IgM
Hillbrow children	White	194	7	(3.6)	166	2.4	14.4	76.5
Sowetan children	Black	358	29	(8.1)	250	9	30.5	86.5
Patients	Black	17	6	(35.3)	13	61.5	84.6	92.3
Patient contacts	Black	58	6	(10.3)	50	26	18	72

Data taken from the thesis of Dr Lynne D. Liebowitz accepted by the Faculty of Medicine, University of the Witwatersrand, for the Doctor of Philosophy in Medicine degree at Johannesburg in 1990.

serogroup A meningococcal IgA was significantly more likely to be found in the sera of the patients (61.5%) than in the sera of healthy children living in Soweto (9%) or Hillbrow (2.4%). All 12 patients who were more than 4 years old at the time of meningococcal dissemination were colonised with one or more cross-reacting organisms (6/12), had raised serum anti-meningococcal IgA (8/9), or both (3/9). Four children who had raised serum anti-meningococcal IgA carried serogroup A meningococci without sickening.

IgA-mediated susceptibility to meningococcal dissemination occurs at the height of the IgA response to enteric bacteria[49,158]. The height of the response may be related to the size of the immunising inoculum. Each individual has a biological set point for serum IgA that varies very little[49]; however, relatively minor interferences with hepatic clearance, such as those that accompany mild alcohol ingestion, can elevate serum IgA levels. Alcohol intake therefore increases the risk that individuals with biological set points at or near the upper limit of 'normal' will sicken during an epidemic[49,158–160]. Therefore the duration of IgA-mediated susceptibility is a function of the individual's biological set point, the height of his or her serum IgA immune response, and the rate of hepatic clearance[158] of serum IgA.

Acquisition of IgA-mediated susceptibility and the epidemiology of meningococcal disease

The silent faecal/oral spread of an enteric 'priming' organism nicely accounts for the epidemiology of epidemic meningococcal disease[1]. Meningococcal disease spreads in hyperendemic waves that are punctuated by focal outbreaks of varying size that involve older children and young adults and that are restricted to single, demographically discrete subpopulations. In developed areas the affected population is usually socio-economically deprived when compared with surrounding groups, and the outbreaks do not spread to these coterminous, demographically separable, populations[1,133]. In underdeveloped countries focal outbreaks coalesce into widespread, diffuse epidemics.

Neither the slow, orderly, and contiguous spread of hyperendemic waves and diffuse epidemics, nor the time/space circumscription of focal outbreaks is consistent with the concept that aerosol transmission of the meningococcus is the principal determinant of its epidemic behaviour. Epidemics of other common respiratory pathogens are explosive, moving quickly through a population to involve all the susceptible individuals and then dying out. Nor can they be explained by the introduction into the population of an epidemic serotype, as the epidemic strain is always present in the affected population before the onset of the epidemic and consistently carried by those living in surrounding unaffected areas during the outbreak. Both aspects of meningococcal epidemiology can be explained by the introduction of a bacterium that has the same surface antigens as the meningococcus, but that is spread by the faecal–oral route among the very young and those with poor sanitation.

The dynamics of meningococcal disease epidemiology

If a strain of *N. meningitidis* can express its epidemic potential in a population only when it co-circulates with a non-pathogenic enteric organism that makes an identical surface antigen, transmission of the meningococcus in the absence of a priming organism results in commensal colonisation of those with circulating lytic antibodies that augments and broadens population immunity. In the absence of the meningococcus, transmission of the priming organism results in inapparent colonisation and an appropriate immune response. Only with fortuitous co-colonisation by both organisms will the temporal kinetics of the IgA response to the priming organism be such that susceptibility will be induced in individuals who lack lytic antibody directed against alternative, non-shared antigens.

Transmission of the priming organism determines the spatial extent of the epidemic, since faecal–oral transmission requires closer contact than aerosol transmission and is more easily interrupted. For any rate of transmission of the priming organism, the rate and extent of meningococcal transmission determines the magnitude of the epidemic, since disease can occur only in newly colonised (and newly susceptible) individuals.

Thus, the epidemiology of epidemic meningococcal disease is a function of the rate of faecal/oral transmission of IgA-inducing enteric organisms, the rate of aerosol transmission of a potentially pathogenic meningococcus, and the prevalence, antigenic specificity and isotypic diversity of meningococcal antibodies in a population.

Other mechanisms for the absence of serum lytic activity and the epidemiology of meningococcal disease

The induction of IgA accounts only for epidemic disease in older children and adults. Endemic disease and epidemic disease in those aged less than four years are accounted for by the various other mechanisms by which effective MAC deposition is avoided.

Fixed population attributes

Regardless of other factors, successful maintenance of the commensal relationship by immune lysis requires an intact complement system. Individuals with isolated primary deficiencies of all five terminal components have developed disseminated neisserial infections, both meningococcal and gonococcal. The susceptibility to fulminant meningococcal disease of men with sex-linked deficiencies of properdin emphasises the importance of initiation of complement activation through the ACP for successful lysis of a meningococcus[35,111].

Several systemic diseases may cause secondary deficiencies of complement components, primarily the early components of the classical pathway[160]. Systemic lupus erythematosus (SLE), nephrotic syndrome and multiple myeloma are most commonly associated with meningococcal dissemination caused by this mechanism. Complement deficiency in these diseases may result from unchecked consumption (SLE) or renal protein wasting (nephrotic syndrome). The mechanism in multiple myeloma is unknown.

The first and most commonly described immune defect in individuals sickening with disseminated meningococcal disease is hypogammaglobulinaemia, primarily isolated IgM deficiency. The fact that IgM deficiency is easily determined probably accounts for the disproportionate number of reports of it in the literature. In fact, it is a rare cause of susceptibility[1].

Genetic deficiencies clearly account for a significant but unknown proportion of endemic meningococcal disease. Estimates of the contribution of complement deficiencies to total disease burden range from 10% to 25%[160]. Whereas hypogammaglobulinaemia would affect children only after the catabolism of maternally transferred antibody, complement deficiencies should affect neonates and infants as well. Since infants who develop meningococcal disease are seldom investigated for immune deficiencies, the proportion of them with complement defects is unknown.

Polysaccharide/complement interactions

The anticomplementary effects of capsular polysaccharides account for endemic disease only in neonates and infants. Because subcapsular immunity can be transferred from mother to infant, risk is not uniform. The period of risk is limited by the rapid increase in the vascular volume of the newborn (and therefore in the total number of circulating complement molecules) and the development of autonomous immunity to subcapsular antigens. Because the serogroup B capsule is particularly effective in down-regulating complement, this serogroup accounts for the greatest proportion of disease in the very young; the effect of the serogroup B capsule is augmented by the absence of maternally transferred antibody[161,162].

ACKNOWLEDGEMENTS

The Centre for Immunochemistry of the University of California San Francisco is supported by The Public Health Service of the United States of

America (Grants AI 21620, AI 21171 AI22998); and The Research Service of the US Department of Veterans Affairs. I would like to thank Drs Ryohei Yamasaki, Randa Hamadeh, Ping Zhou, Brad Gibson, Gary Jarvis, Middy Estabrook, Songqing Zhao, Janice Kim and the rest of the staff of the Centre for Immunochemistry for the use of their ideas and work and for their support. This is paper No. 78 from the Centre for Immunochemistry of the University of California San Francisco.

REFERENCES

1. Griffiss JM. Epidemic meningococcal disease. Synthesis of a hypothetical immunoepidemiologic model. Rev Infect Dis 1982; 4: 159–72.
2. Moulder JW. Comparative biology of intracellular parasitism. Microbiol Rev 1985; 49: 298–337.
3. Bliska JB, Galan JE, Falkow S. Signal transduction in the mammalian cell during bacterial attachment and entry. Cell 1993; 73: 903–20.
4. McGee ZA, Stephens DS, Hoffman LH, Schlech WF, Horn RG. Mechanisms of mucosal invasion by pathogenic *Neisseria*. Rev Infect Dis 1983; 5: S708–14.
5. Stephens DS, McGee ZA. Attachment of *Neisseria meningitidis* to human mucosal surfaces: influence of pili and type of receptor cell. J Infect Dis 1981; 143: 525–32.
6. Stephens DS, Farley MM. Pathogenic events during infection of the human nasopharynx with *Neisseria meningitidis* and *Haemophilus influenzae*. Rev Infect Dis 1991; 13: 22–33.
7. Gubish ER, Chen KCS, Buchanan TM. Attachment of gonococcal pili to lectin-resistant clones of chinese hamster ovary cells. Infect Immun 1982; 37: 189–94.
8. Isberg RR. Discrimination between intracellular uptake and surface adhesion of bacterial pathogens. Science 1991; 252: 934–8.
9. Hultgren SJ, Abraham S, Caparon M, Falk P, Geme JWS, Normark S. Pilus and nonpilus bacterial adhesins: assembly and function in cell recognition. Cell 1993; 73: 887–901.
10. Nassif X, Lowy J, Stenberg P, O'Gaora P, Ganji A, So M. Antigenic variation of pilin regulates adhesion of *Neisseria meningitidis* to human epithelial cells. Mol Microbiol 1993; 8: 719–25.
11. Rudel T, van Putten JPM, Gibbs CP, Has R, Meyer TF. Interaction of two variable proteins (PilE and PilC) required for pilus-mediated adherence of *Neisseria gonorrhoeae* to human epithelial cells. Mol Microbiol 1992; 6: 3439–50.
12. Craven DE, Peppler MS, Frasch CE, Mocca LF, McGrath PP, Washington G. Adherence of isolates of *Neisseria meningitidis* from patients and carriers to human buccal epithelial cells. J Infect Dis 1980; 142: 556–68.
13. Stephens DS, Edwards KM, Morris F, McGee A. Pili and outer membrane appendages on *Neisseria meningitidis* in the cerebrospinal fluid of an infant. J Infect Dis 1982; 146: 568–9.
14. Devoe IW, Gilchrist JE. Pili on meningococci from primary cultures of nasopharyngeal carriers and cerebrospinal fluid of patients with acute disease. J Exp Med 1975; 141: 297–305.
15. Stephens DS, Whitney AM, Rothbard J, Schoolnik GK. Pili of *Neisseria*

meningitidis. Analysis of structure and investigation of structural and antigenic relationships to gonococcal pili. J Exp Med 1985; 161: 1539–53.

16. Pinner RW, Spellman PA, Stephens DS. Evidence for functionally distinct pili expressed by Neisseria meningitidis. Infect Immun 1991; 59: 3169–75.

17. Makino S, van Putten JPM, Meyer TF. Phase variation of the opacity outer membrane protein controls invasion by Neisseria gonorrhoeae into human epithelial cells. EMBO J 1991; 10: 1307–15.

18. Shaw JH, Falkow S. Model for invasion of human tissue culture cells by Neisseria gonorrhoeae. Infect Immun 1988; 56: 1625–32.

19. Hart CA, Rogers TRF. Meningococcal disease. J Med Microbiol 1993; 39: 3–25.

20. Stephens DS, Whitney AM, Schoolnik GK, Zollinger WD. Common epitopes of pilin of Neisseria meningitidis. J Infect Dis 1988; 158: 332–42.

21. Frasch CE, Zollinger WD, Poolman JT. Serotype antigens of Neisseria meningitidis and a proposed scheme for designation of serotypes. Rev Infect Dis 1985; 7: 504–10.

22. Simon D, Rest RF. Escherichia coli expressing a Neisseria gonorrhoeae opacity-associated outer membrane protein invade human cervical and endometrial cell lines. Proc Natl Acad Sci USA 1992; 89: 5512–16.

23. Weel JFL, Hopman CTP, van Putten JPM. In situ expression and localization of Neisseria gonorrhoeae opacity proteins in infected epithelial cells: apparent role of Opa proteins in cellular invasion. J Exp Med 1991; 57: 1395–1405.

24. Blake MS. Functions of the outer membrane proteins of Neisseria gonorrhoeae. In: Jackson GG, Thomas H, eds. The Pathogenesis of Bacterial Infections. Berlin: Springer-Verlag, 1985; 51–66 (Bayer Symposium VIII).

25. Mandrell RE, Griffiss JM, Macher BA. Lipooligosaccharides (LOS) of Neisseria gonorrhoeae and Neisseria meningitidis have components that are immunochemically similar to precursors of human blood group antigens. Carbohydrate sequence specificity of the mouse monoclonal antibodies that recognize crossreacting antigens on LOS and human erythrocytes. J Exp Med 1988; 168: 107–26.

26. Mandrell RE. Further antigenic similarities of Neisseria gonorrhoeae lipooligosaccharides and human glycosphingolipids. Infect Immun 1992; 60: 3017–20.

27. Brooks GF, Olinger L, Lammel CJ, Bhat KS, Calvello CA, Palmer ML et al. Prevalence of gene sequences coding for hypervariable regions of Opa (protein II) in Neisseria gonorrhoeae. Mol Microbiol 1991; 5: 3063–72.

28. Lammel CJ, Dekker NP, Mandrell RE, Griffiss JM, Brooks GF. The role of Opa in adherence of gonococci to HEC-1-B cells and to human fallopian tube tissues. In: Achtman M, Kohl P, Marchal C, Morelli G, Siler A, Thiesen B, eds. Neisseriae 1990. Berlin: Walter de Gruyter, 1991; 615–20.

29. Rest RF, Lee N, Bowden C. Stimulation of human leukocytes by protein II+ gonococci is mediated by lectin-like gonococcal components. Infect Immun 1985; 50: 116–22.

30. Olyhoek AJM, Sarkari J, Bopp M, Morelli G, Achtman M. Cloning and expression in Escherichia coli of opc, the gene for an unusual class 5 outer membrane protein from Neisseria meningitidis. Microb Path 1991; 11: 249–57.

31. Rosenqvist E, Høiby EA, Wedege E, Kusecek B, Achtman M. The 5c protein of Neisseria meningitidis is highly immunogenic in humans and induces bactericidal antibodies. J Infect Dis 1993; 167: 1065–73.

32. Achtman M, Wall RA, Bopp M. Variation in class 5 protein expression by serogroup A meningococci during a meningitis epidemic. J Infect Dis 1991; 164: 375–82.

33. Virji M, Makepeace K, Ferguson DJP, Achtman M, Sarkari J, Moxon ER.

Expression of the Opc protein correlates with invasion of epithelial and endothelial cells by *Neisseria meningitidis*. Mol Microbiol 1992; 6: 2785–95.

34. Gotschlich EC, Goldschneider I, Artenstein MS. Human immunity to the meningococcus. V. The effect of immunization with meningococcal group C polysaccharide on the carrier state. J Exp Med 1969; *129*: 1385–95.

35. Ross SC, Densen P. Complement deficiency states and infections: epidemiology, pathogenesis and consequences of neisserial and other infections in an immune deficiency. Medicine (Baltimore) 1984; *63*: 243–73.

36. Goldschneider I, Gotschlich EC, Artenstein MS. Human immunity to the meningococcus. I. The role of humoral antibodies. J Exp Med 1969; *129*: 1307–26.

37. Goldschneider I, Gotschlich EC, Artenstein MS. Human immunity to the meningococcus. II. Development of natural immunity. J Exp Med 1969; *129*: 1327–48.

38. Heist GD, Solis-Cohen S, Solis-Cohen M. A study of the virulence of meningococci for man and of human susceptibility to meningococcic infection. J Immunol 1922; 7: 1.

39. Gold R, Winkelhake JL, Mars RS, Artenstein MS. Identification of an epidemic strain of group C *Neisseria meningitidis* by bactericidal serotyping. J Infect Dis 1971; *124*: 593–7.

40. Griffiss JM. Bactericidal activity of meningococcal antisera: blocking by IgA of lytic antibody in human convalescent sera. J Immunol 1975; *114*: 1779–84.

41. Petersen BH, Graham JA, Brooks GF. Human deficiency of the eighth component of complement: the requirement of C8 for serum *Neisseria gonorrhoeae* bactericidal activity. J Clin Invest 1976; *57*: 283–90.

42. Griffiss JM, Bertram MA. Immunoepidemiology of meningococcal disease in military recruits. II. Blocking of serum bactericidal activity by circulating IgA early in the course of invasive disease. J Infect Dis 1977; *136*: 733–9.

43. Nicholson A, Lepow IH. Host defense against *Neisseria meningitidis* requires a complement-dependent bactericidal activity. Science 1979; *205*: 298–9.

44. Jarvis GA, Vedros NA. Sialic acid of group B *Neisseria meningitidis* regulates alternative complement pathway activation. Infect Immun 1987; *55*: 174–80.

45. Griffiss JM, Brandt BL, Broud DD, Altieri PL, Berman SL. Relationship of dose to the reactogenicity and immunogenicity of meningococcal polysaccharide vaccines in adults. Milit Med 1985; *150*: 529–33.

46. Gotschlich EC, Goldschneider I, Artenstein MS. Human immunity to the meningococcus. IV. Immunogenicity of group A and group C meningococcal polysaccharides in human volunteers. J Exp Med 1969; *129*: 1367–84.

47. Zollinger WD, Mandrell RE, Altieri P, Berman S, Lowenthal J, Artenstein MS. Safety and immunogenicity of a *Neisseria meningitidis* type 2 protein vaccine in animals and humans. J Infect Dis 1978; *137*: 728–39.

48. Griffiss JM, Goroff DK. IgA blocks IgM and IgG-initiated immune lysis by separate molecular mechanisms. J Immunol 1983; *130*: 2882–5.

49. Griffiss JM. Biologic function of the serum IgA system: modulation of complement-mediated effector mechanisms and conservation of antigenic mass. Ann NY Acad Sci 1983; *409*: 697–707.

50. Käyhty H, Jousimies-Somer H, Peltola H, Mäkelä PH. Antibody response to capsular polysaccharides of groups A and C *Neisseria meningitidis* and *Haemophilus influenzae* type b during bacteremic disease. J Infect Dis 1981; *143*: 32–41.

51. Griffiss JM. Serotypes and serogroups of *Neisseria meningitidis* causing disease in a single city. Med Trop (Mars) 1983; *45*: 53.

52. Griffiss JM, Brandt BL, Gregory D, Filice GA, Counts CW. Epidemic group A meningococcal disease in the Pacific Northwest: an immunologic paradox (abstract). Clin Res 1977; 25: 376.

53. Bhattacharjee Ak, Jennings HJ, Kenny CP, Martin A, Smith ICP. Structural determination of the polysaccharide antigens of *Neisseria meningitidis* serogroups Y, W135 and BO. Can J Biochem 1976; 54: 1–8.

54. Griffiss JM, Schneider H, Mandrell RE, Yamasaki R, Jarvis GA, Kim JJ et al. Lipooligosaccharides: the principal glycolipids of the neisserial outer membrane. Rev Infect Dis 1988; Dis 1988; 10: S287–95.

55. Mandrell RE, Lesse AJ, Sugai JV, Shero M, Griffiss JM, Cole JA et al. In vitro and in vivo modification of *Neisseria gonorrhoeae* lipooligosaccharide epitope structure by sialylation. J Exp Med 1990; 171: 1649–64.

56. Jennings HJ, Lugowski C, Ashton FE. The structure of an R-type oligosaccharide core obtained from some lipopolysaccharides of *Neisseria meningitidis*. Carbohydr Res 1983; 121: 233–41.

57. Yamasaki R, Bacon BE, Schneider H, Griffiss JM. Structural determination of oligosaccharides derived from lipooligosaccharide F62 of *Neisseria gonorrhoeae* by chemical, enzymatic and two-dimensional NMR methods. Biochemistry 1991; 30: 10566–75.

58. John CM, Griffiss JM, Apicella MA, Mandrell RE, Gibson BW. The structural basis for pyocin-resistance in *Neisseria gonorrhoeae* lipooligosaccharides. J Biol Chem 1991; 266: 19303–11.

59. Gibson BW, Webb JW, Yamasaki R, Fisher SJ, Burlingame AL, Mandrell RE et al. Structure and heterogeneity of the oligosaccharides from lipopolysaccharides of a pyocin-resistant *Neisseria gonorrhoeae*. Proc Natl Acad Sci USA 1989; 86: 17–21.

60. Phillips NJ, John CM, Reinders LG, Griffiss JM, Apicella MA, Gibson BW. Structural models for the cell surface lipooligosaccharide (LOS) of *Neisseria gonorrhoeae* and *Haemophilus influenzae*. Biomed Mass Spectrom 1990; 19: 731–45.

61. Gibson BW, Melaugh W, Phillips N, Apicella MA, Campagnari AA, Griffiss JM. Investigation of the structural heterogeneity of lipooligosaccharides from pathogenic *Haemophilus* and *Neisseria* species and R-type lipopolysaccharides from *Salmonella typhimurium* by electrospray mass spectrometry. J Bacteriol 1993; 175: 2702–12.

62. Gibson BW, Schneide H, John CM, Mandrell RE, Griffiss JM. Relationship of Lacto-N-tetraose to the gonococcal LOS receptor for lytic serum IgM. Abstracts, 89th Annual Meeting of the American Society for Microbiology, New Orleans, Louisiana, USA: Am Soc Micobiol 1989; 34: Abs B-21.

63. Griffiss JM, Brandt BL, Engstrom J, Schneider H, Zollinger W, Gibson BW. Meningococcal lipooligosaccharide serotypes are structurally related. Abstracts, 93rd Annual Meeting of the American Society for Microbiology, Atlanta, Georgia, USA: Am Soc Micobiol 1993; 156: Abs B-358.

64. Kerwood DE, Schneider H, Yamasaki R. Structural analysis of lipooligosaccharide produced by *Neisseria gonorrhoeae* strain MS11MK (variant A). Biochemistry 1992; 32: 12760–8.

65. Tsai CM, Civin CI. Eight lipooligosaccharides of *Neisseria meningitidis* react with a monoclonal antibody which binds lacto-N-neotetraose (Galβ1–4GlcNAcβ1–3Galβ1–4Glc) Infect Immun 1991; 59: 3604–9.

66. Gu XX, Tsai CM. Preparation, characterization, and immunogenicity of meningococcal lipooligosaccharide-derived oligosaccharide-protein conjugates. Infect Immun 1993; 61: 1873–80.

67. Schneider H, Griffiss JM, Mandrell RE, Jarvis GA. Elaboration of a 3.6 kDa lipooligosaccharide, antibody against which is absent from human sera, is associated with serum resistance of *Neisseria gonorrhoeae*. Infect Immun 1985; 50: 672–7.

68. Kimm JJ, Mandrell RE, Hu Z, Apicella MA, Poolman JT, Griffiss JM. Electromorphic characterization and description of conserved epitopes of the lipooligosaccharides of group A *Neisseria meningitidis*. Infect Immun 1988; 56: 2631–8.

69. Estabrook MM, Mandrell RE, Apicella MA, Griffiss JM. Measurement of the human immune response to meningococcal lipooligosaccharides antigens by using serum to inhibit monoclonal antibody binding to purified lipooligosaccharide. Infect Immun 1990; 58: 2204–13.

70. Estabrook MM, Baker CJ, Griffiss JM. The immune response of children to meningococcal lipooligosaccharides during disseminated disease is directed primarily against two monoclonal antibody-defined epitopes. J Infect Dis 1993; 167: 966–70.

71. Di Fabio JL, Michon F, Brisson JR, Jennings HJ. Structure of the L1 and L6 core oligosaccharide epitopes of *Neisseria meningitidis*. Can J Chem 1990; 68: 1029–34.

72. Mandrell RE, Kim JJ, John CM, Gibson BW, Sugai JV, Apicella MA et al. Endogenous sialylation of the lipooligosaccharide of *Neisseria meningitidis*. J Bacteriol 1991; 173: 2823–32.

73. Schneider H, Griffiss JM, Boslego JW, Hitchcock PJ, Zahos KM, Apicella MA. Expression of paragloboside-like lipooligosaccharides may be a necessary component of gonococcal pathogenesis in men. J Exp Med 1991; 174: 1601–5.

74. Kannagi R, Fukuda MN, Hakomori SI. A new glycolipid antigen isolated from human erythrocyte membranes reacting with antibodies directed to globo-N-tetraosylceramide (globoside). J Biol Chem 1982; 257: 4438–42.

75. Watanabe K, Hakomori SI. Gangliosides of human erythrocytes. A novel ganglioside with a unique N-acetylneuraminosyl-(2→)-N-acetylgalactosamine structure. J Biochem 1979; 5502–4.

76. Estabrook MM, Christopher NC, Griffiss JM, Baker CJ, Mandrell RE. Sialylation and human neutrophil killing of group C *Neisseria meningitidis*. J Infect Dis 1992; 166: 1079–88.

77. Frosch M, Weisgerber C, Meyer TF. Molar characterization and expression in *Escherichia coli* of the gene complex encoding the polysaccharide capsule of *Neisseria meningitidis* group B. Proc Natl Acad Sci USA 1989; 86: 1669–73.

78. Mandrell RE, Griffiss JM, Smith H, Cole JA. Distribution of a lipooligosaccharide-specific sialytransferase in pathogenic and non-pathogenic *Neisseria*. Microb Path 1993; 14: 315–27.

79. Poolman JT, Hopman CTP, Zanen HC. Colony variants of *Neisseria meningitidis* 2996 (B:2b:P1.2): influence of class 5 outer membrane proteins and lipopolysaccharides. J Med Microbiol 1985; 19: 203–9.

80. Mandrell RE, Smith H, Jarvis GA, Griffiss JM, Cole JA. Detection and some properties of the sialytransferase implicated in the sialylation of lipopolysaccharide of *Neisseria gonorrhoeae*. Microb Path 1993; 14: 307–13.

81. Yamasaki R, Griffiss JM, Quinn KP, Mandrell RE. Neuraminic acid is $\alpha2 \rightarrow 3$ linked in the lipooligosaccharide of *Neisseria meningitidis* serogroup B strain 6275. J Bacteriol 1993; 175: 4565–8.

82. Jarvis GA, Griffiss JM. Human IgA$_1$ initiates complement-mediated killing of *Neisseria meningitidis*. J Immunol 1989; 143: 1703–9.

83. Hostetter MK, Gordon DL. Biochemistry of C3 and related thiolester proteins

in infection and inflammation. Rev Infect Dis 1987; 9: 97–109.

84. Daoudaki ME, Becherer JD, Lambris JD. A 34-amino acid peptide of the third component of complement mediates properdin binding. J Immunol 1988; 140: 1577–80.

85. Eads MM, Levy NJ, Baker CJ, Kasper DL, Nicholson-Weller A. Antibody independent activation of C1 by type 1a group B streptococci. J Infect Dis 1982; 146: 665–72.

86. Clas F, Loos M. Antibody-independent binding of the first component of complement (C1) and its subcomponent C1q to the S and R forms of Salmonella minnesota. Infect Immun 1981; 31: 1138–44.

87. Pangburn MK, Fishelson Z, Müller-Eberhard HJ. Characterization of the initial C3 convertase of the alternative pathway of human complement. J Immunol 1984; 132: 1430–4.

88. Edwards MS, Nicholson-Weller A, Baker CJ, Kasper DL. The role of specific antibody in alternative complement pathway-mediated opsonophagocytosis of type III, group B streptococcus. J Exp Med 1978; 151: 1275–87.

89. Fothergill LD, Wright J. Influenzal meningitis: the relation of age incidence to the bactericidal power of blood against the causal organism. J Immunol 1933; 24: 273–84.

90. Fierer J, Finley F. Deficient serum bactericidal activity against Escherichia coli in patients with cirrhosis of the liver. J Clin Invest 1979; 63: 912–21.

91. Fearon DT, Austen KF. The alternative pathway of complement – a system for host resistance to microbial infection. N Engl J Med 1980; 303: 259–63.

92. Hammerschmidt S, Ebeling O, Frosch M. Relative contribution of sialic acid as component of capsular polysaccharide and lipooligosaccharide of Neisseria meningitidis. Abstracts of the 8th International Pathogenic Neisseria Conference, Cuernavaca, Mexico: Inst. Nac. de Salud Publ. 1992; Abs II-27, p171.

93. Meri S, Pangburn MK. Discrimination between activators and nonactivators of the alternative pathway of complement: regulation via a sialic acid/polyanion binding site on factor H. Proc Natl Acad Sci USA 1990; 87: 3982–6.

94. Masson L, Holbein BE, Ashton FE. Virulence linked to polysaccharide production in serogroup B Neisseria meningitidis. FEMS Microbiol Lett 1982; 13: 187–90.

95. Craven DE, Shen KT, Frasch CE. Natural bactericidal activity of human serum against Neisseria meningitidis isolates of different serogoups and serotypes. Infect Immun 1982; 37: 132–7.

96. Ninno VLD, Chenier VK. Activation of complement by Neisseria meningitidis. FEMS Microbiol Lett 1981; 12: 55–60.

97. Pluschke G, Mayden J, Achtman M, Levine RP. Role of the capsule and the O antigen in resistance of O18:K1 Escherichia coli to complement-mediated killing. Infect Immun 1983; 42: 907–13.

98. Edwards MS, Kasper DL, Jennings HJ, Baker CJ, Nicholson-Weller A. Capsular sialic acid prevents activation of the alternative complement pathway by type III, Group B streptococci. J Immunol 1982; 128: 1278–83.

99. Griffiss JM, Schecter S, Eads MM, Yamasaki R, Jarvis GA. Regulation of complement activation on bacterial surfaces. In: Kohler H, LoVerde PT, eds. Vaccines: New Concepts and Developments. Harlow, England: Longman Scientific & Technical, 1988; 167–76.

100. Varki A, Kornfeld S. An autosomal dominant gene regulates the extent of 9–0 acetylation of murine erythrocyte sialic acid. A probable explanation for the variation in capacity to activate the human alternative complement pathway. J

Exp Med 1980; *152*: 532–44.

101. Griffiss JM, Brandt BL, Broud DD, Goroff DK, Baker CJ. Immune response of infants and children to disseminated infections with *Neisseria meningitidis*. J Infect Dis 1984; *150*: 71–9.

102. Koistinen V. Effect of complement-protein-C3b density on the binding of complement factor H to surface bound C3b. Biochem J 1991; *280*: 255–9.

103. Parsons NJ, Andrade JRC, Patel PV, Cole JA, Smith H. Sialylation of lipopolysaccharide and loss of absorption of bactericidal antibody during conversion of gonococci to serum resistance by cytidine 5′-monophospho-N-acetyl neuraminic acid. Microb Path 1989; *7*: 63–72.

104. Fox AJ, Jones DM, Scotland SM, Rowe B, Smith A, Brown MRW *et al.* Serum killing of meningococci and several other gram-negative bacterial species is not decreased by incubating them with cytidine-5′-monophospho-N-acetyl neraminic acid. Microb Path 1989; *7*: 317–8.

105. Densen P, Weiler JM, Griffiss JM, Hoffman LF. Familial properdin deficiency and fatal meningococcemia. N Engl J Med 1987; *316*: 922–6.

106. Sung SJ, Nelson RS, Silverstein SC. Yeast mannans inhibit binding and phagocytosis of zymosan by mouse peritoneal macrophages. J Cell Biol 1983; *96*: 160–6.

107. Schneider H, Hale TL, Zollinger W, Seid RC, Hammack CA, Griffis JM. Heterogeneity of molecular size and antigenic expression within the lipooligosaccharides of individual strains of *Neisseria gonorrhoeae* and *Neisseria meningitidis*. Infect Immun 1984; *45*: 544–9.

108. Schneider H, Griffiss JM, Williams GD, Pier GB. Immunological basis of serum resistance of *Neisseria gonorrhoeae*. J Gen Microbiol 1982; *128*: 13–22.

109. Joiner KA, Warren KA, Brown EJ, Swanson J, Frank MM. Studies on the mechanism of bacterial resistance to complement-mediated killing. IV. C5b-9 forms high molecular weight complexes with bacterial outer membrane constituents on serum-resistant but not on serum-sensitive *Neisseria gonorrhoeae*. J Immunol 1983; *131*: 1443–51.

110. Griffiss JM, Jarvis GA, Schneider H, O'Brien JP, Eads MM. Lysis of *Neisseria gonorrhoeae* initiated by binding of normal human IgM to a hexosamine-containing lipooligosaccharide epitope is augmented by strain-specific, properdin binding-dependent alternative complement pathway activation. J Immunol 1991; *147*: 298–305.

111. Sjöholm AG, Braconier JH, Söderström C. Properdin deficiency in a family with fulminant meningococcal infections. Clin Exp Immunol 1982; *50*: 291–7.

112. Konno T, Hirai H, Tamura N. Binding of activated properdin to untreated erythrocytes. Immunology 1978; *34*: 207–15.

113. Jennings HJ, Rosell KG, Kasper DL. Structural determination and serology of the native polysaccharide antigen of type III group B streptococcus. Can J Biochem 1980; *58*: 112–20.

114. Borsos T, Circolo A. Binding and activation of C1 by cell bound IgG: activation depends on cell surface hapten density. Mol Immunol 1983; *20*: 433–8.

115. Apicella MA, Mandrell RE, Shero M, Wilson M, Griffiss JM, Brooks GF *et al.* Modification by sialic acid of *Neisseria gonorrhoeae* lipooligosaccharide epitope expression in human urethral exudates: an immunoelectron microscope analysis. J Infect Dis 1990; *162*: 506–12.

116. Hamadeh RH, Zhou P, Griffiss JM. Human IgG that kill group B and C *Neisseria meningitidis* bind non-sialylated lipooligosaccharides (LOS). Clin Res 1993; 250A.

117. Zhao S, Griffiss JM, Kim JJ, Jarvis GA. Human antibodies that kill group A

Neisseria meningitidis are directed at α Lactosyl determinants on lipooligosaccharides of M_r < 4,500. Abstracts, 93th Annual Meeting of the American Society for Microbiology, Atlanta, Georgia, USA: Am Soc Microbiol, 1993; Abs B-367, p156.

118. Stein DC, Petricoin EF, Griffiss JM, Schneider H. Use of transformation to construct Neisseria gonorrhoeae strains with altered lipooligosaccharides. Infect Immun 1988; 56: 762–5.

119. Schreiber RD, Pangburn MK, Lesavre PH, Müller-Eberhard HJ. Initiation of the alternative pathway of complement: recognition of activators by bound C3b and assembly of the entire pathway from six isolated proteins. Proc Natl Acad Sci USA 1978; 75: 3948–52.

120. Zollinger WD, Mandrell RE, Griffiss JM, Altieri P, Berman S. Complex of meningococcal group B polysaccharide and type 2 outer membrane protein immunogenic in man. J Clin Invest 1979; 63: 836–48.

121. Mandrell RE, Zollinger WD. Measurement of antibodies to meningococcal group B polysaccharide; low avidity binding and equilibrium binding constants. J Immunol 1982; 129: 2172–8.

122. Zollinger WD, Mandrell RE. Bactericidal activity of human antibody and murine monoclonal antibody to the meningococcal group B polysaccharide: importance of the complement source. Infect Immun 1983; 40: 257–64.

123. Zollinger WD, Mandrell RE, Griffiss JM. Enhancement of immunologic activity by non-covalent complexing of meningococcal group B polysaccharide and outer membrane proteins. In: Robbins JB, Hill JC, Sadoff JV, eds. Seminars in Infectious Disease. Vol. 4. New York: Thieme-Stratton Inc. 1982; 254–262 (Bacterial Vaccines).

124. Eddie DS, Schulkind ML, Robbins JB. The isolation and biologic activities of purified secretory IgA and IgG anti-Salmonella typhimurium 'O' antibodies from rabbit intestinal fluid and colostrum. J Immunol 1971; 106: 181–90.

125. Russell-Jones GJ, Ey PL, Reynolds BL. The ability of IgA to inhibit the complement-mediated lysis of target red blood cells sensitized with IgG antibody. Mol Immunol 1980; 17: 1173–80.

126. Musher DM, Goree A, Baughn RE, Birdsall HH. Immunoglobulin A from bronchopulmonary secretions blocks bactericidal and opsonising effects of antibody to nontypable Haemophilus influenzae. Infect Immun 1984; 45: 36–40.

127. Apicella MA, Westerink MAJ, Morse SA, Schneider H, Rice PA, Griffiss JM. Bactericidal antibody response of normal human serum to the lipooligosaccharide of Neisseria gonorrhoeae. J Infect Dis 1986; 153: 520–6.

128. van Epps DE, Williams RC. Suppression of leukocyte chemotaxis by human IgA myeloma components. J Exp Med 1976; 144: 1227–42.

129. Wilton JMA. Suppression by IgA of IgG mediated phagocytosis by human polymorphonuclear leukocytes. Clin Exp Immunol 1978; 34: 423–8.

130. Jarvis GA, Griffiss JM. IgA modulation of IgG-initiated complement activation. Abstracts of the 86th Annual Meeting of the American Society for Microbiology. 1986: Abstr B-161.

131. Kim JJ, Zhou D, Mandrell RE, Griffiss JM. Effect of exogenous sialylation of the lipooligosaccharide of Neisseria gonorrhoeae on opsonophagocytosis. Infect Immun 1992; 60: 4439–42.

132. Rest RF, Frangipane JV. Growth of Neisseria gonorrhoeae in CMP-N-acetylneuraminic acid inhibits nonopsonic (opacity-associated outer membrane protein-mediated) interactions with human neutrophils. Infect Immun 1992; 60: 989–97.

133. Broud DD, Griffiss JM, Baker CJ. Heterogeneity of serotypes of *Neisseria meningitidis* that cause endemic disease. J Infect Dis 1984; *140*: 465–70.

134. Feigin RD, Baker CJ, Herwaldt LA, Lampe RM, Mason EO, Whitney SE. Epidemic meningococcal disease in an elementary school. N Engl J Med 1982; *307*: 1255–7.

135. Artenstein MS, Brandt BL, Tramont EC, Branche WC, Fleet HD, Cohen RL. Serologic studies of meningococcal infection and polysaccharide vaccination. J Infect Dis 1971; *124*: 277–88.

136. Filice GA, Hayes PS, Counts GA, Griffiss JM, Fraser DW. Risk of group A meningococcal disease: bacterial interference and cross-reactive bacteria among mucosal flora. J Clin Microbiol 1985; *22*: 152–6.

137. Gold R, Goldschneider I, Lepow ML, Draper TF, Randolph M. Carriage of *Neisseria meningitidis* and *Neisseria lactamica* in infants and children. J Infect Dis 1978; *137*: 112–21.

138. Blakebrough IS, Greenwood BM, Whittle HC, Bradley AK, Gilles HM. The epidemiology of infections due to *Neisseria meningitidis* and *Neisseria gonorrhoeae* in a northern Nigerian community. J Infect Dis 1982; *146*: 626–37.

139. Hu Z, Wang JF. Epidemiological investigation of carrier rates of *Neisseria lactamica* and *Neisseria meningitidis* in different regions of China. In: Hu Z, ed. *National Epidemiology of Cerebrospinal Meningitis: Collected Research.* Beijing, People's Republic of China: National Acute Infectious Respiratory Disease Advisory Committee, 1986: 68–71.

140. Jiang ZP. Carriage of *Neisseria lactamica* and *Neisseria meningitidis* in populations of Shandong Province. In: Hu Z, ed. *National Epidemiology of Cerebrospinal Meningitis: Collected Research.* Beijing, People's Republic of China: National Acute Infectious Respiratory Disease Advisory Committee, 1986: 71–5.

141. Kim JJ, Mandrell RE, Griffiss JM. *Neisseria lactamica* and *Neisseria meningitidis* share lipooligosaccharide epitopes, but lack common capsular and class 1, 2, and 3 protein epitopes. Infect Immun 1989; *57*: 602–8.

142. Griffiss JM, Broud DD, Silver CA, Artenstein MS. Immunoepidemiology of meningococcal disease in military recruits. I. A model for serogroup independency of epidemic potential as determined by serotyping. J Infect Dis 1977; *136*: 176–86.

143. Griffiss JM, Kim JJ. Antigenic specificity of natural bactericidal activity for serogroup B and C strains of *Neisseria meningitidis* in human sera. In: Poolman JT, Zanen H, Mayer T, Heckels J, Mäkelä PH, Smith H, Beuvery C, eds. *Gonococci and Meningococci.* Nijhoff, Dordrecht, The Netherlands: 1988; 523–7.

144. Griffiss JM, Goroff DK. Immunological cross-reaction between a naturally occurring galactan, agarose, and an LPS locus for immune lysis of *Neisseria meningitidis* by human sera. Clin Exp Immunol 1981; *43*: 20–7.

145. Griffiss JM. Human serum IgA and susceptibility to disseminated meningococcal disease. In: Robbins JB, Hill JC, Sadoff JV, eds. *Bacterial Vaccines.* New York: Thieme-Stratton Inc, 1982; 13–18 (Seminars in Infectious Disease, Vol 4).

146. Zahos KM, Kind P, Griffiss JM, Schneider H. Induction of human paragloboside antibodies by gonococcal LOS during urethritis. Abstracts, 32nd Interscience Conference on Antimicrobial Agents and Chemotherapy, Anaheim, CA, USA: Am Soc Microbiol 1992: Abstr 1289; p. 325.

147. Tsai CM, Mocca LF, Frasch CE. Immunotype epitopes of *Neisseria meningitidis* lipooligosaccharide types 1 through 8. Infect Immun 1987; *55*: 1652–6.

148. Reller LB, MacGregor RR, Beaty HN. Bactericidal antibody after colonization with *Neisseria meningitidis*. J Infect Dis 1973; *127*: 56–62.

149. Griffiss JM, Brandt BL, Jarvis GA. Nature immunity to *Neisseria meningitidis*. In:

Vedros NAO ed. *Evolution of Meningococcal Disease*. Vol II. Boca Raton: CRC Press Inc, 1987; 99–119.
150. Winstanley FP, Blackwell CC, Weir DM, Kinane DF. Gonorrhoea, a predisposing factor for meningococcal disease? Lancet 1983; *ii*: 1135.
151. Glode MP, Robbins JB, Liu TY, Gotschlich EC, Ørskov I, Ørskov F. Cross-antigenicity and immunogenicity between capsular polysaccharides of group C *Neisseria meningitidis* and of *Escherichia coli* K92. J Infect Dis 1977; *135*: 94–102.
152. Lowell GH, Smith LF, Griffiss JM, Brandt BL. IgA-dependent monocyte-mediated antibacterial activity. J Exp Med 1980; *152*: 452–7.
153. Greenwood BM, Greenwood AM, Bradley AK, Williams K, Hassan-King M, Shenton FC *et al*. Factors influencing susceptibility to meningococcal disease during an epidemic in The Gambia, West Africa. J Infect 1987; *14*: 167–84.
154. Countes GW, Gregory DF, Spearman JG, Lee BA, Filice GA, Holmes KK *et al*. Group A meningococcal disease in the U.S. Pacific Northwest: epidemiology, clinical features, and effect of a vaccination control program. Rev Infect Dis 1984; *6*: 640–8.
155. Filice GA, Englender SJ, Jacobson JA, Jourden JL, Burns DA, Gregory D *et al*. Group A meningococcal disease in skid rows: epidemiology and implications for control. Am J Public Health 1984; *74*: 253–4.
156. Guirguis N, Schneerson R, Bax AD, Egan W, Robbins JB, Shiloach J *et al*. *Escherichia coli* K51 and K93 capsular polysaccharides are cross-reactive with the group A capsular polysaccharide of *Neisseria meningitidis*. J Exp Med 1986; *162*: 1837–51.
157. Liebowitz LD. The possible role of enteric cross-reacting bacteria inducing susceptibility to group A meningococcal disease. PhD Thesis, University of the Witwatersrand, South Africa, 1990.
158. Griffiss JM. Protective and permisive antibodies in bacterial sepsis. In: Root RK, Sande MA, eds. *Septic Shock*. 1985: 135–46 (Root RK, Sande MA, eds. Contemporary Issues in Infectious Diseases, Vol 4).
159. Kaplan NM, Braude AI. *Haemophilus influenzae* infection in adults. Arch Intern Med 1958; *101*: 515–23.
160. Ellison RT, Kohler PF, Curd JG, Judson FN, Reller LB. Prevalence of congenital or acquired complement deficiency in patients with sporadic meningococcal disease. N Engl J Med 1983; *308*: 913–16.
161. Reid KBM, Porter RR. The proteolytic activation systems of complement. Ann Rev Biochem 1981; *50*: 433–64.
162. Baker CJ, Griffiss JM. Influence of age on serogroup distribution of endemic meningococcal disease. Pediatrics 1983; *71*: 923–6.

4
Pathogenesis of Meningococcal Infections

PETTER BRANDTZAEG
Department of Pediatrics, Ulleval University Hospital, Oslo, Norway

INTRODUCTION

Since the isolation of *Neisseria meningitidis* in 1887, studies have gradually disclosed a complex interrelationship between intruding meningococci and the host, involving molecular mimicry and circumvention of immune recognition. Clinical and laboratory observations of meningococcal patients combined with extensive *in vitro* studies of *N. meningitidis*, human tissue and cell culture studies and, recently, targeted genetic manipulation have been employed to study the various steps from initial mucosal colonisation to life-threatening illness. However, detailed studies of the bacterium–host interaction at a molecular level have been severely hampered by the lack of a suitable standardised animal model since *N. meningitidis* is an obligate human pathogen.

In this chapter, aspects of the three principal stages in the development of meningococcal disease, as proposed by Herrick in 1918, will be reviewed, namely mucosal colonisation and penetration, the bacteraemic state, and the localised inflammatory response[1]. Over eight months Herrick treated 265 patients with meningococcal infections and concluded: 'It soon became apparent, however, that the disease with which we were dealing was not a primary meningitis but a meningococcic sepsis with a secondary meningeal localisation. As the epidemic continued and our study widened, this opinion became firmly fixed'[1]. Research conducted since then has affirmed this view.

Meningococcal Disease. Edited by Keith Cartwright © 1995 John Wiley & Sons Ltd

COLONISATION AND INVASION

Mucosal colonisation

Meningococcal infection starts with colonisation of the upper respiratory tract—mainly the mucosa of the nasopharynx and the tonsils. Meningococci are transferred in droplets from a (usually asymptomatic) carrier to the recipient. The distance between the two is one of several largely unknown factors influencing the transmission rate[2–4]. Crowding facilitates transmission and is considered to be one of several factors contributing to the high attack rate among fresh military recruits[5].

Observations during epidemics[6,7] and in infected laboratory workers (Brandtzaeg P, unpublished observations) suggest that invasive disease often develops shortly after the pathogenic clone has been transmitted to a new host. Some patients experience mild upper respiratory symptoms 1–2 days prior to developing generalised disease[1], but most individuals are asymptomatic during nasopharyngeal colonisation. Preceding viral infections, inhalation of dry, dusty air, and exposure to passive smoking among children have been associated with invasive meningococcal disease[8–12]. However, Artenstein et al. did not find any association between acute respiratory infections and systemic meningococcal disease among army recruits[13].

IgA protease and disease-causing strains

In common with other potentially invasive oropharyngeal bacteria such as Streptococcus pneumoniae and Haemophilus influenzae, N. meningitidis strains produce extracellular IgA_1 proteases of two specificities[14,15]. Secretory IgA_2 is not inactivated[16]. The biological significance of these IgA_1 proteases is not clear[16], but they are not produced by non-pathogenic oropharyngeal bacteria such as N. lactamica.

N. meningitidis adherence to non-ciliated epithelial cells

In a series of studies employing human nasopharyngeal tissue cultures Stephens et al. found that encapsulated, piliated meningococci adhere selectively to the microvilli on non-ciliated epithelial cells[17–22]. Fresh isolates of pathogenic strains possessed class I and II pili which facilitated attachment to the epithelium[23–26]. Non-capsulated strains adhered better than capsulated parent strains. As well as adhering to epithelial cells, meningococci also caused down-regulation of ciliary activity at a distance, suggesting that soluble products inducing ciliostasis are released[21]. The nature of these products is presently unknown; purified meningococcal lipopolysaccharides (LPS) did not induce epithelial cell damage or cioliostasis in the same experimental model. Locally produced inflammatory mediators such as tumour necrosis factor α (TNF-α) or interleukin-1β (IL-1β) are candidate molecules which may induce some or all of these effects. Inocula of 10^6 colony forming units (CFUs) were needed to produce a sustained microbial proliferation in this model[21]. In partially encapsulated non-piliated strains the class 5 outer membrane protein Opc may facilitate adherence to endothelial cells *in vitro*[27].

Mucosal penetration

After mucosal adherence followed by a period of adaptation and local proliferation, meningococci can initiate a parasite-directed endocytosis by non-ciliated epithelial cells[17-21]. Encapsulated meningococci are transported through the cell in large membrane-bound phagocytic vacuoles whereas non-capsulated strains apparently traverse the cytoplasm without vacuoles[22]. Within 24 hours meningococci are observed in the submucosa in close proximity to local immune cells and blood vessels[22]. Although pili facilitate adhesion to endothelial cells[28,29], they are down-regulated in the migration of meningococci from the mucosa to deeper tissues.

The immune response induced by N. meningitidis colonisation

Mucosal colonisation by *N. meningitidis* initiates a general immune response[6,7,30]. Serial studies of army recruits, a group at high risk of developing meningococcal infections, show a significant increase in specific and cross-reacting antibodies within 14 days of mucosal colonisation[6,7]. Lack of bactericidal antibodies predisposes to systemic meningococcal disease (SMD) whereas their presence confers protection[7,30].

The exact mechanisms leading to a general immune response through mucosal colonisation are not known but observations made in Stephens' nasopharynx tissue model suggest that parasite-directed endocytosis of non-pathogenic *N. meningitidis* and *N. lactamica* may be a regular occurrence[17-22].

Transition from submucosa to the vascular bed

In an unknown percentage of colonised persons, pathogenic *N. meningitidis* strains, characterised by encapsulation and a specific configuration of outer membrane molecules, are not adequately contained by the local immune system. After mucosal penetration and presumably a phase of adaptation, the bacteria gain access to the circulation. The polysaccharide capsule may partly protect invading meningococci by down-regulating the complement-mediated phagocytic capacity of local macrophages and granulocytes[31]. Locally produced IgA may block or reduce the bactericidal effect of IgG and

IgM[32]. Pili increase the adherence of pathogenic meningococci to cultured human umbilical vein endothelial cells (huvecs) but capsulation has no influence on the parasite–endothelium interaction in the huvec model[29]. However, huvecs may not entirely simulate the properties of the endothelium in nasopharyngeal capillaries and veins since endothelial cell characteristics may vary according to the anatomical site[32a].

In the vascular compartment the intruding meningococcus may either be neutralised by the combined actions of circulating antibodies, complement and phagocytic cells or may reveal a capacity to multiply within the circulation, initiating the bacteraemic stage. Knowledge of this early bacteraemic phase is scanty.

In many patients developing SMD the exact time of the first symptoms indicating invasion can be defined fairly accurately. Fever, rigors, general malaise and nausea are common initial symptoms. In experimental human endotoxinaemia these symptoms can be reproduced by inflammatory mediators, notably TNF-α, IL-1β, IL-6 and IL-8, whose release is elicited by LPS[33–38]. The minimum pyrogenic dose of *Escherichia coli* 0113 LPS needed to elicit fever in man is 0.5–1 ng per kilo body weight given as an intravenous bolus[39]. After a latent period of 30–90 minutes—the time needed for transcription and synthesis of TNF-α and other cytokines—symptoms become increasingly apparent in healthy volunteers[33–38]. Observations in experimental human endotoxinaemia suggest that cytokines are synthesised in, and released from, tissue macrophages, primarily Kupffer cells, although spleen and lung macrophages and circulating monocytes may also contribute[40]. One nanogram of purified LPS represents approximately the amount of LPS found in 10^5 bacteria[41].

Bacteraemia

Systemic meningococcal infection is a bacteraemic disease with secondary infection of skin, meninges and other parts of the body[1]. *N. meningitidis* can be isolated from blood cultures in a majority of untreated patients with SMD[1,42]. Based on observations of more than 300 cases, Herrick concluded that symptoms and signs of generalised disease appeared concurrently with meningococcaemia and preceded symptoms of meningitis by 24 to 48 hours in most patients[1,43]. In extreme cases this bacteraemic stage lasted several weeks before meningitis finally developed[1].

The number of bacteria per millilitre of blood has been correlated with disease severity in children[44–47]. More than 1000 CFUs were present in seven of 15 patients with meningitis and in four of 10 cases of meningococcaemia, two of whom died[47]. However, when a quantitative blood culture technique (1.1 ml of blood) was used in 14 adult patients with distinct meningitis or with meningococcaemia without meningitis or shock, only three patients had detectable bacteria, with counts ranging from 23 to 240 CFUs per millilitre of blood[42]. Conventional blood cultures (6 × 5 ml of blood) collected from 11 of the 14 patients were all positive[42]. This observation suggests that bacteraemia was low grade, i.e. < 1 CFU per millilitre of blood in most of these young adults with meningococcal meningitis or mild systemic disease without meningitis. In two young adults with severe persistent septic shock, multiple organ failure and disseminated intravascular coagulation, 500 and 800 CFUs of *N. meningitidis* respectively were detected on admission[42]. Fulminant septicaemia in an adolescent was associated with 10^5 CFUs per millilitre of blood, whereas a co-primary case who presented with meningitis without shock symptoms had negative quantitative blood culture[46]. The number of CFUs appears to be higher in young children than in adults with meningoccaemia and higher numbers of CFUs are associated with a more severe clinical presentation.

Direct visualisation of meningococci in peripheral blood

Intra- and extracellular meningococci in buffy coat preparations have usually been associated with a fulminating course and fatal outcome[48–50]. However, abundant meningococci have been visualised in peripheral blood in a patient with meningitis without development of septic shock or multiple organ failure[51]. Visualisation of bacteria in peripheral blood reflects a much higher number of bacteria than usually observed in bacteraemia[52].

Circulating endotoxin as a marker of disease severity

Since the end of the last century it has been clear that pathogenic bacteria including *N. meningitidis* contained a toxic filtrable agent closely connected to the bacterial cell wall[53–68]. Netter and Debré reviewed the scientific data in 1911 and stated that endotoxin represented the main toxic agent[59]. This statement has never really been challenged although direct proof has been lacking until recently.

Measurements of circulating endotoxin in patients with life-threatening meningococcaemia were first attempted in the late 1970s using the classical limulus amoebocyte lysate (LAL) test[69–73]. The results failed to show any direct relationship between detectable plasma endotoxin and disease outcome[69,70]. Studies carried out after the sensitivity of the LAL assay had been improved and the test made quantitative[74] showed high levels of endotoxin in lethal cases with irreversible septic shock[75,76]. In a study of 45 consecutive confirmed cases, increasing levels of circulating endotoxin were associated with an increasing fatality rate[42] (Figure 4.1). Contrary to observations made in other gram-negative infections, comparatively high levels of LPS, e.g. 110–600 ng/l (1.1–6.0 endotoxin units (EU/ml)) were

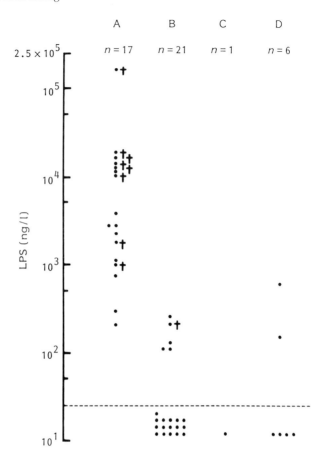

Figure 4.1   *The LPS levels of 45 consecutively admitted patients with meningococcal infections. A, patients with fulminant septicaemia characterised by septic shock, multiple organ failure, severe DIC and minimal CSF pleocytosis (< 100 × 10⁶/l leucocytes). B, patients with meningitis (> 100 × 10⁶/l leucocytes) without persistent septic shock and multiple organ failure. C, one patient with meningitis and persistent septic shock without multiple organ failure. D, patients with meningogoccaemia without shock, multiple organ failure or meningitis. † Death. Dashed line indicates detection limit (25 ng/l)*

measured in individual patients without the development of circulatory collapse and multiple organ failure[42,77,78]. However, of 15 patients with LPS levels ≥ 700 ng/l, all developed persistent septic shock, renal impairment and disseminated intravascular coagulation with an ultimate fatality rate of 53%[42].

The physicochemical characteristics of circulating, native endotoxin

In the LAL assay endotoxin is detected in biological fluids by its ability to activate the coagulation cascade of the horseshoe crab, *Limulus polyphemus*[71]. LPS, comprising lipid A (Figure 4.2), the core region and a terminal polysaccharide chain of variable length, is an amphipathic molecule tending to form large aggregates in aqueous solutions[79]. Human plasma contains various molecules with the ability to complex with LPS, primarily lipoproteins but also complement factors, antibodies, albumin and the recently characterised acute phase protein, lipopolysaccharide binding protein (LBP)[80-84]. Several of these proteins appear to have a detoxifying effect, i.e. they down-regulate the biological effects of LPS and represent 'physiological buffer systems' in the circulation of mammals.

Studies of circulating native meningococcal LPS collected from cases of SMD with fulminant septicaemia indicate that LAL activity is connected to structures with a high sedimentation coefficient[85]. Electron microscopic studies of sediments (100 000 *g* for one hour) from such plasmas showed fragments of bacterial outer membrane (Figure 4.3). Analysis of plasma by gas chromatography and mass spectrometry confirmed the presence of 3-hydroxy-lauric acid, a marker of neisserial LPS[86]. There was close agreement between quantitative estimates of 3-hydroxy-lauric acid and LAL activity, confirming the presence of circulating meningococcal LPS and not LPS absorbed from the bowel in these profoundly hypotensive patients[85].

Lipoproteins, particularly high density lipoprotein (HDL), appear to

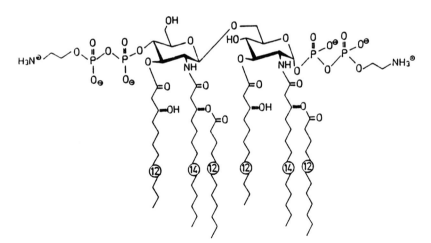

Figure 4.2 *Lipid A representing the toxic moiety of meningococcal lipopolysaccharides. Published with permission from the Journal of Bacteriology (Kulshin et al. 1992; 174: 1793)*[86]

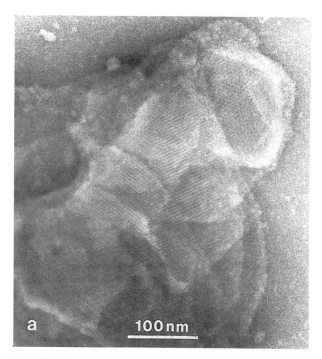

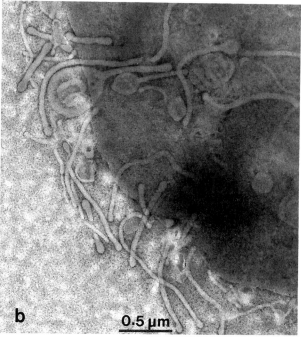

neutralise purified LPS injected into experimental animals[80-84]. HDL and low density lipoprotein (LDL) may not play the same detoxifying role in fulminant meningococcal endotoxinaemia, perhaps because native LPS circulates more as membrane fragments than as single molecules[85].

Production and elimination of native LPS

The level of LPS in an untreated meningococcal patient is a consequence of rapid proliferation of *N. meningitidis* surpassing the host's capacity to eliminate whole bacteria and LPS-containing material. In cases of fulminant meningococcaemia high levels of LPS are detected within 12 hours of the first symptoms, suggesting a doubling time of less than 60 minutes, since the half-life of native LPS is approximately 120–180 minutes[42,87]. In patients with other clinical presentations the ability of meningococci to multiply in the bloodstream appears to be more restricted, as judged by the much lower LPS levels[42,88].

The half-life $(T_{1/2})$ of biologically active meningococcal LPS has been estimated at 1–3 hours (mean 2 hours) during the first 4–6 hours of antibiotic treatment[42]. Subsequently, the $T_{1/2}$ appears to increase to 4–9 hours (mean 6 hours). van Deuren *et al.* found the $T_{1/2}$ of meningococcal LPS to be 3 hours in a group of patients treated intermittently with plasmapheresis[87]. In one patient with fulminant meningococcaemia LPS elimination was monitored for 39 hours until the child died. The levels declined steadily from 10 500 ng/l (105 EU/ml) one hour after initiation of antibiotic treatment to 100 ng/l (1 EU/ml) immediately before the patient expired (Figure 4.4). Elimination continued despite progressive deterioration of the child's clinical condition.

The influence of bactericidal antibiotics on LPS plasma levels

It has long been debated whether bactericidal antibiotics might increase the circulating level of free LPS and as a consequence, up-regulate the inflammatory reaction[89-91]. Serial measurements of plasma LPS in meningococcal patients show a consistent pattern of rapidly decreasing levels of free LPS when compared with levels in the initial sample immediately before

Figure 4.3 *(Opposite) Transmission electron micrographs of negatively stained (0.5% phosphotungstic acid pH 7.0) bacterial membranes found after ultracentrifugation at 103,000 × g for 60 minutes. (a) Microbial unit membrane showing typical moiré pattern from overlapping membrane fragments (× 200,000). (b) Part of a microbe with multiple long membrane protrusions representing outer membrane vesicles detected in one patient's plasma (× 30,000). Reproduced from the Journal of Clinical Investigation (1992; 89: 816)[85], by copyright permission of the American Society for Clinical Investigation*

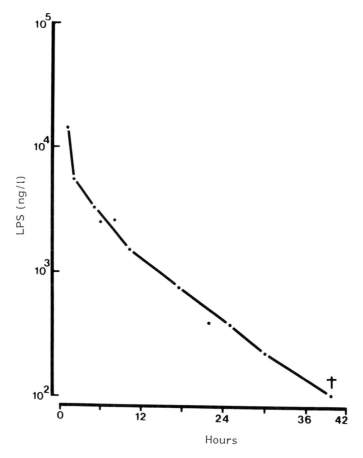

Figure 4.4   The elimination of native LPS in a boy aged 18 months until death. Elimination continued in spite of deterioration of the general condition and failing circulation

bactericidal antibiotic treatment[42] (Figure 4.5). The capacity to eliminate native LPS clearly surpasses the LPS-releasing capacity of antibiotics in meningococcal patients. More importantly, many of the LPS-activated mediator systems which contribute to the multiple organ dysfunction are down-regulated shortly after antibiotics are infused[92-100].

THE INTRAVASCULAR INFLAMMATORY RESPONSE

When LPS-containing material gains access to the circulation, a plethora of inflammatory reactions are activated, ultimately causing organ malfunc-

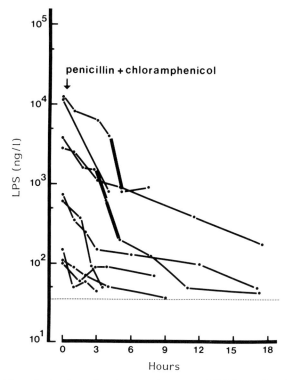

Figure 4.5 *The elimination of native meningococcal LPS from the circulation in nine patients. The first plasma samples were collected immediately before the antibiotic treatment was initiated. Reproduced with permission from the Journal of Infectious Diseases (Brandtzaeg et al. 1989; 159: 195)*[42]. *© 1989 by the University of Chicago. All rights reserved*

tion[101,102]. LPS levels in cases of fulminant meningococcal septicaemia are among the highest ever detected in human plasma[42,75,76,87,88]. The intravascular inflammatory response can be divided into activation of fluid phase cascade systems, the release of intercellular mediators from cells adjacent to circulating plasma, and to the altered function of various cells in the vascular wall. In meningococcal infection major cascade systems including the coagulation, fibrinolysis, complement and kallikrein–kinin systems, as well as the production of different cytokines, are all apparently triggered and up-regulated simultaneously by native LPS in a dose-dependent manner[98,103].

The haemorrhagic diathesis in meningococcal infections

The combination of haemorrhagic rash, fever and nuchal rigidity led to the recognition of SMD as a clinical entity. Later, haemorrhagic skin lesions became the hallmark of epidemic cerebrospinal fever; skin haemorrhages increasing in size with disease severity still represent an important diagnostic marker[1,104-107]. The haemorrhagic lesions are caused by at least two different processes occurring together, namely activation of the coagulation system and localised vessel wall damage.

Activation of the coagulation system

If small doses (2–4 ng/kg) of purified *E. coli* LPS are given as a bolus injection to healthy volunteers to create a transitory endotoxinaemia with maximum plasma LPS levels of 13 ng/l, the coagulation system is activated[36]. Prothrombin activation peptides F_1 and F_2 and thrombin–antithrombin III (TAT) complexes can be identified in the circulation in the next 4–6 hours, indicating formation of the prothrombinase complex (activated coagulation factor X combined with activated factor V assembled on a lipid membrane)[36]. Activation of the plasma contact system via factor XII (Hageman factor) could not be detected in the same experiment, suggesting that procoagulant activity was induced primarily by generation of tissue factor, presumably on circulating monocytes[36]. In a similar human experiment employing TNF-α instead of LPS, activation of the extrinsic, but not the intrinsic, coagulation pathway was demonstrated; TNF-α may act cooperatively with LPS[108].

Generation of procoagulant activity on circulating monocytes

Extensive disseminated intravascular coagulation (DIC) is often observed in patients with severe SMD. In such patients a significant increase (60–300 fold) in tissue factor activity in monocytes has been documented in samples collected on hospital admission[109]. High tissue factor activity is associated with fatal outcome, suggesting that monocytes, stimulated by circulating bioactive LPS, are the direct cause of the DIC. TNF-α and anaphylatoxins split off during complement activation may furthermore, synergistically stimulate tissue factor expression[92,110-112]. Tissue factor activity was rapidly down-regulated in a single patient who was followed over several days[109].

Activation of the plasma contact system

In fulminant SMD there is triggering of the contact activation system[98,103]. Functional levels of plasma kallikrein inhibitor and α2-antiplasmin are inversely related to plasma LPS levels, indicating that the most extensive consumption of these inhibitors occurs in patients with the most extensive coagulopathy[103]. Whether activation of Hageman factor (factor XII) plays a quantitatively important role in the coagulopathy of fulminant meningococcal septicaemia remains to be clarified.

Common coagulation pathway activation and thrombin generation

Low functional levels of coagulation factor V have been documented in several studies of coagulation activation in fulminant meningococcal septicaemia[113-115]. When the prothrombinase complex has been generated, prothromin is converted to thrombin, splitting fibrinogen to fibrin and several smaller peptides including fibrinopeptide A (FPA). FPA can be used as a direct marker of thrombin activity as it has a $T_{1/2}$ in the circulation of 1–2 minutes. FPA levels have been measured in 31 patients with confirmed SMD. Ten were in deep septic shock with signs of multiple organ failure and extensive DIC, as judged by thrombocytopenia, prolonged partial thromboplastin time, increased thrombin clotting time, reduced fibrinogen levels and increased fibrin degradation products (FDP)[93]. On admission to hospital levels of FPA were significantly higher in patients with deep septic shock and LPS levels > 700 ng/l than in patients with lower (< 700 ng/l) or undetectable (< 25 ng/l) plasma levels of LPS[93]. Plasma FPA levels declined with time (Figure 4.6). All patients were treated with fresh frozen plasma. In two patients treated with plasmapheresis FPA levels doubled during the centrifugation procedure, indicating renewed thrombin generation as a consequence of this procedure[93].

Functional levels of natural coagulation inhibitors as markers of coagulopathy and disease severity

Low functional levels of antithrombin III (AT-III) and protein C (PC) may reflect disease severity in life-threatening meningococcal infections[116,117]. Significantly lower levels of AT-III and PC were found in 13 patients developing septic shock and multiple organ failure than in 26 patients without multiple organ failure[93]. Furthermore, the functional levels of AT-III and PC were inversely correlated with levels of LPS in plasma on admission[98]. In sequentially collected samples from individual patients, PC levels reached a nadir within 36 hours in survivors with shock. In patients who ultimately died, PC levels continued to decline despite extensive transfusion with fresh frozen plasma containing protein C[93].

The longitudinal profile of AT-III was more variable in shock patients. Declining levels were observed for more than 7 days in some of the surviving patients. All survivors with multiple organ failure regained levels within the normal range by 6 weeks[93].

Tissue factor pathway inhibitor (TFPI) previously called external pathway inhibitor (EPI) or lipoprotein associated coagulation inhibitor (LACI), is a recently identified natural coagulation inhibitor[118-120]. It is presently the

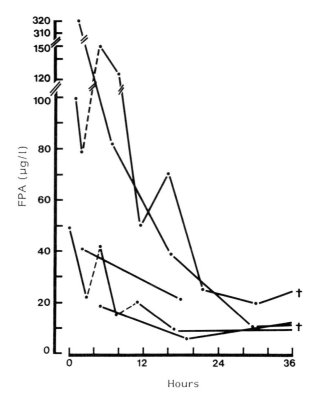

Figure 4.6   Fibrinopeptide A (FPA) in sequentially collected plasma samples in five patients with meningococcal infections, revealing a down-regulation of thrombin activity with time. Dotted lines indicate the effect of plasmapheresis on FPA formation. Reproduced from Thrombosis Research (Brandtzaeg et al.[93]p. 459), copyright 1989, with kind permission from Pergamon Press Ltd, Headington Hill Hall, Oxford OX3 0BW, UK

only identified protein regulating the complex formation of activated factor VII (FVIIa), tissue factor and activated factor X (FXa).

Interestingly, during the first days of meningococcal septic shock, TFPI increased significantly as opposed to the decreases observed in AT-III and PC levels[93]. This 'paradoxical' rise of TFPI may represent release related to endothelial cell damage induced by the intravascular inflammatory response. Vascular endothelial cells are assumed to be the main site of production of TFPI[118,119]. Despite high levels of functional TFPI, extensive coagulopathy persists, presumably induced by activation of the extrinsic coagulation pathway. Animal experiments suggest that TFPI may antagonise low levels of factor VIIa–tissue factor complex formation, but cannot counteract extensive external pathway activation[120]. An interesting observation in individual patients is that while levels of TFPI increased, levels of FPA decreased[93].

Activation and inhibition of the fibrinolytic system

In patients with severe meningococcal coagulopathy and septic shock, low levels of plasminogen and α2-antiplasmin, combined with high levels of fibrin degradation products (FDP) in blood samples collected on admission indicate that extensive activation of the fibrinolytic system occurs before hospital admission[94]. However, on admission, plasma samples from these patients show significant inhibition of fibrinolysis[97]. This functional inhibition is associated with high levels of plasminogen activator inhibitor-1 (PAI-1)[94]. The levels of immunoreactive PAI-1 reflect the disease severity. Levels > 360 μg/l in plasma samples collected on or shortly after admission predicted correctly the development of severe persistent septic shock with renal impairment in 12 of 13 patients, whereas none of 25 patients who did not develop this clinical entity had PAI-1 levels > 260 μg/l on admission. Five patients with PAI-1 levels of > 1850 μg/l all died. Levels of plasminogen activator inhibitor-2 (PAI-2) were not markedly elevated[94].

PAI-1 levels peaked on, or shortly after, initiation of antibiotic and fluid treatment and then declined rapidly[94]. The falling levels of PAI-1 as measured by an immunoassay, paralleled a decrease in functional levels[94,97]. Our observations in meningococcal patients are in accordance with results in human volunteers given a bolus intravenous injection (2–4 ng/kg) of LPS[36,121]. The fibrinolytic system was initially activated at the same time as the coagulation system, as shown by increased levels of circulating tissue plasminogen activator (t-PA) and plasmin–antiplasmin complexes. Subsequently, plasmin activity was down-regulated by the appearance of PAI-1[121]. Functionally active TNF-α preceded detectable t-PA in the circulation, suggesting that t-PA was partly induced by TNF-α[36]. This has been confirmed by infusion of TNF-α in cancer patients and healthy volunteers[122,123].

The coagulation system is clearly triggered by the very high plasma levels of meningococcal LPS in cases of fulminant septicaemia. Circulating monocytes appear to up-regulate surface exposed tissue factor and thereby initiate activation of the extrinsic coagulation pathway. Activation of the plasma contact system via the Hageman factor (factor XII) may also contribute to intrinsic coagulation pathway activation *in vivo*. High levels of thrombin activity are present, converting fibrinogen to fibrin. Subnormal levels or absence of fibrinogen caused by excessive consumption are commonly observed in the most severe cases whereas abnormally high levels of fibrinogen associated with an acute phase response are found in patients with milder disease[107] (Figure 4.7).

The fibrinolytic system is activated early, as indicated by low plasma levels of α2-antiplasmin. Fibrinolytic activity is, however, down-regulated by the appearance of functional active PAI-1. The result is a procoagulant state which is reflected in formation of microthrombi in the skin, the extremities and in the adrenals[124-126]. The excessive consumption of coagulation factors results in a haemorrhagic diathesis and local tissue haemorrhages.

The vessel wall is altered in these lethal or near-lethal cases. There is abnormal capillary leakage[127]. Various molecules derived from endothelial cells (PAI-1 and TFPI) can be detected in plasma in above-normal concentrations[93,94]. At least two molecules participating in the inflammatory reaction (bioactive TNF-α and granulocyte elastase) may inflict damage on the endothelial surface[92,98-100,103,128-132]. Whereas TNF-α may exert its influence on the entire endothelial lining of the vascular tree, release of elastase appears at first to be associated with margination of neutrophils in small vessels. Whether tissue factor is up-regulated on the endothelial cells *in vivo* has yet to be demonstrated. The stripping away of endothelial cell surface molecules which normally exert an anticoagulant effect (heparan sulphates, other negatively charged molecules, tissue factor pathway

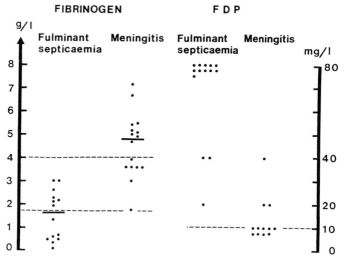

Figure 4.7 *Fibrinogen and fibrin degradation products (FDPs) in 30 patients clinically characterised as fulminant meningococcal septicaemia or meningococcal meningitis. Bars indicate mean values and the dotted lines denote the normal reference levels (fibrinogen 1.7–4.0 g/l, FDP < 10 mg/l)*

inhibitor etc.), together with reduced levels of prostacyclin, render the surface of the vessel wall more procoagulant even without exposure to tissue factor. However, despite compelling evidence for an association between severe coagulopathy and multiple organ dysfunction, two clinical studies failed to show benefit for heparin treatment[133,134].

Complement activation

The cooperative action of specific antibodies and a normal functioning complement system are cornerstones in protecting man from invasive *N. meningitidis*[135–137]. Complement defects have long been associated with an increased risk of acquiring meningococcal infection. Paradoxically, defects in the terminal complement cascade (C5–C9) are associated with reduced case fatality, whereas the rare patients with properdin defects located in the alternative activation pathway often suffer lethal infection[135–140]. Several studies show that significant complement activation occurs in patients developing overwhelming meningococcal septicaemia[141,142]. In the process of complement activation anaphylatoxins (C3a, C4a, C5a) are formed, exhibiting potent inflammatory effects and causing vasodilation and leakage. Furthermore, generation of the membrane attack complex (MAC) at the surface of bacteria may induce a significant release of LPS[143]. Observation in one C6 deficient patient infected with serogroup Y meningococci, treated initially with penicillin and later with fresh frozen plasma as well, suggested that complement truly exerts a LPS-releasing effect *in vivo*[144].

Knowledge about complement activation patients with SMD has recently been extended by the use of a new generation of immunoassays detecting neoepitopes exposed during activation of the complement cascade[145–148]. Employing these sensitive methods, complement activation at C3 and C5b-9 levels can be documented even in mild cases[110]. Increasing severity is associated with significantly higher levels of C3 activation products and terminal complement complex (TCC)[110]. The highest levels were found among the fatal shock patients[110]. In 32 surviving patients the median time to reach peak levels was 7 hours. Among patients with meningitis, significant C3 activation could be detected during the first 36 hours but not 6 days after admission, when compared with baseline samples collected 6 weeks after admission. In several shock patients who died, massive complement activation occurred, suggesting dysfunction of counter-regulatory mechanisms. The degree of complement activation on admission predicted ultimate survival or death. Five of seven patients with initial C3 activation products (C3 act) > 98 arbitrary units (AU) per ml died, compared with only two of 32 patients with C3act < 98 AU/ml. Six of seven patients with TCC levels > 12.7 AU/ml died as opposed to one of 32 with lower levels[110].

Further analyses of neoepitope exposure on complement factors B and C4 has helped to elucidate the relative importance of the classical and alternative complement pathways in SMD. The alternative pathway was activated significantly during the initial phase and activation was most pronounced in patients with fulminant disease. However, activation of the classical pathway did occur in many patients indicating that both classical and alternative pathways were activated together (Brandtzaeg P and Mollnes TE, unpublished results). Anaphylatoxins are known to up-regulate tissue factor expression, thereby linking activation of both the complement and coagulation systems[111,112].

CIRCULATING CYTOKINES AS MARKERS OF DISEASE SEVERITY

High levels of cytokines notably TNF-α, IL-1, IL-6 and IL-8 are detected in the circulation of SMD patients developing septic shock, multiple organ failure and disseminated intravascular coagulation[92,95,98−100,103,128−132]. Much attention has lately been given to these pro-inflammatory molecules as important mediators of organ dysfunction and as potential targets for new therapeutic interventions.

Circulating tumour necrosis factor α (TNF-α)

An association between serum TNF-α and the development of severe septic shock was first described in meningococcal patients[128]. In 79 patients, 10 of 11 deceased versus eight of 68 surviving patients had detectable bioactive TNF-α in serum samples collected on admission, a highly significant difference. Circulatory collapse was the primary cause of death in 10 of the 11 nonsurvivors. In a second study, seven of eight non-survivors compared with five of 32 survivors had detectable TNF activity[103]. The latter study also showed a significant association between plasma LPS levels and bioactive TNF-α[103]. Bioactive TNF-α was present in 12 of 13 patients (of whom seven died) with LPS > 700 ng/l and increased with increasing LPS concentrations, but in none of 27 patients (of whom one died owing to brain oedema) with LPS < 700 ng/l. Combined, these two studies comprising 119 SMD patients, revealed that all eight patients with TNF-α levels of greater than 100 ng/l died, compared with 11 of 110 with TNF-α levels less than 100 ng/l. Therefore, not only the presence, but also the absolute serum levels of bioactive TNF-α were related to outcome in SMD.

In patients with severe infectious purpura—mainly meningococcal infections—increasing levels of TNF-α detected by immunoassay correlate with increasing levels of IL-1, interferon gamma, decreasing levels of fibrinogen and increasing clinical severity[129]. Soluble TNF receptors (sTNF-RI and sTNF-RII), which may function as important circulating TNF-neutralising agents, increased with increasing TNF levels up to 500 ng/l in shock patients[131]. Above this level, little increase in soluble receptors occurred, suggesting an upper limit for production and consequently a larger fraction of bioavailable TNF, capable of damaging vessel walls and facilitating development of septic shock.

Circulating levels of bioactive TNF-α reach their maximum on or a few hours after hospital admission; thereafter TNF-α disappears from the circulation with a half-life of approximately 70 minutes[92]. In some patients a secondary increase is observed, unrelated to LPS levels[92].

Interleukin-1 (IL-1) in the circulation

Girardin *et al.* found that IL-1 was present in seven of 33 patients tested with an immunoassay[129]. The levels increased in line with clinical severity. In 20 patients tested with a functional cell assay (induction of IL-2 production), only three had detectable IL-1 activity[92]. These patients were characterised by exceptionally high levels of LPS (300, 170 and 12.5 μg/l respectively) and all died a few hours after hospital admission[92,100]. TNF-α and IL-1 each potentiate the lethal effect of the other cytokines, a phenomenon first observed in these three SMD patients and verified subsequently in animal experiments[149].

Most studies on experimental human endotoxinaemia have not been able to show increasing levels of IL-1[33,36]. However, Cannon *et al.*, employing an immunoassay, documented increasing IL-1 levels after the TNF-α peak[37]. This might also be the case in fulminant meningococcaemia. In two septic shock patients who died, maximum IL-1 activity occurred appoximately 4 hours after admission, whereas TNF-α levels were highest on admission.

Human monocytes stimulated with meningococcal LPS produce both IL-1α and IL-1β; the former is retained within the cell whereas the latter is secreted[150]. In 12 severe septic shock patients of whom six died, there was no difference in immunoreactive IL-1α levels between survivors and non-survivors although the former group had median LPS levels six times lower than the latter[100]. Indirectly, these resultrs suggest that IL-1 activity in the most severely shocked patients is due to IL-1β. In shock patients there is a 2–3 fold increase in immunoreactive IL-1α during the first 12 hours[100]. Plasma samples remained functionally inactive when tested for their ability to induce IL-2, suggesting that plasma IL-1α was complexed with IL-1 inhibitors. The role of IL-1 receptor antagonist in meningococcal infections has not been elucidated so far.

Circulating interleukin-6 (IL-6)

Of the cytokines investigated so far, IL-6 increases most significantly during SMD[92]. In SMD patients with lethal septic shock IL-6 levels 10 000 times higher than TNF-α have been documented, and 1000-fold increases over baseline levels are regularly observed[92]. Production of IL-6 is stimulated by LPS, TNF-α and IL-1[36,108]. In human LPS experiments TNF-α peaks before IL-6[34,36]. Recombinant TNF-α infused into human volunteers induces a significant IL-6 response[151]. The IL-6 response can be partly blocked in experimental endotoxinaemia in baboons by infusing anti-TNF-α antibodies[152]. Whereas up-regulation of TNF-α can be blocked by pretreatment of human volunteers with pentoxyfylline—a phosphodiesterase inhibitor—this is not the case for induction of IL-6[34]. These observations indicate a complex mechanism for initiation and modulation of IL-6 production. In 10 septic shock patients with LPS levels ranging from 0.8 to 300 μg/l, IL-6 levels correlated strongly with LPS ($r = 0.94$, $p = 0.0002$)[92]. Furthermore, in 69 SMD patients IL-6 was positively correlated with levels of TNF-α ($r = 0.62$, $p = 0.0001$), suggesting that both molecules participate in the regulation of IL-6 production *in vivo*[92,100,103]. Peak levels were noted on, or some hours after, admission. The half-life was approximately 100 minutes[92].

Unlike TNF-α and IL-1, IL-6 is not considered to be a toxic molecule. Levels measured on hospital admission do, however, show a strong association with disease severity, LPS levels and outcome[92,100,103,132,153]. IL-6 is a major pyrogen, an important inducer of acute phase responses, and is probably an important regulator of the inflammatory response.

Circulating interleukin-8 (IL-8)

IL-8, previously known as neutrophil activating peptide-1, up-regulates various functions of the neutrophil granulocyte. In human volunteers given a bolus injection of endotoxin, IL-8 peaks after TNF-α and reveals kinetics similar to IL-6[38,95]. Cyclo-oxygenase inhibitors augment its release, suggesting a negative feedback loop involving cyclo-oxygenase products, as has been observed for TNF-α. Patients with fulminant meningococcal septicaemia and high LPS levels have significantly higher levels of IL-8 than other SMD presentations[95]. IL-8 levels are positively correlated with those of TNF-α ($r = 0.64$, $p < 0.001$) and IL-6 ($r = 0.83$, $p < 0.001$)[95].

IL-8, leucopenia and the activation of the neutrophil granulocyte

Leucopenia in meningococcaemia is usually observed in fulminant cases. It is caused by margination, i.e. adherence of neutrophils to capillary walls. By using neutrophil elastase–α1-antitrypsin complexes in plasma as markers of neutrophil activation and release, we have observed maximum elastase release concomitantly with the most pronounced leucopenic phase and maximum IL-8 release (Brandtzaeg P, unpublished results). We assume that several adhesion molecules are up-regulated on the intraluminal endothelial surface and on the granulocytes simultaneously, facilitating close contact and thereby possibly inducing tissue damage through release of various proteases and toxic oxygen metabolites. IL-8 may participate actively in the up-regulation of adhesion molecules, notably intercellular adhesion molecule-1 (ICAM-1) which interacts with the β_2-selectin (CD18) on granulocytes[154].

Cytokines in the compartmentalised inflammatory response

By comparing levels of cytokines collected simultaneously in blood and CSF samples, it is possible to observe the contours of a compartmentalised inflammatory response induced by high levels of LPS either in the circulation or in the subarachnoid space[95,99,153]. In cases of fulminant septicaemia, significantly higher levels of TNF-α, IL-6 and IL-8 are generated in the circulation than in the CSF; the converse is also true, reflecting the main sites of bacterial proliferation in septicaemia and meningitis respectively.

ORGAN DYSFUNCTION RELATED TO INTRAVASCULAR INFLAMMATION

In fulminant meningococcal septicaemia many organ systems, particularly the circulation, the kidneys, the lungs and the haematological system (cells and plasma components) are affected simultaneously leading to variable degrees of dysfunction commonly designated multiple organ failure.

Circulatory failure

Persistent circulatory collapse is the single most important cause of death in fulminant meningococcaemia[42,69,70,76,87,105-107,124,126,130,133,134,155-158]. Previously thought to be caused by adrenal haemorrhage, most researchers today consider circulatory failure to be due to a combination of altered vascular tone, i.e. vasodilation, and myocardial failure induced by the intravascular inflammatory response[155-158]. Though initial vascular resistance was increased or normal in one group of children studied[158], other workers have found persistently low peripheral vascular resistance after fluid resuscitation and an initial high cardiac output subsequently declining to a hypodynamic circulation in non-surviving children and young adults (Brandtzaeg P, unpublished results) (Figure 4.8). Despite the use of

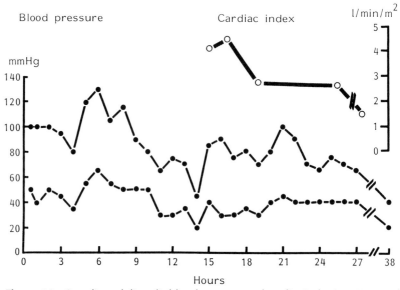

Figure 4.8 *Systolic and diastolic blood pressure and cardiac index in a 12 year old girl. She died 39 hours after hospital admission in spite of intensive care treatment including plasmapheresis performed once shortly after admission. The measurements revealed a persistent low peripheral vascular resistance in spite of vasoactive and inotropic drugs. Initially the circulation was hyperdynamic but gradually became hypodynamic. The peripheral resistance remained low until she died*

vasoconstrictor drugs, vascular resistance remains low in many patients. Ultimately, several such patients die with a ventricular arrhythmia[42].

Myocarditis with visualisation of meningococci in heart tissue has been documented by several authors[124,126,157]. Heart failure was therefore regarded as a consequence of direct invasion of bacteria in the heart. However, myocarditis has not been a common finding at post mortem examination in lethal septic shock cases caused by B15:P1.16 or C2a:P1.2 clones[42] (Brandtzaeg P, unpublished results). At present, myocardial failure in septic shock is regarded as a dysfunction of myocytes induced by unidentified myocardial depressant factors[159]. TNF-α and nitric oxide NO$^-$ are candidate molecules and LPS may, without involvement of mediators, alter myocardial cell metabolism.

Persistent vasodilatation is caused by an imbalance between forces causing dilatation and those causing contraction of the peripheral vasculature. A myriad of mediators have been identified which participate in regulation of vessel tone. Several vasodilating substances have been identified in the circulation of patients with fulminant meningococcal septic shock: vasoactive intestinal peptide (VIP), anaphylatoxins, e.g. C3a and C5a, bradykinin, TNF-α and IL-1[92,96,103,110,128,129,160]. Counter-regulatory mechanisms are, however, also activated, notably release of adrenaline, noradrenaline, cortisol and endothelin-1[160] (Brandtzaeg P, unpublished results). Recently, induction of nitric oxide synthase generating NO^- from L-arginine in endothelial cells has been implicated in the pathogenesis of LPS-induced septic shock[161,162].

Capillary leakage syndrome

Patients with fulminant meningococcal septicaemia are known to have a severe capillary leak syndrome which may be related to the effect of circulating bioactive TNF-α and IL-8 in addition to locally produced cytokines[100,158]. The tissue toxic effect is thought to be mediated in part through activated neutrophils. In one study decreasing levels of albumin on admission were associated with disease severity[127]. The syndrome is most clearly demonstrated by the amount of albumin needed to maintain an adequate serum level in fulminant septic shock[158]. After a few days treatment, patients show signs of excessive extravascular fluid accumulation.

Renal failure

Renal failure in SMD is closely associated with high LPS levels in plasma, septic shock and disseminated intravascular coagulation[42,93,94]. Patients with plasma LPS levels > 700 ng/l who developed persistent septic shock all had impaired renal function[42]. Clinical severity as judged by outcome (death or survival) was reflected in the initial renal function in that non-survivors became anuric within a few hours whereas most surviving patients maintained reduced kidney function which later recovered[42].

Serum creatinine can be used as a marker of endotoxinaemia and clinical severity in SMD patients[42]. However, the high serum creatinine levels generated within a few hours in the most fulminant cases cannot be explained fully by renal failure and reduced excretion alone. Serum creatinine levels two to three times above upper normal limits suggest increased breakdown of muscle proteins[42].

Peritoneal or haemodialysis or continuous haemofiltration are often used in the acute phase of fulminant meningococcal sepsis. The long-term prognosis for renal function is generally good[42]. However, a minority of shock patients never regain full kidney function.

There has been little research into the disease mechanism which results in endotoxin-induced renal failure in human septic shock[163–165]. The prevailing view is that structural and functional abnormalities of the proximal tubules are the pathological correlates of septic acute renal failure[164]. The pronounced reduction in glomerular filtration rate observed in such cases cannot be explained solely by a modest reduction in renal blood flow. Post mortem studies of fatal meningococcal cases have documented widespread thrombosis in glomeruli and necrosis of tubules, findings which have also been detected in the baboon septic shock model[124,126,165]. However, fibrin deposits in glomeruli were not present in non-survivors with pronounced DIC in a recent study[42] (and Brandtzaeg P, unpublished results). Ongoing fibrinolysis from death to post mortem examination—a time span of 12–18 hours—may explain this discrepancy. However, moderate fibrin deposition was observed in subcutaneous vessels of the same group of patients (Brandtzaeg P, unpublished results).

Adult respiratory distress syndrome

Adult respiratory distress syndrome (ARDS) is an acute inflammatory capillary leak syndrome of the lungs[166]. Patients become hypoxic and tachypnoeic. Chest X-ray shows diffuse, patchy lung infiltrates and pulmonary compliance is reduced[166,167]. Neutrophils have long been implicated in the pathogenesis[166,167]. In man, the site of granulocyte margination during the initial phase of leucopenia caused by overwhelming SMD is not known. The lungs may be a possible target organ. This hypothesis is supported by observations in the baboon septic shock model[168]. Damage to adjacent tissue by the release of a variety of toxic antibacterial substances from adherent neutrophils has been proposed as one mechanism which may lead to lung capillary damage and ARDS[168].

In meningococcal infection ARDS is found mainly in patients with high levels of LPS[42]. The development of ARDS is closely associated with fatal circulatory collapse[42]. The exact molecular mechanism leading to lung capillary leakage are unknown. ARDS can develop in severely and persistently neutropenic patients, indicating that pathogenic mechanisms unrelated to leucocytes must also operate[169]. Ferguson and Chapman noted signs of congestion, oedema and interstitial haemorrhages in the lung, but no accumulation of granulocytes in the capillaries in acute lethal cases of meningococcal septicaemia was seen[124]. We have observed children dying of circulatory collapse fulfilling all criteria of severe ARDS with and without significant intravascular granulocyte accumulation in the inter-alveolar septa (Brandtzaeg P, unpublished results). A complex interplay of LPS, cytokines, other inflammatory mediators, adhesion molecules and leucocytes may perhaps act together to alter the integrity of the lung capillary endothelium.

Adrenal haemorrhages

Massive adrenal haemorrhage, often referred to as suprarenal apoplexy, was long thought to be the most important cause of circulatory collapse in lethal cases of meningococcaemia[49,50,170–176]. However, in a carefully conducted study of 16 fulminant cases, Ferguson and Chapman stated: 'The term

"Waterhouse–Friderichsen syndrome" should be discontinued as evidence shows the condition to be one of general bacterial toxaemia, and the occurrence of massive haemorrhage into the adrenal glands is not necessary to produce the peripheral vascular collapse which, is so prominent in these cases'[124]. Adrenal haemorrhage is, however, detectable in a large percentage of cases developing fatal circulatory collapse[124,126,172–176] (Plate 1).

Why overwhelming infections cause haemorrhage in the adrenals has not yet been established. The phenomenon is also observed in septic shock in primates[177]. In SMD it is clearly related to high circulating levels of native endotoxin and various cytokines, disseminated intravascular coagulation (DIC), formation of fibrin thrombi and consumption of coagulation factors causing haemorrhagic diathesis. However, components related to the local vascular system must also be involved since massive tissue haemorrhage is not a universal phenomenon in these patients. The abundant capillary system in the adrenal cortex may be of importance[173]. Haemorrhage starts in the inner zona reticularis and may extend outwards to the zona glomerulosa while the medulla may escape[124,173,176]. The capillaries are often distended and congested with erythrocytes. Multiple fibrin thrombi have been visualised in some post mortem series although they have been completely lacking in others[124,126,173,176].

Cortisol levels are usually within, or above, the normal range when a patient dies due to septic shock, although pathologically low levels have been recorded in a few cases[178–182] (Brandtzaeg P, unpublished results). Adrenal haemorrhage can be visualised in living patients with the use of modern ultrasonography[182,183]. Addison's disease must be exceedingly rare, if ever described, in survivors of fulminant meningococcal septicaemia. This astonishing fact is even more remarkable today when a higher percentage of fulminant cases survive. The adrenals clearly have a significant regenerative capacity.

Petechiae and ecchymoses

Haemorrhagic skin lesions are the hallmark of, although not pathognomonic of, meningococcal infection. Lesions vary in size from pinpoint spots to massive ecchymoses several centimetres in diameter[104,184–188]. Individual lesions are usually slightly larger than purpuric lesions caused by thrombocytopenia and 'innocent' vasculitis related to common infections. They are purple or slightly bluish, may appear all over the body, but with a certain predilection for the extremities. The size of individual lesions is associated with underlying coagulopathy and vascular damage. Large confluent ecchymoses reflect a severe disease state, massive DIC and haemorrhagic diathesis and are associated with significant mortality[113–115,189–192].

In their classical description Hill and Kinney stated that: 'The fundamental pathologic lesion in the skin in meningococcaemia is diffuse vascular damage'[125]. The endothelial cells appeared swollen, protruded into the lumen and could in some cases be seen lying free in the vessel. Meningococci were visualised within the endothelium and within leucocytes. Necrotic endothelial cells and diapedesis of erythrocytes led to perivascular haemorrhage. Fibrin and platelet thrombi with early signs of leucocyte infiltration occluded a variable degree of the lumen. There was a diffuse dilatation and engorgement of blood vessels through the dermis[125]. Hardman describes a similar picture of haemorrhagic vasculitis and fibrin plugging of arterioles and capillaries[126]. However, Ferguson and Chapman observed diffuse haemorrhage without recognisable changes in the vessels in one patient, and focal capillary thromboses in another[124]. We have observed significant perivascular haemorrhage without any signs of acute vasculitis or massive alteration of endothelial cells as judged by light microscopy. Moderate amounts of intravascular fibrin were present (see Plate 2) but not platelet thrombi (Brandtzaeg P, unpublished results).

It has long been known that meningococci can be visualised in, and cultivated from, haemorrhagic skin lesions[125,185,193,194]. Meningococci probably form a local nidus in and around the vessel wall of the dermis during the bacteraemic state. Local endothelial cells are damaged, facilitating the formation of a local thrombus and/or extravasation of erythrocytes. In some cases the process develops into a marked vasculitis whereas in others, haemorrhage occurs without evidence of leucocyte infiltration. Extensive ecchymoses are clearly related to pronounced consumption coagulopathy, low levels of essential coagulation factors and thus haemorrhagic diathesis.

The predilection of meningococci for the vessels of the dermis remains to be explained. Localised haemorrhages are seen on serosal surfaces including the peritoneum, pleura and epicardium but never to the same extent as in skin. Specific characteristics of the skin vasculature, slow local blood flow and a slightly lower body temperature may contribute to the unusual distribution of skin lesions.

Muscular infarction

Serial measurements of creatine kinase (CK) and CK isoenzymes show that patients with fulminant septicaemia and DIC have biochemical evidence of significant muscle infarctions (Brandtzaeg P, unpublished data). In certain cases rhabdomyolysis may contribute to renal failure and may explain the high creatinine levels seen early on in these cases[42]. Disseminated intravascular thrombosis in muscles as in other organs is the most likely cause. CK isoenzyme analyses have not shown involvement of heart muscles and the moderately elevated levels of serum glutamic oxaloacetic transferase (SGOT) and serum glutamic pyruvic transaminase (SGPT) are presumably

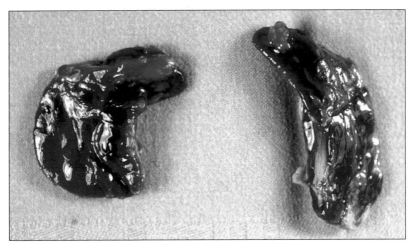

Plate 1 *Adrenals with massive haemorrhage in a 2 year old girl with fatal meningococcal septic shock and DIC. Kidneys, liver and lungs were, however, all free of gross haemorrhage*

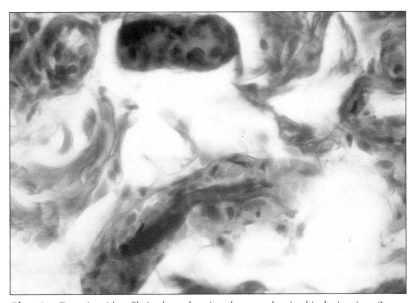

Plate 2 *Dermis with a fibrin thrombus in a haemorrhagic skin lesion in a 2 year old girl with fatal meningococcal septic shock and DIC. Stained by the method of Lendrum. By courtesy of Dr Tove Eeg Larsen, Department of Pathology, Ullevål University Hospital*

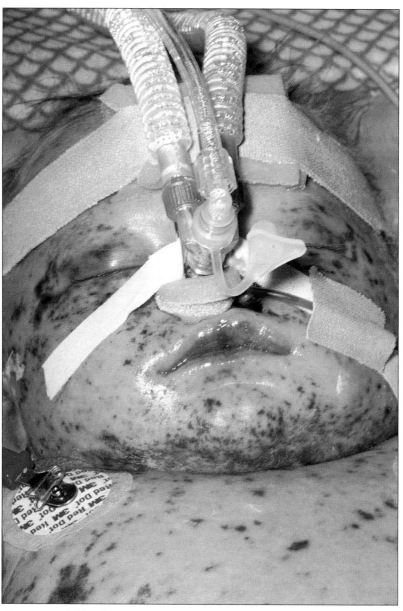

Plate 3 A child with meningococcal shock. Following resuscitation with colloid, gross oedema is seen in all tissues

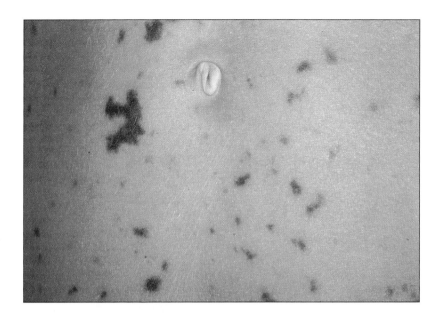

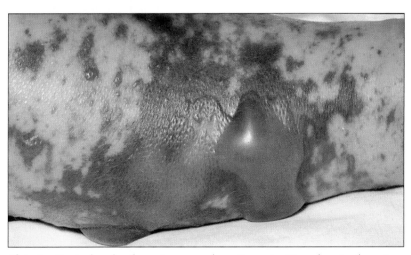

Plate 4 *Typical rash of meningococcal septicaemia. Top: fine erythematous macules are present in some areas. In others, petechiae are seen, progressing to the typical, jagged edged purpuric lessions. Bottom: fulminant meningococcal septicaemia. Confluent purpuric areas have formed with blistering and necrosis*

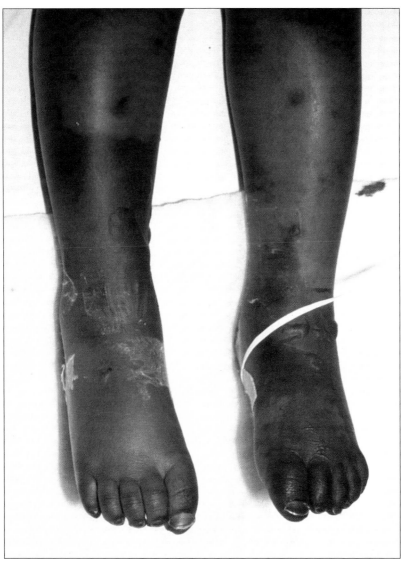

Plate 5 Peripheral limb ischaemia due to meningococcal septicaemia. A clear line of demarcation is present in the right leg, below which perfusion is absent. The left leg shows areas of confluent purpura and gangrene of the toes

derived primarily from the muscles and not heart or liver since gammaglutamyl transferase (GT) remains normal (Bradtzaeg P, unpublished data). Infarction of muscle may explain the intense 'flu-like' symptoms with muscle pain experienced by many patients in the early sepsis phase.

Arthritis

Acute septic arthritis occurs occasionally as the primary manifestation of SMD, accompanied by bacteraemia and sometimes by other clinical signs of meningococcal infection[195-198]. Arthritis in one or occasionally several larger joints may also be the sole organ manifestation of an intermittent, sometimes chronic, low-grade bacteraemia[195,199]. Schaad, reviewing the literature, found that septic arthritis occurred in approximately 5% of children and 11% of adults with SMD[195]. Bacterial characteristics may be important, since primary septic arthritis has been a rare occurrence during the prevailing B15:P1.7,16 meningococcal epidemic in Western Europe (Brandtzaeg P, unpublished data).

Meningococci may also induce an immune complex arthritis developing several days after initiation of antibiotic treatment[195,199]. A drop in complement C3 levels and a concomitant rise in complement split products in serum suggest activation of the complement system. As levels of immune complexes in serum do not differ from SMD patients without joint involvement, arthritis may be induced by locally produced immune complexes[199].

Pericarditis

During the bacteraemic state seeding of the pericardium with meningococci may occur[200-205]. Pericarditis evolves rapidly and life-threatening cardiac tamponade may occasionally be the sole manifestation of infection[202,205]. *N. meningitidis* strains of serogroup C have been particularly implicated[204,205]. Patients are febrile, nauseated and often complain of epigastric pain, symptoms which may easily be mistaken for those of an acute abdomen if other signs of a disseminated meningococcal infection are lacking[205]. Blood cultures may be negative but cultivation and microscopical examination of the exudate provide the correct diagnosis[205]. Locally formed immune complexes may prolong the inflammation[205].

Other rare organ manifestations in meningococcaemia

In the pre-antibiotic era panophthalmitis, endocarditis, pneumonia, pleurisy, peritonitis and otitis media were occasionally observed[1]. More recently, urogenital infections and symptoms suggesting acute gastroenteritis have been added to the list of less common manifestations[206].

PATHOPHYSIOLOGY OF MENINGITIS

Transition of meningococci from the vascular bed to the meninges

How and where meningococci cross the blood–brain barrier in man is not known. In young baboons a localised inflammation in the choroid plexus is an early event in the development of primate meningitis[207]. Herrick observed in 1918 that CSF collected by lumbar puncture shortly before death in several patients did not yield *N. meningitidis*, whereas CSF aspirated from the lateral ventricles immediately after death, from the same patients, contained significant numbers of bacteria[1]. He regarded the choroid plexus, which has an extraordinarily high blood flow, as the most likely portal of entry. In one post mortem examination he described leucocyte infiltration of the choroid plexus as the only evidence of CSF infection[43]. Ferguson and Chapman remarked on a focal inflammatory reaction and hyaline thrombi in the choroid plexus in four of six patients examined who had no overt evidence of meningitis[124]. If these observations are correct, initial infection of the central nervous system may start as a ventriculitis, spreading subsequently to the subarachnoid space.

Indirect evidence suggests that a tissue tropism exists, permitting *N. meningitidis* to adhere readily to the cerebrovascular endothelium. Meningococci appear to have a predilection for the meninges and for the skin. The nature of the cellular interactions are known. Adhesins located on pili or other surface exposed structures of *N. meningitidis* are candidate molecules which may interact with complementary carbohydrate moieties on the luminal side of the cerebrovascular endothelium. *In vitro*, piliated *N. meningitidis* strains adhere better to endothelial cells than non-piliated variants[25,26,29]. The class 5 outer membrane protein Opc, which is expressed on many disease-causing meningococci, represents an additional subcapsular structure associated with increased *in vitro* adherence[27]. Close contact apparently increases the cytopathogenic effect of microbial components on endothelial cells and may contribute to the loosening of the tight junctions of the brain endothelium.

Inflammation and changes in the blood–brain barrier

After adhering to endothelial cells, meningococci traverse the vessel walls. This probably occurs in small veins or capillaries[154,208]. Locally produced inflammatory mediators such as TNF-α, IL-1β induced by increasing levels of LPS in CSF may play a role in increasing the permeability of the blood–brain barrier[154,208]. Though meningococci may gain access to the subarachnoid space via the choroid plexus, animal experiments employing labelled albumin suggest that the influx of proteins—mainly albumin—occurs along the arachnoid veins by opening of the tight junctions[209].

The very early stages of human subarachnoid infection have been studied in patients with fulminant meningococcal septicaemia without clinical signs of meningitis[88]. *N. meningitidis* could be cultivated in 50% of such cases although all patients had minimal pleocytosis ($< 100 \times 10^6$ leucocytes/l of CSF)[42]. Levels of protein in CSF were normal or slightly elevated (≤ 0.66 g/l) and all had a normal CSF/blood glucose ratio[88]. These patients with fulminant meningococcal septicaemia were characterised by exceptionally high levels of LPS in plasma (median 3800, range 750–14 000 ng/l) and low levels of LPS in CSF (median 40, range < 25–165 ng/l), indicating very rapid intravascular bacterial proliferation, whereas bacterial growth in CSF remained very limited as judged by low CSF LPS levels. There may be a time lag between initial bacteraemia and seeding of the meninges in these cases, a phenomenon recognised much earlier by Herrick[1].

Despite high levels of LPS, bioactive TNF-α, IL-8, anaphylatoxins and massive bradykinin production in plasma, the cerebral vasculature still appears intact at this stage of the disease. However, after significant bacterial proliferation in CSF has occurred, generating inflammatory mediators and inducing a massive inflammatory response in the subarachnoid space, the cerebral endothelium becomes leaky. In patients with distinct pleocytosis ($> 10^6$ leucocytes/l of CSF), high levels of LPS (median 2500, range < 25–500 000 ng/l), abnormal high levels of protein and low CSF:plasma glucose ratios were present[88], suggesting that inflammation surrounding the vessels in the arachnoid may have a more pronounced influence on endothelial integrity than intravascular inflammation.

Microbial proliferation in CSF

Increasing levels of bacteria or LPS in CSF in bacterial meningitis are associated with increasing disease severity, as judged by clinical symptoms, laboratory parameters and outcome[210–213]. In experimental animals including young primates, a dose–response relationship exists between the levels of cell wall components and the inflammatory response[214–216]. This also appears to be the case in meningococcal meningitis. Increasing levels of LPS are associated with increasing levels of protein in CSF and a decrease in the blood:CSF glucose ratio, which is related to increasingly anaerobic brain metabolism[88]. The levels of leucocytes, initially predominantly neutrophils, are not significantly correlated with LPS levels although there is a trend towards correlation[88].

Cytokine response in experimental meningococcal meningitis

In rabbits, TNF-α, IL-1 and IL-6 are released into CSF in a coordinated and compartmentalised manner after injections with purified meningococcal LPS or live meningococci into the subarachnoid space[217] (Figure 4.9). TNF-α can be detected within 30 minutes, followed by IL-1 and IL-6. Rising protein levels are detected one hour after the injection and precede the influx of neutrophils which starts 2 hours after the challenging dose. Although this experiment does not entirely simulate the *in vivo* situation with gradually increasing levels of bacteria shedding outer membrane material and spontaneously undergoing lysis, it suggests that TNF-α is an early inflammatory mediator and may partially trigger the induction of IL-1 and IL-6.

Leakage of albumin starts at the same time as levels of TNF-α begin to rise sharply, and precedes the maximum release of IL-1 and the influx of neutrophils[217]. Therefore early inflammatory mediators, notably TNF-α and IL-1, may exert a disrupting effect on the endothelial lining which is independent of the cytotoxic action of neutrophils. TNF-α and IL-1 may enhance endothelial leakage cooperatively.

Cytokine release in meningococcal meningitis

In patients developing meningococcal meningitis LPS levels in CSF are 100 to 1000 times higher than those detected in simultaneously collected plasma samples[88]. This compartmentalised bacterial growth is reflected in the levels of inflammatory mediators. Bioactive TNF-α in CSF was detected in 55% of 44 patients with meningitis but in only 19% of 16 patients with meningococcal septic shock or mild systemic disease without significant pleocytosis[217]. Levels of TNF-α were also significantly higher among patients with meningitis than in patients with other clinical presentations[217].

Bioactive IL-1 revealed the same pattern of distribution as TNF-α, i.e. 50% positive samples among patients with distinct meningitis and 15% in patients with shock or bacteremia[217]. Bioactive IL-6 was present in the CSF of 41 of 42 cases of distinct meningitis at a median level of 154 ng/ml and in all 16 cases of septic shock or bacteraemia, but at a significantly lower median level (42 ng/ml)[217]. The detection rate and levels of immuno-reactive IL-8 in CSF did not show significant variations between the different clinical presentations[95].

In these studies of CSF comprising 60 patients infected with serogroup B and C meningococci, a particular cytokine release pattern is thus apparent. TNF-α and IL-1 can be detected in approximately 50%, and IL-6 and IL-8 in almost 100% of meningitis cases. The differences in detection rate may reflect the different release kinetics of the various cytokines indicating a longer-lasting response for IL-6 and IL-8. The latter two cytokines are not as strictly compartmentalised as TNF-α and IL-1 since they could also be detected in CSF collected from patients with minimal pleocytosis, although at a lower level for IL-6[69].

Levels of TNF-α in CSF could be significantly correlated with levels of

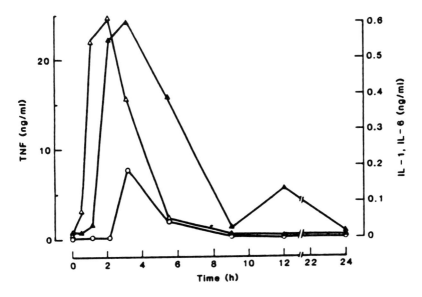

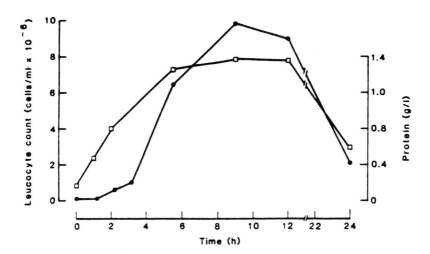

Figure 4.9 *TNF-α (△), IL-1 (▲), IL-6 (○) (top), protein (□) and leucocyte count (●) (bottom) in cerebrospinal fluid from a rabbit with experimental meningococcal meningitis. Meningococcal LPS was injected into the subarachnoid space at time point 0. Data from one rabbit is shown. Similar results were obtained in 10 independent experiments with LPS doses varying from 0.001 to 1 mg. Injections of LPS-free saline did not induce detectable levels of TNF-α, IL-1 or IL-6. Reproduced from the Journal of Experimental Medicine (1989; 170: 1859)[217], by copyright permission of the Rockefeller University Press*

IL-1, IL-6 and IL-8 suggesting a coordinated release pattern[217]. TNF-α may partly induce or up-regulate the production of the other three cytokines. Levels of IL-1 were significantly associated with the levels of IL-6 but not with IL-8[95]. IL-6 was associated with IL-8[95,217].

LPS, protein, glucose and leucocyte levels in CSF

In a series of 30 patients, increasing levels of LPS in CSF were associated with increasing protein levels and decreasing blood:CSF glucose ratio[88]. In an earlier study, levels of TNF-α, IL-1 and IL-6 were positively correlated with both parameters[217]. LPS, TNF-α, IL-1 and IL-8 levels were not significantly associated with the numbers of CSF leucocytes in these studies[88,95,99,217].

CSF from patients with meningococcal meningitis contains chemotactic substances[218,219]. In 38 patients with serogroup A and C *N. meningitidis* studied in Nigeria, the mean complement C3 level was 8.8% of the pooled human serum level[218]. In individual patients, C3 levels are associated with CSF protein levels but not with C3 serum levels. Passive diffusion may account for the presence of C3 in the CSF. In six CSF samples with high C3 levels, significant amounts of breakdown products were detectable suggesting that anaphylatoxins (C3a, C4a, C5a) may be generated locally[218]. Chemotactic activity was present in most of 35 CSF samples collected from Nigerian patients with meningococcal meningitis. Heat inactivation and fractionation studies suggested that the activity was related to a protein with molecular mass in the range of 10–80 kDa[219].

In vitro data and animal experiments suggest that the transition of neutrophils from the intraluminal side of the cerebral vasculature to the subarachnoid space involves several adhesion molecules regulated by cytokines and other inflammatory mediators. According to the prevailing hypothesis, P-selectin and E-selectin on the endothelial cell surface and L-selectin on the neutrophil surface, all belonging to the selectin superfamily, are up-regulated within a few minutes of being stimulated by locally produced IL-1 and TNF-α[154]. Later, selectins are down-regulated and replaced by ICAM-1 (belonging to the immunoglobulin superfamily) which interacts with CD18 (β_2 integrin) on neutrophils, a process which is under control of locally produced IL-8. The tight junctions of the endothelium are widened, facilitating leucocyte diapedesis[154]. The importance of β_2 integrins in the influx of leucocytes into the subarachnoid space has been elegantly demonstrated in a rabbit meningitis model. Pretreatment with anti-CD18 antibodies led to a significant reduction in leucocyte migration, reduced brain oedema and increased survival compared with controls[220].

The available data suggest that when meningococci have gained access to the subarachnoid space in man, increasing levels of bacterial cell wall components, primarily LPS, elicit increasing cytokine release. The effects on the cerebral vasculature result in protein and leucocyte influx, altered brain glucose metabolism, brain oedema and impaired cerebral circulation. Untreated, most patients die due to cerebral oedema and ischnemia.

CONCLUSIONS

Harrick stated that 'no other infection so quickly slays'[1]. Few doctors with much experience of meningococcal disease would disagree. We still lack a basic understanding of the bacterium–host interaction which enables meningococci to undergo massive intravascular proliferation within hours in fully immunocompetent hosts. Crucial meningococcal surface epitopes recognised as self by the host immune system may play an important role, but can hardly explain the diversity of disease manifestations among different patients infected with seemingly identical meningococcal clones[221]. The individual antibody profile is surely of importance in modulating the disease development.

Observations during the last century clearly established systemic meningococcal disease as a bacteraemic illness. *N. meningitidis* reveals a variable capacity for intravascular growth and seeding of various organs. Extensive local bacterial proliferation and thus LPS production induce a significant inflammatory response, causing the different clinical manifestations. The overwhelming endotoxinaemia which is generated in some patients, and the capacity of certain clones to cause large epidemics, will remain a continuing challenge to the medical community until we have produced effective vaccines capable of protecting future generations.

REFERENCES

1. Herrick WW. Early diagnosis and intravenous serum treatment of epidemic cerebrospinal meningitis. JAMA 1918; *71*: 612–17.
2. Meningococcal Disease Surveillance Group. Meningococcal disease: secondary attack rate and chemoprophylaxis in the United States 1974. JAMA 1976; *235*: 261–5.
3. Feigin RD, Baker CJ, Herwaldt LA, Lampe RM, Mason EO, Whitney SE. Epidemic meningococcal disease in an elementary-school classroom. N Engl J Med 1982; *307*: 1255–7.
4. Griffiss JMcL, Bertram MA. Epidemic meningococcal disease: synthesis of a hypothetical immunoepidemiologic model. Rev Infect Dis 1982; *4*: 159–72.
5. Berild D, Gedde-Dahl TW, Abrahamsen T. Meningococcal disease in the Norwegian armed forces in 1967–79. NIPH Ann 1980; *3*: 23–30.
6. Edwards EA, Devine LF, Sengbusch CH, Ward HW. Immunological investigations of meningococcal disease. III. Brevity of group C acquisition prior to disease occurrence. Scand J Infect Dis 1977; *9*: 105–10.

7. Goldschneider I, Gotschlich EC, Artenstein MS. Human immunity to the meningococcus. II. Development of natural immunity. J Exp Med 1969; *129*: 1327–48.
8. Young LS, LaForce FM, Head JJ, Feeley JC, Bennett JV. A simultaneous outbreak of meningococcal and influenza infections. N Engl J Med 1972; *287*: 5–9.
9. Moore PS, Hierholzer J, DeWitt W, Gauan K, Djoré D, Lippeveld T, Plikaytis B, Broome CV. Respiratory viruses and mycoplasma as cofactors for epidemic group A meningococcal meningitis. JAMA 1990; *264*: 1271–5.
10. Cartwright KAV, Jones DM, Smith AJ, Stuart JM, Kaczmarski EB, Palmer SR. Influenza A and meningococcal disease. Lancet 1991; *338*: 554–7.
11. Hubert B, Watier L, Garnerin P, Richardson S. Meningococcal disease and influenza-like syndrome: a new approach to an old question. J Infect Dis 1992; *166*: 542–5.
12. Hanenberg B, Tønjum T, Rodahl K, Gedde-Dahl TW. Factors preceding the onset of meningococcal disease with special emphasis on passive smoking, stressful events, physical fitness and general symptoms of ill health. NIPH Ann 1983; *6* 169–73.
13. Artenstein MS, Rust JH, Hunter DH, Lamson TH, Buescher EL. Acute respiratory disease and meningococcal infections in army recruits. JAMA 1967; *201*: 1004–8.
14. Mulks MH, Plaut AG, Feldman HA, Frangione B. IgA proteases of two distinct specificities are released by *Neisseria meningitidis*. J Exp Med 1980; *152*: 1442–7.
15. Mulks MH, Plaut AG. IgA protease production as a characteristic distinguishing pathogenic from harmless neisseriaceae. N Engl J Med 1978; *299*: 973–6.
16. Bleich HL, Boro ES. Microbial IgA proteases. N Engl J Med 1978; *298*: 1459–63.
17. Stephens DS. Gonococcal and meningococcal pathogenesis as defined by human cell, cell culture, and organ culture assays. Clin Microbiol Rev 1989; *2*: S104–11.
18. Stephens D, McGee ZA. Attachment of *Neisseria meningitidis* to human mucosal surfaces: influence of pili and type of receptor cell. J Infect Dis 1981; *143*: 525–32.
19. Stephens DS, Edwards KM, Morris F, McGee ZA. Pili and outer membrane appendages on *Neisseria meningitidis* in the cerebrospinal fluid of an infant. J Infect Dis 1982; *146*: 568.
20. Stephens DS, Hoffman LH, McGee ZA. Interaction of *Neisseria meningitidis* with human nasopharyngeal mucosa: attachment and entry into columnar epithelial cells. J Infect Dis 1983; *148*: 369–76.
21. Stephens DS, Farley MM. Pathogenic events during infection of the human nasopharynx with *Neisseria meningitidis* and *Haemophilus influenzae*. Rev Infect Dis 1991; *13*: 22–33.
22. Stephens DS, Spellman PPA, Swartley JS. Effect of the (α2-8)-linked polysialic acid capsule on adherence of *Neisseria meningitidis* to human mucosal cells. J Infect Dis 1993; *167*: 475–9.
23. DeVoe IW, Gilchrist JE. Pili on meningococci from primary cultures of nasopharyngeal carriers and cerebrospinal fluid of patients with acute disease. J Exp Med 1975; *141*: 197–205.
24. Stephens DS, Whitney AM, Schoolnik GK, Zollinger WD. Common epitopes of pilin of *Neisseria meningitidis*. J Infect Dis 1988; *158* 332–42.
25. Heckels JE. Structure and function of pili of pathogenic neisseria species. Clin Microbiol Rev 1989; *2*: S66–73.
26. Virji M, Alexandrescu C, Ferguson DJP, Saunders JR, Moxon ER. Variations in

the expression of pili: the effect on adherence of *Neisseria meningitidis* to human epithelial and endothelial cells. Mol Microbiol 1992; *6*: 1271–9.

27. Virji M, Makepeace K, Ferguson DJP, Achtman M, Sakari J, Moxon ER. Expression of the Opc protein correlates with invasion of epithelial and endothelial cells by *Neisseria meningitidis*. Mol Microbiol 1992; *6*: 2785–95.

28. Kristiansen BE, Sørensen B, Simonsen T, Spanne O, Lund V, Bjorvatn B. Isolates of *Neisseria meningitidis* from different sites in the same patient: phenotypic and genomic studies, with special reference to adherence, piliation, and DNA restriction endonuclease pattern. J Infect Dis 1984; *150*: 389–96.

29. Virji M, Kayhty H, Ferguson DJP, Alexandrescu C, Heckels JE, Moxon ER. The role of pili in the interactions of pathogenic *Neisseria* with cultured human endothelial cells. Mol Microbiol 1991; *5*: 1831–41.

30. Goldschneider I, Gotschlich EC, Artenstein MS. Human immunity to the meningococcus. I. The role of human antibody. J Exp Med 1969: *129*: 1307–26.

31. Jarvis GA, Vedros NA. Sialic acid of group B *Neisseria meningitidis* regulates alternative complement pathway activation. Infect Immun 1987; *55*: 174–80.

32. Griffiss JM, Bertram MA. Immunoepidemiology of meningococcal disease in military recruits. II. Blocking of serum bactericidal activity by circulating IgA early in the course of invasive disease. *J Infect Dis* 1977; *136*: 733–9.

32a. Drake TA, Cheng J, Chang A, Taylor FB. Expression of tissue factor, thrombomodulin, and E-selectin in baboons with lethal *Escherichia coli* sepsis. Am J Pathol 1993; *142*: 1458–70.

33. Michie HR, Manogue KR, Spriggs DR, Revhaug A, O'Dwyer S, Dinarello CA, Cerami A, Wolff SH, Wilmore DW. Detection of circulating tumor necrosis factor after endotoxin administration. N Engl J Med 1988; *318*: 1481–6.

34. Zabel P, Wolter DT, Schönharting MM, Schade UF. Oxpentifylline in endotozaemia. Lancet 1989; *ii*: 1474–7.

35. Fong Y, Moldawer LL, Marano M, Wei H, Tatter SB, Clarick RH *et al.* Endotoxemia elicits increased circulating β_2-INF/IL-6 in man. J Immunol 1989; *142*: 2321–4.

36. van Deventer SJH, Büller HR, ten Cate JW, Aarden LA, Hack E, Sturk A. Experimental endotoxemia in humans: analysis of cytokine release and coagulation, fibrinolytic, and complement pathways. Blood 1990; *76*: 2520–6.

37. Cannon JC, Tompkins RG, Gelfand JA, Michie HR, Stanford GG, van der Meer JWM *et al.* Circulating interleukin-1 and tumor necrosis factor in septic shock and experimental endotoxin fever. J Infect Dis 1990; *161*: 79–84.

38. Martich GD, Danner RL, Ceska M, Suffredini AF. Detection of interleukin 8 and tumor necrosis factor in normal humans after intravenous endotoxin: the effect of antiinflammatory agents. J Exp Med 1991; *173*: 1021–4.

39. Elin RJ, Wolff SM, McAdam KPWJ, Chedid L, Audibert F, Bernard C, Oberling F. Properties of reference *Escherichia coli* endotoxin and its phthalylated derivative in humans. J Infect Dis 1981; *144*: 329–36.

40. Fong Y, Marano MA, Moldawer LL, Calvano SE, Kenny JS, Allison AC *et al.* The acute splanchnic and peripheral tissue metabolic response to endotoxin in humans. J Clin Invest 1990; *85*: 1896–1904.

41. Berry LJ. Introduction. In: Berry LJ, ed. *Handbook of Endotoxin, Volume 3: Cellular Biology of Endotoxin*. Amsterdam: Elsevier Science Publishers, 1985; 17–21.

42. Brandtzaeg P, Kierulf P, Gaustad P, Skulberg A, Bruun JN, Halvorsen S *et al.* Plasma endotoxin as predictor of multiple organ failure and death in systemic meningococcal disease. J Infect Dis 1989; *159*: 195–204.

43. Herrick WW. Extrameningeal meningococcal infections. Arch Intern Med

1919; 23: 409–18.
44. La Scolea LJ, Dryja D, Sullivan TD, Mosovich L, Ellerstein N, Neter E. Diagnosis of bacteremia in children by quantitative direct plating and a radiometric procedure. J Clin Microbiol 1981; 13: 478–82.
45. La Scolea LJ, Dryja D. Quantitation of bacteria in cerebrospinal fluid and blood of children and its diagnostic significance. J Clin Microbiol 1984; 19: 187–90.
46. Zwahlen A, Waldvogel FA. Magnitude of bacteremia and complement activation during Neisseria meningitidis infection: Study of two co-primary cases with different clinical presentation. Eur J Clin Microbiol 1984; 3: 439–41.
47. Sullivan TD, La Scolea LJ. Neisseria meningitidis bacteremia in children: quantitation of bacteremia and spontaneous clinical recovery without antibiotic therapy. Pediatrics 1987; 80: 63–7.
48. Boone JT, Hall WW. Meningococcal septicemia with report of case showing organism in direct blood smear. US Nav Med Bull 1935; 33: 446–51.
49. Thomas HM. Meningococcic meningitis and septicemia. JAMA 1943; 123: 264–72.
50. Boger WP. Fulminating meningococcemia. N Engl J Med 1944; 231: 385–7.
51. Young EJ, Cardella TA. Meningococcemia diagnosed by peripheral blood smear. JAMA 1988; 260: 992.
52. Yagupsky P, Nolte FS. Quantitative aspects of septicemia. Clin Microbiol Rev 1990; 3: 269–79.
53. Pfeiffer R. Untersuchungen über das Choleragift. Zeitschr Hyg Infektionskr 1892; 11: 393–9.
54. Centanni E. Untersuchung über das Infectionsfieber. Das Fiebergift der Bacterien. Deutsch Med Wschr 1894; 20: 148–50.
55. Centanni E, Bruschettini A. Untersuchungen über das Infectionsfieber. Das Antitoxin des Bacterienfiebers. Deutsch Med Wschr 1894; 20: 270–2.
56. Flexner S. Experimental cerebrospinal meningitis and its serum treatment. JAMA 1906; 47: 560–6.
57. Kolle W, Wassermann A. Versuche zur Gewinnung und Wertbestimmung eines Meningococcenserums. Deutsch Med Wschr 1906; 32: 609–12.
58. Jochmann G. Versuche zur Serodiagnostik und Serotherapie der epidemischen Genickstarre. Deutsch Med Wschr 1906; 32: 788–93.
59. Netter A, Debré R. La méningite Cérébro-spinale. Paris: Masson et Cie, 1911; 47–82, 245–82.
60. Flexner S. The results of the serum treatment in thirteen hundred cases of epidemic meningitis. J Exp Med 1913; 17: 553–76.
61. Scherp HW. Neisseria and neisserial infections. Ann Rev Microbiol 1955; 9: 319–34.
62. Ducker TB. The pathogenesis of meningitis. Arch Neurol 1968; 18: 123–28.
63. Davis CE, Arnold K. Role of meningococcal endotoxin in meningococcal purpura. J Exp Med 1974; 140: 159–70.
64. Davis CE, Ziegler EJ, Arnold KF. Neutralization of meningococcal endotoxin by antibody to core glycolipid. J Exp Med 1978; 147: 1007–17.
65. DeVoe IW, Gilka F. Disseminated intravascular coagulation in rabbits: synergistic activity of meningococcal endotoxin and materials egested from leukocytes containing meningococci. J Med Microbiol 1976; 9: 451–8.
66. DeVoe IW, Gilka F, Gilchrist JE, Yu E. Pathology of rabbits treated with leukocyte-degenerated meningococci in combination with meningococcal endotoxin. Infect Immun 1977; 16: 271–9.
67. DeVoe IW. The meningococcus and mechanisms of pathogenicity. Microbial

Rev 1982; 46: 162–90.

68. Verheul AFM, Snippe H, Poolman JT. Meningococcal lipopolysaccharides: virulence factor and potential vaccine component. Microbial Rev 1993; 57: 34–49.

69. Lewis LS. Prognostic factors in acute meningococcaemia. Arch Dis Child 1979; 54: 44–8.

70. Tubbs HR. Endotoxin in meningococcal infections. Arch Dis Child 1980; 55: 808–10.

71. Levin J, Tomasulo PA, Oser RS. Detection of endotoxin in blood and demonstration of an inhibitor. J Lab Clin Med 1970; 75: 903–11.

72. Levin J, Poore TE, Zauber NP, Oser RS. Detection of endotoxin in the blood of patients with sepsis due to gram-negative bacteria. N Engl J Med 1970; 283: 1313–16.

73. Levin J, Poore TE, Young NS, Margolis S, Zauber NP, Townes AS, Bell WR. Gram-negative sepsis: detection of endotoxemia with the Limulus test. Ann Intern Med 1972; 76: 1–7.

74. Iwanaga S, Morita T, Harada T. Chromogenic substrates for horseshoe crab clotting enzyme, its application for the assay of bacterial endotoxin. Haemostasis 1978; 7: 183–8.

75. Harthug S, Bjorvatn B, Østerud B. Quantitation of endotoxin in blood from patients with meningococcal disease using a Limulus lysate test in combination with chromogenic substrate. Infection 1983; 11: 192–5.

76. Bjorvatn B, Bjertnaes L, Fadnes HO, Flaegstad T, Gutteberg TJ, Kristiansen BE *et al.* Meningococcal septicaemia treated with combined plasmapheresis and leukapheresis or with blood exchange. Br Med J 1984; 288: 439–41.

77. van Deventer SJH, Buller HRA, ten Cate JW, Sturk A, Pauw W. Endotoxaemia: an early predictor of septicaemia in febrile patients. Lancet 1988; i; 605–9.

78. Danner RL, Elin RL, Husseini JM, Wesley RA, Reilly JM, Parillo JE. Endotoxemia in human septic shock. Chest 1991; 99: 169–75.

79. Rietschel ET, Seydel U, Zähringer U, Schade U, Brade L, Loppnow H *et al.* Bacterial endotoxin: molecular relationship between structure and activity. Infect Dis Clin N Am 1991; 5: 753–79.

80. Skarnes RC. *In vivo* distribution and detoxification of endotoxins. In: Berry LJ, ed. *Cellular Biology of Endotoxin.* Amsterdam: Elsevier Science Publishers, 1985; 56–81.

81. Ulevitch RJ, Johnston AR, Weinstein DB. New function for high density lipoproteins. Their participation in intravascular reactions of bacterial lipopolysaccharides. J Clin Invest 1979; 64: 1516–24.

82. Harris HW, Grunfeld C, Feingold KR, Rapp JH. Human very low density lipoproteins and chylomicrons can protect against endotoxin-induced death in mice. J Clin Invest 1990; 86: 696–702.

83. Flegel WA, Wolpl A, Mannel DN, Northoff N. Inhibition of endotoxin-induced activation of human monocytes by human lipoproteins. Infect Immun 1989; 57: 2237–45.

84. Tesh VL, Vukajlovich SW, Morrison DC. Endotoxin interactions with serum proteins, relationship to biological activity. In: Levin J, Büller HR, ten Cate JW, van Deventer SJH, Sturk A, eds. *Bacterial Endotoxins: Pathophysiological Effects, Clinical Significance, and Pharmacological Control.* New York: Alan R. Liss, 1988; 47–62.

85. Brandtzaeg P, Bryn K, Kierulf P, Øvstebø R, Namork E, Ase B *et al.* Meningococcal endotoxin in lethal septic shock plasma studied by gas chromatography, mass-spectrometry, ultracentrifugation, and electron micro-

scopy. J Clin Invest 1992; *89*: 816–23.
86. Kulshin VA, Zähringer U, Lindner B, Frasch CE, Tsai C-M, Dmitriev BA *et al.* Structural characterization of the lipid A component of pathogenic *Neisseria meningitidis*. J Bacteriol 1992; *174*: 1793–1800.
87. van Deuren M, Santman FW, van Dalen R, Sauerwein RW, Span LFR, van der Meer JWM. Plasma and whole blood exchange in meningococcal sepsis. Clin Infect Dis 1992; *15*: 424–30.
88. Brandtzaeg P, Øvstebø R, Kierulf P. Compartmentalization of lipopolysac-charide-production correlates with the clinical presentation in meningococcal disease. J Infect Dis 1992; *166*: 650–2.
89. Buxton Hopkin DA. Frapper fort ou frapper doucement: a gram-negative dilemma. Lancet 1978; *ii*: 1193–4.
90. Shenep JL, Mogan KA. Kinetics of endotoxin release during antibiotic therapy for experimental gram-negative bacterial sepsis. J Infect Dis 1984; *150*: 380–8.
91. Andersen BM, Solberg O, The endotoxin-liberating effect of antibiotics on meningococci in vitro. Acta Pathol Microbiol Scand Sect B 1980; *88*: 231–6.
92. Waage A, Brandtzaeg P, Halstensen A, Kierulf P, Espevik T. The complex pattern of cytokines in serum from patients with meningococcal septic shock. J Exp Med 1989; *169*: 333–8.
93. Brandtzaeg P, Sandset M, Joø GB, Øvstebø R, Kierulf P, Abilgaard U. The quantitative association of plasma endotoxin, antithrombin, protein C, extrinsic coagulation pathway inhibitor and fibrinopeptide A in systemic meningococcal disease. Thromb Res 1989; *55*: 459–70.
94. Brandtzaeg P, Joø GB, Brusletto B, Kierulf P. Plasminogen activator inhibitor 1 and 2, alpha-2-antiplasmin, plasminogen, and endotoxin levels in systemic meningococcal disease. Thromb Res 1990; *57*: 271–8.
95. Halstensen A, Ceska M, Brandtzaeg P, Redl H, Naess A, Waage A. Interleukin-8 in serum and cerebrospinal fluid from patients with meningococcal disease. J Infect Dis 1993; *167*: 471–5.
96. Brandtzaeg P, Øktedalen O, Kierulf P, Opstad PK. Elevated VIP and plasma endotoxin in human gram-negative septic shock. Regulatory Peptides 1989; *24*: 37–44.
97. Engebretsen LF, Kierulf P, Brandtzaeg P. Extreme plasminogen activator inhibitor and endotoxin values in patients with meningococcal disease. Thromb Res 1986; *42*: 713–16.
98. Brandtzaeg P, Kierulf P. Endotoxin and meningococcemia; intravascular inflammation induced by native endotoxin in man. In: Ryan JL, Morrison DC, eds. *Bacterial Endotoxic Lipopolysaccharides, volume 2 Immunopharmacology and Pathophysiology*. Boca Raton: CRC Press, 1992; 327–46.
99. Brandtzaeg P, Halstensen A, Kierulf P, Espevik T, Waage A. Molecular mechanisms in the compartmentalized inflammatory response presenting as meningococcal meningitis or septic shock. Microb Pathog 1992; *13*: 423–31.
100. Brandtzaeg P. Cytokines in overwhelming Gram-negative bacteremia. In: Schlag G, Redl H, Traber DL, eds. *Shock, Sepsis and Organ Failure*. Berlin: Springer Verlag, 1993; 369–411.
101. Morrison DC, Ulevitch RJ. The effects of bacterial endotoxins on host mediation systems. Am J Pathol 1978; *93*: 527–617.
102. Morrison DC, Ryan JL. Endotoxins and disease mechanisms. Ann Rev Med 1987; *38*: 417–32.
103. Brandtzaeg P, Waage A, Mollens TE, Øktedalen O, Kierulf P. Severe septic shock involves more than tumor necrosis factor. In: Sturk A, van Deventer SJH,

ten Cate JW, Büller HR, Thijs LG, Levin J, eds. *Bacterial Endotoxins: Cytokine Mediators and New Therapies for Sepsis.* New York: Wiley-Liss, 1991; 25–42.

104. Brandtzaeg P, Dahle JS, Høiby EA. The occurrence and the feature of hemorrhagic skin lesions in 115 cases of systemic meningococcal disease. NIPH Ann 1983; *6*: 183–90.

105. Halstensen A, Pedersen SH, Haneberg B, Bjorvatn B, Solberg CO. Case fatality of meningococcal disease in Western Norway. Scand J Infect Dis 1987; *19*: 35–42.

106. Wong VJ, Hitchcock W, Mason WH. Meningococcal infections in children: a review of 100 cases. Pediatr Infect Dis J 1989; *8*: 224–7.

107. Giraud T, Dahainaut JF, Schremmer B, Regnier B, Desjara P, Loirat P *et al.* Adult overwhelming meningococcal purpura. Arch Intern Med 1991; *151*: 310–6.

108. van der Poll T, Büller HR, ten Cate H, Wortel CH, Bauer KA, van Deventer SJH *et al.* Activation of coagulation after administration of tumor necrosis factor to normal subjeccts. N Engl J Med 1990; *322*: 1622–7.

109. Østerud B, Flaegstad T. Increased tissue thromboplastin activity in monocytes of patients with meningococcal infection: related to unfavourable prognosis. Thromb Haemostas 1983; *49*: 5–7.

110. Brandtzaeg P, Mollnes TE, Kierulf P. Complement activation and endotoxin levels in systemic meningococcal disease. J Infect Dis 1989; *160*: 58–65.

111. Prydz H, Allison AC, Schorlemmer HU. Further link between complement activation and blood coagulation. Nature 1977; *270*: 173–4.

112. Østerud B, Eskeland T. The mandatory role of complement in the endotoxin-induced synthesis of tissue thromboplastin in blood monocytes. FEBS Lett 1982; *149*: 75–9.

113. McGehee WG, Rapaport SI, Hjort PF. Intravascular coagulation in fulminant meningococcemia. Ann Intern Med 1967; *67*: 250–60.

114. Dennis LH, Cohen RJ, Schachne SH, Conrad ME. Consumptive coagulopathy in fulminant meningococcemia. JAMA 1968; *205*: 133–5.

115. Evans RW, Glick B, Kimball F, Lobell M. Fatal intravascular consumption coagulopathy in meningococcal sepsis. Am J Med 1969; *46*: 910–18.

116. Powars DR, Rogers ZR, Patch MJ, McGhee WG, Francis RB. Purpura fulminans in meningococcemia: association with acquired deficiencies of protein C and S. N Engl J Med 1987; *317*: 571–2.

117. Fourrier F, Lestavel P, Chopin C, Marey A, Goudemand J, Rime A *et al.* Meningococcemia and purpura fulminans in adults: acute deficiencies of protein C and S and early treatment with antithrombin III concentrated. Intensive Care Med 1990; *16*: 121–4.

118. Rapaport SI. The extrinsic pathway inhibitor: a regulator of tissue factor-dependent blood coagulation. Thromb Haemostas 1991; *66*: 6–15.

119. Sandset PM, Abildgaard U. Extrinsic pathway inhibitor. The key to feedback control of blood coagulation initiated by tissue thromboplastin. Haemostasis 1991: *21*: 219–39.

120. Sandset PM, Warn-Cramer BJ, Rao VML, Maki SL, Rapaport SI. Depletion of extrinsic pathway inhibitor (EPI) sensitizes rabbits to disseminated intravascular coagulation induced with tissue factor: Evidence supporting a physiologic role for EPI as a natural anticoagulant. Proc Natl Acad Sci USA 1991; *88*: 708–12.

121. Suffredini AF, Harpel PC, Parrillo JE. Promotion and subsequent inhibition of plasminogen activation after administration of intravenous endotoxin to normal subjects. N Engl J Med 1989; *320*: 1165–72.

122. van Hinsbergh VWM, Bauer KA, Kooistra T, Kluft C, Dooijewaard G, Sherman ML *et al.* Progress of fibrinolysis during tumor necrosis factor

infusions in humans. Concomitant increase in tisue-type plasminogen activator, plasminogen activator inhibitor type-1, and fibrin(ogen) degradation products. Blood 1990; 76: 2284–9.

123. van der Poll T, Levi M, Büller HR, van Deventer SJH, de Boer JP, Hack Ce et al. Fibrinolytic response to tumor necrosis factor in healthy subjects. J Exp Med 1991; 174: 729–32.

124. Ferguson JH, Chapman OD. Fulminating meningococcic infections and the so-called Waterhouse–Friderichsen syndrome. Am J Pathol 1948; 24: 763–95.

125. Hill WR, Kinney TD. The cutaneous lesions in acute meningococcemia. JAMA 1947; 134: 513–18.

126. Hardman JM. Fatal meningococcal infections: the changing pathologic picture in the '60s. Milit Med 1968; 133: 951–64.

127. Kahn A, Brachet E. Accroissement de la perméabilité vasculaire lors de l'endotoxinémie chez l'enfant. Pathol Biol (Paris) 1980; 28: 449–51.

128. Waage A, Halstensen A, Espevik T. Association between tumour necrosis factor in serum and fatal outcome in patients with meningococcal disease. Lancet 1987; i: 355–7.

129. Girardin E, Gray GE, Dayer JM; Roux-Lombard P, The J5 study group, Lambert PH. Tumor necrosis factor and interleukin-1 in serum of children with severe infectious purpura. N Engl J Med 1988; 319: 397–400.

130. Girardin E, J5 Study Group. Treatment of severe infectious purpura in children with human plasma from donors immunized with Escherichia coli J5: a prospective double-blind study. J Infect Dis 1992; 165: 695–701.

131. Girardin E, Roux-Lombard P, Grau GE, Suter P, Gallati H, The J5 Study Group, Dayer J-M. Imbalance between tumour necrosis factor-alpha and soluble TNF receptor concentrations in severe meningococcaemia. Immunology 1992; 76: 20–3.

132. Waage A, Brandtzaeg P, Espevik T, Halstensen A. Current understanding of the pathogenesis of Gram-negative shock. Infect Dis Clin N Am 1991; 5: 781–91.

133. Manios SG, Kanakoudi F, Maniati E. Fulminant meningococcemia; heparin therapy and survival rate. Scand J Infect Dis 1971; 3: 127–33.

134. Haneberg B, Gutterberg TJ, Moe PJ, Østerud B, Bjorvatn B, Lehmann EH. Heparin for infants and children with meningococcal septicemia. NIPH Ann 1983; 6: 43–7.

135. Ross SC, Densen P. Complement deficiency states and infection: epidemiology, pathogenesis and consequences of Neisseria and other infections in an immuno deficiency. Medicine (Baltimore) 1984; 63: 243–73.

136. Densen P. Interaction of complement with Neisseria meningitidis and Neisseria gonorrhoeae. Clin Microbiol Rev 1989; 2: S11–17.

137. Figueroa JE, Densen P. Infectious diseases associated with complement deficiencies. Clin Microbiol Rev 1991; 4: 359–95.

138. Sjøholm AG, Braconier JH, Soderstrom C. Properdin deficiency in a family with fulminant meningococcal infections. Clin Exp Immunol 1982; 50: 291–7.

139. Densen P, Weiler JM, Griffiss JM, Hoffmann LG. Familial properdin deficiency and fatal meningococcemia. N Engl J Med 1987; 316: 922–6.

140. Sjøholm AG, Kuijper EJ, Tijssen CC, Jansz A, Bol P, Spanjaard L, Zanen HC. Dysfunctional properdin in a Dutch family with meningococcal disease. N Engl J Med 1988; 319: 33–7.

141. Greenwood BM, Onyewotu II, Whittle HC. Complement and meningococcal infection. Br Med J 1976; i: 797–9.

142. Beatty DW, Ryder CR, Heese HDV. Complement abnormalities during an

epidemic of group B meningococcal infection in children. Clin Exp Immunol 1986; *64*: 465–70.

143. Frank MM, Joiner K, Hammer C. The function of antibodies and complement in the lysis of bacteria. Rev Infect Dis 1987; *9*: S537–45.

144. Lehner PJ, Davies KA, Walport MJ, Cope AP, Würzner R, Orren A, Morgan BP, Cohen J. Meningococcal septicaemia in a C6-deficient patient and effects of plasma transfusion on lipopolysaccharide release. Lancet 1992; *ii*: 1379–81.

145. Mollnes TE, Lachmann PJ. Activation of the third component of complement (C3) detected by a monoclonal anti-C3'g' neoantigen antibody in a one-step enzyme immunoassay. J Immunol Meth 1987; *101*: 201–7.

146. Mollnes TE, Lea T, Frøland SS, Harboe M. Quantification of the terminal complement complex in human plasma by an enzyme-linked immunosorbent assay based on monoclonal antibodies against a neoantigen of the complex. Scand J Immunol 1985; *22*: 197–202.

147. Mollnes TE. Early- and late-phase activation of complement evaluated by plasma levels of C3d,g and the terminal complement complex. Complement 1985; *2*: 156–64.

148. Mollnes TE, Harboe M. Neoepitope expression during complement activation. Immunologist 1993; *1*: 43–9.

149. Waage A, Espevik T. Interleukin 1 potentiates the lethal effect of tumor necrosis factor α/cachectin in mice. J Exp Med 1988; *167*: 1987–92.

150. Cavaillon JM, Munoz C, Fitting C, Couturier C, Haeffner-Cavaillon N. Signals involved in interleukin-1 production induced by endotoxins. In: Nowotny A, Spitzer JJ, Ziegler EJ, eds. *Cellular and Molecular Aspects of Endotoxin Reactions.* Amsterdam: Elsevier Science Publishers, 1990; 257–67.

151. van der Poll T, van Deventer SJH, Hack CE, Wolbink GJ, Aarden LA, Büller HR *et al.* Effects on leukocytes following injection of tumor necrosis factor into healthy humans. Blood 1992; *79*: 693–8.

152. Fong Y, Tracey KJ, Moldawer LL, Hesse DG, Manogue KB, Kenney JS, Lee AT, Kuo GC, Allison AC, Lowry SF, Cerami A. Antibodies to cachectin/tumor necrosis factor reduce interleukin 1 beta and interleukin 6 appearance during lethal bacteremia. J Exp Med 1989; *170*: 1627–33.

153. Waage A, Halstensen A, Espevik T, Brandtzaeg P. Compartmentalization of TNF and IL-6 in meningitis and septic shock. Mediat Inflam 1993; *2*: 23–5.

154. Quagliarello VJ, Scheld WM. Bacterial meningitis: pathogenesis, pathophysiology, and progress. N Engl J Med 1992; *327*: 864–72.

155. Levin S, Painter MB. The treatment of acute meningococcal infection in adult. Ann Intern Med 1966; *64*: 1049–56.

156. Boucek MM, Boerth RC, Artman M, Graham TP, Boucek RJ. Myocardial dysfunction in children with acute meningococcemia. J Pediatr 1984; *105*: 538–42.

157. Monsalve F, Rucabado L, Salvador A, Bonastre J, Cuñat J, Ruano M. Myocardial depression in septic shock caused by meningococcal infection. Crit Care Med 1984; *12*: 1021–3.

158. Mercier JC, Beaufils F, Hartman JF, Azéma D. Hemodynamic patterns of meningococcal shock in children. Crit Care Med 1988; *16*: 27–33.

159. Parrillo JE. Pathogenetic mechanisms of septic shock. N Engl J Med 1993; *328*: 1471–7.

160. Romijn JA, Godfried MH, Wortel C, Sauerwein HP. Hypoglycemia, hormones and cytokines in fatal meningococcal septicemia. J Endocrinol Invest 1990; *13*: 743–7.

161. Moncada S, Higgs EA. Endogenous nitric oxide: physiology, pathology and

clinical relevance. Eur J Clin Invest 1991; *21*: 361–74.
162. Vane JR, Änggård EE, Botting RM. Regulatory functions of the vascular endothelium. N Engl J Med 1990; *323*: 27–36.
163. Wardle N. Acute renal failure in the 1980s: the importance of septic shock and endotoxaemia. Nephron 1982; *30*: 193–200.
164. Myers BD, Moran SM. Hemodymically mediated acute renal failure. N Engl J Med 1986; *314*: 97–105.
165. Voss BL, De Bault LE, Blick KE, Chang ACK, Stiers DL, Hinshaw LB, Taylor FB. Sequential renal alterations in septic shock in the primate. Circ Shock 1991; *33*: 142–55.
166. Repine JE. Scientific perspectives on adult respiratory distress syndrome. Lancet 1992; *i*: 466–9.
167. Martin MA, Silverman HJ. Gram-negative sepsis and the adult respiratory distress syndrome. Clin Infect Dis 1992; *14*: 1213–28.
168. Dormehl IC, Maree M, Cromarty D, Böckmann H, Jacobs L, van Rensburg E, Kilian J. Investigation by scintigraphic methods of neutrophil kinetics under normal and septic shock conditions in the experimental baboon model. Eur J Nucl Med 1990; *16*: 643–47.
169. Ognibene FP, Martin SE, Parker MM, Schlesinger T, Roach P, Burch C *et al.* Adult respiratory distress syndrome in patients with severe neutropenia. N Engl J Med 1986; *315*: 547–51.
170. Waterhouse R. A case of suprarenal apoplexy. Lancet 1911; *i*: 577–8.
171. Friderichsen C. Nebennierenapoplexie bei kleinen Kindern. Jb Kinderheilk 1918; *87*: 109–25.
172. Bernhard WG, Jordan AC. Bilateral adrenal hemorrhage (Waterhouse-Friderichsen syndrome) associated with meningococcal septicemia. J Lab Clin Med 1944; *29*: 357–65.
173. Martland HS. Fulminating meningococcic infection with bilateral massive adrenal hemorrhage (the Waterhouse-Friderichsen syndrome). Arch Path 1944; *37*: 147–58.
174. D'Agati VC, Marangoni BA. The Waterhouse-Friderichsen syndrome. N Engl J Med. 1945; *232*: 1–7.
175. Banks HS. Meningococcosis: a protean disease. Lancet 1948; *ii*: 637–40, 677–81.
176. Thomison JB, Shapiro JL. Adrenal lesions in acute meningococcemia. Arch Pathol 1957; *63*: 527–31.
177. Taylor FB, Chang A, Ruf W, Morrissey JH, Hinshaw L, Catlett R *et al.* Lethal *E coli* septic shock is prevented by blocking tissue factor with monoclonal antibody. Circ Shock 1991; *33*: 127–34.
178. Visser HKA. The adrenal cortex in childhood; pathological aspects. Arch Dis Child 1966; *41*: 113–36.
179. Migeon CJ, Kenny FM, Hung W, Voorhess ML, Lawrence B, Richards C. Study of adrenal function in children with meningitis. Pediatr 1967; *40*: 163–83.
180. Zachmann M, Fanconi A, Prader A. Plasma corticol in children with fulminating meningococcal infection. Helv Paediatr Acta 1974; *29*: 245–50.
181. Bosworth DC. Reversible adrenocortical insufficiency in fulminant meningococcemia. Arch Intern Med 1979; *139*: 823–4.
182. Enriquez G, Lucaya J, Dominguez P, Aso C. Sonographic diagnosis of adrenal hemorrhage in patients with fulminant meningococcal septicemia. Acta Paediatr Scand 1990; *79*: 1255–8.
183. Sarnaik AP, Sanfilippo DJ, Slovis TL. Ultrasound diagnosis of adrenal hemorrhage in meningococcemia. Pediatr Radiol. 1988; *18*: 427–8.

184. Netter A, Debré R. *La méningite cérébro-spinale*. Paris: Masson et Cie, 1911; 102–3.
185. McLean S, Caffey J. Endemic purpuric meningococcus bacteremia in early life. Am J Dis Child 1931; 42: 1053–74.
186. Margaretten W, McAdams AJ. An appraisal of fulminant meningococcemia with reference to the Shwartzman phenomenon. Am J Med 1958; 25: 868–76.
187. Toews WH, Bass JW. Skin manifestations of meningococcal infection. Am J Dis Child 1974; 127: 173–6.
188. Dahle JS. Pathogenesis of hemorrhagic skin lesions in meningococcal disease. NIPH Annal 1983; 6: 49–53.
189. Evans RW, Glick B, Kimball F, Lobell. M. Fatal intravascular consumption coagulopathy in meningococcal sepsis. Am J Med 1969; 46: 910–18.
190. Winkelstein A, Songster CL, Caras TS, Berman HH, West WL. Fulminant meningococcemia and disseminated intravascular coagulation. Arch Intern Med 1969; 124: 55–9.
191. Blum D, Fondu P, Denolin-Reubens , Dubois J. Early heparin therapy in 60 children with acute meningococcemia. Acta Chir Belg 1973: 72: 288–97.
192. Vik-Mo H, Lote K, Nordoy A. Disseminated intravascular coagulation in patients with meningococcal infection: laboratory diagnosis and prognostic factors. Scand J Infect Dis 1978; 10: 187–91.
193. Netter A, Salanier M. Présence des meningocoques dans les éléments purpuriques de l'infection méninogococcique. Compt Rend Soc Biol 1916; 79: 670.
194. Pick L. Histologische und histologisch-bacteriologische Befunde beim petechialen Exanthem der epidemischen Genickstarre. Deutsch Med Wschr 1916; 42: 994–8.
195. Schaad UB. Arthritis in disease due to *Neisseria meningitidis*. Rev Infect Dis 1980; 2: 880–8.
196. Schenfeld L, Gray RG, Poppo MJ, Gaylis NB, Gottlieb NL. Bacterial monoarthritis due to *Neisseria meningitidis* in systemic lupus erythematosus. J Rheumatol 1981; 8: 145–8.
197. Harcup C, Wing E, Schneider S, Pipher A. Primary meningococcal arthritis and pseudogout in an elderly woman. Arthritis Rheum 1983; 26: 1409–11.
198. Andersson S, Krook A. Primary meningococcal arthritis. Scand J Infect Dis 1987; 19: 51–4.
199. Greenwood BM, Onyewotu II, Whittle HC. Complement and meningococcal infection. Br Med J 1976; i: 797–9.
200. Penny JL, Grace WJ, Kennedy RJ. Meningococcic pericarditis: a case report and review of the literature. Am J Cardiol 1966; 18: 281–5.
201. Morse JR, Oretsky MJ, Hudson JA. Pericarditis as a complication of meningococcal meningitis. Ann Intern Med 1971; 74: 212–17.
202. Beal R, Ustach TJ, Ferker AD. Meningococcemia without meningitis presenting as cardiac tamponade. Am J Med 1971; 51: 659–62.
203. Jones C. Pericarditis complicating a case of meningococcal meningitis. Br Heart J 1977; 39: 107–9.
204. Blaser MJ, Reingold AL, Alsever RN, Hightower A. Primary meningococcal pericarditis; a disease of adults associated with serogroup C *Neisseria meningitidis*. Rev Infect Dis 1984; 6: 625–32.
205. van Dorp WT, van Rees C, van der Meer JWM, Thompson J. Meningococcal pericarditis in the absence of meningitis. Infection 1987; 15: 109–10.
206. Ødegaard A. Unusual manifestations of meningococcal infection: a review. NIPH Ann 1983; 6: 59–63.
207. Smith AL, Daum RS, Scheifele D, Syriopolou V, Averill DR, Roberts MC *et al.* Pathogenesis of *Haemophilus influenzae* meningitis. In: Sell SH, Wright PF, eds.

Haemophilus influenzae: Epidemiology, Immunology, and Prevention of Disease. New York: Elsevier Science Publishers, 1982; 89–109.

208. Tunkel AR, Scheld WM. Pathogenesis and pathophysiology of bacterial meningitis. Clin Microbiol Rev 1993; 6: 118–36.

209. Quagliarello VJ, Ma A, Stukenbrok H, Palade GE. Ultrastructural localization of albumin transport across the cerebral microvasculature during experimental meningitis in rats. J Exp Med 1991; 174: 657–72.

210. Feldman WE. Relation of concentration of bacteria and bacterial antigen in cerebrospinal fluid to prognosis in patients with bacterial meningitis. N Engl J Med 1977; 296: 433–5.

211. Dwelle TL, Dunkle LM, Blair L. Correlation of cerebrospinal fluid endotoxinlike activity with clinical and laboratory variables in gram-negative bacterial meningitis in children. J Clin Microbiol 1987; 25: 856–8.

212. Arditi M, Ables L, Yogev R. Cerebrospinal fluid endotoxin levels in children with *H. influenzae* meningitis before and after administration of intravenous ceftriaxone. J Infect Dis 1989; 160: 1005–11.

213. Mertsola J, Kennedy WA, Waagner D, Sáez-Llorens X, Olsen K, Hansen EJ et al. Endotoxin concentrations in cerebrospinal fluid correlate with clinical severity and neurological outcome of *Haemophilus influenzae* type b meningitis. Am J Dis Child 1991; 145: 1099–1103.

214. Scheifele DW, Daun R, Syriopoulou V, Smith AL. CSF endotoxin in primates with *Hemophilus influenzae* b meningitis. Clin Res 1978; 26: 188A.

215. Syrogiannopoulos GA, Hansen EJ, Erwin AL, Munford RS, Rutledge J, Reisch JS et al. *Haemophilus influenzae* b lipooligosaccharide induces meningeal inflammation. J Infect Dis 1988; 157: 237–44.

216. Wispelwey B, Hansen EJ, Scheld WM. *Haemophilus influenzae* outer membrane vesicle-induced blood–brain barrier permeability during experimental meningitis. Infect Immun 1989; 57: 2559–62.

217. Waage A, Halstensen A, Shalaby R, Brandtzaeg P, Kierulf P, Espevik T. Local production of tumor necrosis factor α, interleukin 1, and interleukin 6 in meningococcal meningitis. J Exp Med 1989; 170: 1859–67.

218. Whittle HC, Greenwood BM. Cerebrospinal fluid immunoglobulins and complement in meningococcal meningitis. J Clin Pathol 1977; 30: 720–2.

219. Greenwood BM. Chemotactic activity of cerebrospinal fluid in pyogenic meningitis. J Clin Pathol 1978; 31: 213–16.

220. Tuomanen EI. Saukkonen K, Sande S, Cioffe C, Wright SD. Reduction of inflammation, tissue damage, and mortality in bacterial meningitis in rabbits treated with monoclonal antibodies against adhesion-promoting receptors of leukocytes. J Exp Med 1989; 170: 959–69.

221. Griffiss J McL, Yamasaki R, Estabrook M, Kim JJ. Meningococcal molecular mimicry and the search for an ideal vaccine. Trans Roy Soc Trop Med Hyg 1991; 85: S32–6.

5
Meningococcal Carriage and Disease

KEITH CARTWRIGHT
Public Health Laboratory, Gloucester, UK

INTRODUCTION

The process of development of meningococcal disease can be broken down into a sequence of three events—exposure, followed in some cases by acquisition, followed occasionally by the development of invasive disease[1]. The process is the same whether the invasive disease manifests itself as meningitis, septicaemia, a combination of the two, or as some milder illness. Despite the recognition of these three stages over a period of almost a hundred years, and despite considerable research during this time, we still understand only incompletely the process of acquisition and the ensuing factors which lead in a few cases to the development of invasive disease. There is no clear-cut relationship between meningococcal carriage rates and disease rates. The peak age-specific incidence of meningococcal disease in the USA and Europe is in children aged under one year, whereas carriage rates are at their highest in teenagers and young adults.

MENINGOCOCCAL CARRIAGE
Site of carriage

The human nasopharynx is the natural habitat of the meningococcus. The organisms demonstrate sophisticated structural and functional adaptations to this environment (see Chapter 2), including the production of pili to

Meningococcal Disease. Edited by Keith Cartwright © 1995 John Wiley & Sons Ltd

facilitate adherence to epithelial cell surfaces[2,3]. Recently, meningococcal pili, like their gonococcal equivalents, have been shown to be capable of antigenic variation, such variation markedly affecting adhesiveness and probably providing a means by which the bacteria can evade the host immune system[4]. In common with many other pathogenic oropharyngeal bacteria, meningococci produce an extracellular IgA_1 protease capable of cleaving human secretory IgA_1[5], a major immunoglobulin constituent in bodily secretions[6].

The human nasopharynx is a highly iron-depleted environment. Meningococci, which require iron for growth, have evolved receptors capable of binding human transferrin and lactoferrin. The inability of meningococci to colonise any host other than man may be related to the specificity of these receptors, which will bind only to their respective human substrates[7-9].

Meningococci are usually carried in the nasopharynx; in laboratory studies they show a preference for attachment to epithelial cells from the nasopharynx over epithelium from other sites[2,10]. They are also occasionally isolated from the urethra, but even in sexually active populations urethral carriage appears to be very uncommon and is usually detected in association with evidence of active infection[11,12,13].

Claire Broome's excellent and comprehensive review of the meningococcal carrier state documents the very considerable contributions made by early workers in the field and provides a clear guide to the intricacies of the relationship between meningococcal carriage and disease[14].

Acquisition

The numbers of individuals within a population carrying meningococci at any particular time are determined both by the rate of acquisition and by the duration of carriage. Transmission from person to person takes place during prolonged close contact, probably mediated relatively efficiently by mouth kissing or, less efficiently, by airborne spread and other, less intimate contact. In most settings, acquisition is slow.

In Belgian school children studied after an outbreak, acquisition rates were unaffected by season[15]. In Greenfield's study of 'normal' families, a high carriage rate in adult males was entirely accounted for by this group acquiring meningococci at a rate ten times higher than adult females and twenty times higher than children. However, within family groups meningococci passed from person to person only with some reluctance[16].

There are probably true differences in the transmissibility of meningococci according to their serogroup. For example, the low carriage rate of serogroup B (ET-5) strains in families[17], schools and communities[18], and the protracted nature of outbreaks of disease caused by this organism in

Norway[19] and elsewhere[20] are both consistent with the hypothesis that this clone is of low transmissibility but high virulence. This contrasts with the sometimes conflagrational nature of meningococcal disease associated with clones of serogroup A or serogroup C in open communities in Africa[21] and elsewhere, and in closed or semi-closed communities such as schools and military recruit training establishments in Europe and the USA. High acquisition rates, as observed in this setting[22], are probably more important determinants of disease risk than any particular level of meningococcal carriage[23,24].

Methodological differences in carriage studies

Despite many studies of meningococcal carriage carried out over the last hundred years, it is still difficult to make accurate estimates of the incidence or duration of meningococcal nasopharyngeal carriage. Early studies using non-selective media must have underestimated carriage rates substantially; strain characterisation methods and strain definitions have also changed over the years—the non-pathogenic *Neisseria lactamica* has only been recognised as a separate species since 1969[25]; it would have been classed as a meningococcus until then. Meningococcal classification systems have undergone even greater evolution. The serogrouping classification in current use was formalised as recently as 1950[26] and has been extended on more than one occasion since; serotyping, serosubtyping, and lipo-polysaccharide immunotyping (see Chapter 2) are all more recent developments.

Closed or semi-closed communities such as military recruit camps, boarding schools and prisons behave quite differently from civilian communities with regard to the circulation of meningococci; likewise, the findings of studies in African populations are probably not comparable with those carried out in European or North American communities. The majority of carriage studies have been undertaken in response to an outbreak of disease and comparisons with carriage rates in 'normal' communities may therefore not be valid. During a period of hyperendemic meningococcal disease due to a serogroup B serotype 15 strain in the Faroe Islands, carriage rates of both the outbreak strain and of all meningococci were higher in households with young children in areas of high disease incidence than in similar households in areas with a low disease incidence[27].

Olcén *et al.* showed a higher isolation rate from throat swabs than from pernasal swabs[28], though the former are technically difficult if not impossible to obtain in infants and in many patients with acute meningococcal disease. Swabbing on a single occasion has been shown repeatedly to underestimate the prevalence of carriage by a substantial amount[29–32]. This insensitivity may be due more to variations in the swabbing procedure than to major fluctuations in the numbers of meningococci in the nasopharynx. If there are such major fluctuations in the numbers of nasopharyngeal meningococci, the reasons are not known. The fact that only a proportion of carriers will be identified by a single swab underlines the importance of using epidemiological and not bacteriological criteria to define close contact groups requiring chemoprophylaxis following cases of meningococcal disease. The accuracy of a single negative throat swab in defining freedom from nasopharyngeal meningococcal colonisation is too poor to be relied upon.

The use of selective liquid enrichment culture slightly increases the meningococcal isolation rate from the nasophraynx[32]. Simultaneous carriage of more than one meningococcal strain has been demonstrated occasionally[30,33,34]. Such studies are laborious, requiring the serogrouping and serotyping of multiple 'picks' from each positive culture plate. In each of the above studies the proportion of carriers harbouring more than one strain of meningococcus was less than 5%. Current studies comparing results of conventional bacterial culture of throat swabs with a meningococcus-specific polymerase chain reaction (PCR) may shed more light on the sensitivity of conventional culture techniques and may explain at least some cases of apparently intermittent carriage.

FACTORS AFFECTING CARRIAGE RATES

Organism-related factors

Most meningococci isolated during community-wide surveys of carriage are probably harmless commensals[35]. Even when surveys are carried out in response to outbreaks or clusters of cases of disease, carriage rates of the pathogenic strain may be low[18]. Many strains isolated from the nasopharynx of healthy carriers express little or no capsular polysaccharide and consequently cannot be assigned to a specific serogroup. Encapsulation probably reduces adherence to oropharyngeal epithelial cells[2] and loss of expression of capsular polysaccharide may be an adaptation to long-term pharyngeal carriage[36].

As the invasion of an immunocompetent host is dependent on the expression by the meningococcus of capsular polysaccharide (particularly of serogroups A, B or C), strains which express no capsular polysaccharide (or polysaccharide of serogroups other than A, B or C) have very limited pathogenic potential. They are probably beneficial[37], providing a boost to immunity through expression of other immunogenic surface structures such as class 1 outer membrane proteins, iron-dependent proteins, and lipo-oligosaccharides.

Age and sex

Large prevalence studies in open Western communities show that nasopharyngeal carriage of meningococci is unusual in infancy and early childhood, rises progressively through the first two decades to peak at about 20–25% in late teenage and early adult life and then slowly declines (Figure 5.1)[18,35,38–40]. In Europe, the overall carriage rate is about 10%[18,35]. Some studies have shown no sex difference in carriage rates[16,39,41,42] while others have found males more frequently colonised than females[18,27,35]. The conflicting results might be explained, at least in part, by sex differences in the prevalence of smoking and exposure to smokers in the different study populations (see below).

Season

In view of the marked seasonal variation in meningococcal disease rates in Europe, the Americas and in Africa it is perhaps surprising that a seasonal variation in carriage in civilian communities has not been observed in Nigeria[41,43], India[44], or Belgium[15], or in military recruits in the USA[34].' The

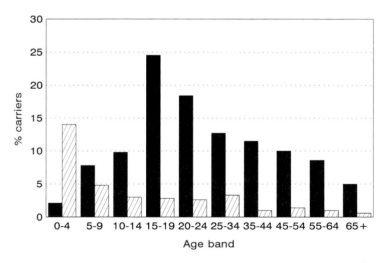

Figure 5.1 *Age specific carriage of* N. meningitidis *and* N. lactamica: *Stonehouse, Gloucestershire, UK (total; subjects: 5,006). Solid columns,* N. meningitidis; *hatched columns,* N. lactamica. *Though most meningococcal disease occurs in children aged 0–4, meningococcal carriage is rare in this age group. The high prevalence of carriage of* N. lactamica *in infants and young children is an important factor in the development of antimeningococcal bactericidal antibodies*

higher incidence of viral respiratory infections in winter months in the northern hemisphere[45] might be expected to increase transmission of meningococci by enhanced dissemination through coughing, but there is no evidence as yet that it does so.

Smoking

A strong, dose-related effect of smoking on risk of meningococcal carriage was first demonstrated in a case–control study in 1989. In carriers of serogoup B (ET-5) strains and in carriers of other meningococci the risk of carriage increased progressively with the numbers of cigarettes smoked each day. Smokers of 20 or more cigarettes per day had an odds ratio for meningococcal carriage of 5.3 relative to non-smokers[46]. Exposure to passive smoking in the home was also independently associated with an increased risk of meningococcal carriage. These associations have been confirmed subsequently by other groups[35,47–49]; smoking appears to predispose to meningococcal carriage regardless of whether healthy populations are studied or communities in which cases of disease have occurred.

Smoking has marked effects on cell-mediated and humoral immunity[50]. It causes a fall in salivary IgA and a rise in IgM concentrations[51]. It also affects the composition of the oral flora[52]. The association between smoking and meningococcal carriage may explain why the adult male subjects in Greenfield's family study had very high carriage and acquisition rates when compared with all other groups in the study[16], and may also explain in part some of the variations in carriage rates observed in other studies. Data on smoking habits has not been recorded in past carriage studies.

Occupation

In a recent Norwegian study of carriage in a randomly sampled population, working outside the home and having an occupation in transportation or industry conferred a modestly increased risk of meningococcal carriage, when corrections for age, gender and smoking were made in a logistic regression analysis[35].

Inhibitory flora

In a study of meningococcal carriers amongst military recruits during World War I, Colebrook noted that when meningococcal numbers fell they were often replaced by abundant pneumococci or streptococci[53]. He went on to confirm that both live pneumococci and bacteria-free filtrates of pneumococcal culture fluids can inhibit meningococcal growth *in vitro*. An alarming attempt to influence the meningococcal carrier state by inoculation of live pneumococcal cultures into the oropharynx was unsuccessful, though at least the subjects were not reported as being any the worse for the experience! Gordon extended these observations, showing that raw saliva is inhibitory to meningococci whereas nasal mucus from normal persons is not[54]. The inhibitory property of saliva was due to its content of live bacteria, mixed salivary streptococci being principally responsible. The lack of inhibition of meningococci by nasal mucus may in part explain why meningococci inhabit the posterior pharyngeal wall, whereas they are not easily isolated from saliva.

The oral and nasopharyngeal flora, both aerobic and anaerobic, are extremely complex. This, in conjunction with the lack of any reproducible and standardised method of quantitation, makes it extremely difficult to measure in anything other than the crudest manner the interactions between meningococci and other components of the nasopharyngeal flora. Colebrook's and Gordon's experiments were carried out with aerobic bacteria only. The inhibitory properties (if any) of the anaerobic oropharyngeal flora have not been investigated.

Some characteristics of aerobic nasopharyngeal bacteria capable of interfering with meningococcal growth were investigated during an outbreak of serogroup A meningococcal disease in 'skid row' populations (mainly homeless adult males) in the western USA[55]. Inhibitory strains amongst the nasopharyngeal flora were found in 45% of control subjects, but were less common (32%) in residents of skid row areas, where cases of disease had occurred, though the numbers of subjects studied were small. Nine different species of nasopharyngeal bacteria capable of inhibiting meningococci were identified; all were gram-positive, and most were commensal streptococci. Inhibitory nasopharyngeal bacteria were isolated from only 1/9 patients with serogroup A meningococcal disease. These interesting findings have not been extended, but the observation that smoking augments the gram-negative oropharyngeal flora at the expense of the gram-positive flora[52] provides one of a number of possible mechanisms by which smoking could increase carriage of meningococci.

Blood group and secretor status

Secretor status is a measure of the genetically determined ability to secrete soluble blood group substances into saliva and other body fluids. Non-secretors were found significantly more frequently than expected in Scottish and Icelandic patients with meningococcal disease[56]. Two subsequent studies carried out by Blackwell and her colleagues showed no association between blood group and meningococcal carriage but gave conflicting results on the influence of secretor status on meningococcal carriage rates. In the first, much larger study there was no difference between the proportion of meningococcal carriers who were non-secretors of blood group antigens and the proportion of non-secretors in the total population studied[57]. In the second there was a slightly higher proportion of non-secretors amongst meningococcal carriers than amongst non-carriers[47].

Tonsillectomy

Kristiansen found 15/62 patients undergoing tonsillectomy acquired nasopharyngeal meningococci in the 3 months after the operation, compared with 0/62 controls[58]. Salivary IgA is transiently reduced after tonsillectomy[59]. However, a history of tonsillectomy was not a risk factor for meningococcal disease in a recent case–control study[60] (though this does not contradict the Norwegian findings).

Virus infection

Viral infections can influence nasopharyngeal carriage of a variety of different bacteria[61,62]. Virus infections either in the community or in the individual might therefore affect meningococcal carriage rates. As meningococci are presumed to pass from individual to individual by prolonged close contact, especially by mouth kissing, meningococcal nasopharyngeal carriers subsequently acquiring viral upper respiratory infections might disseminate meningococci more easily through increased coughing and sneezing. There is evidence to suggest that pneumococcal carriers with 'colds' disseminate pneumococci more effectively than those without colds[63]. Susceptibility to colonisation amongst contacts of meningococcal carriers might also be increased if the contacts were suffering from viral upper respiratory infection with sore throat and coryza. Infection with influenza virus increases adhesion of meningococci to Hep-2 cells[64]. However, the evidence that viruses have any substantial effect on either meningococcal acquisition or carriage is conflicting.

During a simultaneous outbreak of both influenza A infection and meningococcal disease amongst residents of a long-stay residential mental health institution 17% of those with serological evidence of influenza A infection were carriers of the outbreak strain meningococcus compared with none of those lacking influenza A antibodies[65]. Olcén showed a significantly higher meningococcal carriage rate in household contacts of cases who gave a history of recent upper respiratory symptoms than in contacts not giving such a history[66], but it was not clear whether the respiratory symptoms were caused by recent viral infection or whether they might have been provoked by the meningococci themselves.

In US military recruits at Fort Dix, antecedent viral respiratory disease did not influence the rate of meningococcal acquisition[67], and Thomas et al. did not find increased meningococcal carriage rates in new jail bookings who gave a history of colds or flu-like symptoms in the preceding 30 days[48]. These data, and the failure of meningococcal carriage rates to rise in the winter months[15,34] when viral respiratory infections are most prevalent, and the lack of significant seasonal variation in carriage rates in longitudinal African[41] and Indian studies[44] argue, somewhat surprisingly, against any important effect of respiratory virus infection on the rate of meningococcal acquisition or carriage.

Meningococcal vaccination

Vaccination with serogroup C[68] or serogroup A + C[69] polysaccharide reduced carriage rates of serogroup C meningococci in military recruits, but in Africa, serogroup A polysaccharide vaccine appeared to have no effect on carriage of strains of the homologous serogroup[14,70,71].

Closed and semi-closed communities

Carriage rates of outbreak strains and of all meningococci, may be much higher in military recruit training establishments, schools, prisons and other closed or partially-closed communities. Carriage rates of 50% or more, with or without accompanying meningococcal disease, have been recognised for many years in military recruit training camps[34,38,72]. This is probably because of the continuing influx of individuals susceptible to colonisation into an environment where acquisition is facilitated by shared living and sleeping accommodation, high rates of smoking and possibly by high levels of physical stress. As might be expected, carriage rates often, thought not always[73], rise rapidly in the period immediately after recruits enter a training camp; if cases of disease are going to occur they usually do so in the first few weeks of training[74]. However, circulation of meningococcal strains is probably increased indiscriminately, and only a small proportion of strains will have any pathogenic potential. Glover thought that overcrowded sleeping accommodation was an important factor in raising carriage rates[75] but this has been questioned[34]. It seems that overcrowding has to be severe before spread of meningococci is facilitated[76], though in a study carried out in a Los Angeles men's jail, new bookings were significantly more likely to carry serogroup C meningococci if they came from a dwelling with more than two people per home bedroom (odds ratio 8.2, 95% CI 1.5–45.3)[48].

Carriage and transmission within families

High rates of carriage are also observed in family and other close contacts of cases of meningococcal disease[40,66,70,76–79]. In this situation, most isolates from contacts are indistinguishable from the index case strain[66,80,81]. This fact can be exploited to establish the probable identity of the causative strain in cases of meningococcal disease where an isolate from the index case is not available for serogrouping and serotyping[17].

The study of Munford and his coworkers, carried out during an outbreak of serogroup C disease in São Paulo, Brazil, produced a number of interesting and useful results[78]. Carriage rates were higher in contacts sleeping within the house than in other household contacts, although those sleeping in the same room as the index case were no more likely to be carriers than those sleeping elsewhere within the house (in contrast to the finding of Blakebrough and Gilles[79]). Contact carriage rates were highest in households where the index case was an infant, intermediate in households with an index case aged 1–14 years, and lowest in households with an adult case.

This pattern was also observed in an English investigation, mainly of serogroup B disease[17]. It suggests that infants, and to a lesser extent young children, acquire their invasive meningococcal strains from close family contacts, whereas teenage and adult cases more frequently acquire their invading strains from contacts outside the family group. If, after chemoprophylaxis of close contacts, pathogenic meningococci are reintroduced into the family group from unidentified and untreated carriers outside the family, this would explain some failures of chemoprophylaxis.

In most of the family studies cited, parents were the most likely family members to be carriers. Munford concluded that pathogenic meningococci are most frequently introduced into the family unit by a parent, although this pattern of spread did not accord with data in a Swedish study[66], and it may not be the case in Africa[42]. In the Faroe Islands study children aged 0–14 years living in households without cases of meningococcal disease were at significantly higher risk of being outbreak strain carriers if their mothers were colonised with the outbreak serogroup B (ET-5) strain[27].

Perhaps surprisingly, a consistent finding in studies of contacts is that isolation of meningococci from groups of household contacts is the exception rather than the rule; in the majority of cases, regardless of the age of the index case, no carriers are identified amongst the household contact group. This probably reflects the marked insensitivity of conventional culture as a means of detecting meningococcal carriage.

DURATION OF MENINGOCOCCAL CARRIAGE

Point prevalence studies ('snapshots') cannot provide data on duration of carriage. Repeated swabbing of the same individuals over many months provides some indication of the duration of meningococcal carriage, but such longitudinal studies are not without difficulties of design and interpretation.

In most such studies, known carriers have been followed up to establish the point at which the carrier state is terminated. However, it is not possible to make any estimate of the duration of carriage prior to the point at which the subject was enrolled. Defining freedom from carriage is just as difficult. One or more negative swabs may be followed by a positive swab yielding a meningococcus indistinguishable from that last isolated, the inference being that the subject has remained colonised throughout, and that the intervening negative swabs were false negatives[32,82]. In our hands three consecutive negative swabs were necessary to define freedom from carriage of serogroup B (ET-5) meningococci in an asymptomatic adult carrier population.

Several workers have suggested that there may be short-term and long-term carriers[16,32,39,82,83]. Rake's careful study of 24 office and laboratory workers over a 20 month period identified five constant, two intermittent and three transient carriers. One of the constant carriers was shown to be colonised with the same strain of meningococcus continuously for at least 26 months. As this subject was colonised both at the start and at the end of the study period the duration of carriage might have been even greater. No studies of systemic or mucosal immunity have yet been reported which might explain these differences in patterns of carriage, though the gradual but persistent decline in carriage after the third decade indicates that the nasopharynx becomes progressively less receptive to meningococci with the ageing process.

In American and European populations the median duration of carriage has been estimated at between 9 and 10 months[15,16]. Gold's estimate was lower at 4.1 months[39], similar to the duration of carriage observed in Nigeria[41]. The serogroup of the infecting strain appears to affect the duration of carriage; serogroup A strains were lost significantly more rapidly than non-serogroup A strains in the Nigerian study[41], and the behaviour of serogroup C strains in schools and military recruit camps is often more suggestive of a pattern of high acquisition and short duration of carriage.

ACQUISITION AND CARRIAGE OF *NEISSERIA LACTAMICA*

Perhaps surprisingly, meningococci themselves are probably not important in the initial development of protective antibodies. The meningococcal carriage rate is very low in young children at a time when the prevalence of bactericidal antibodies is rising steadily[39,84,85].

Neisseria lactamica is closely related to the meningococcus but is a non-pathogen. It is distinguished from the meningococcus not only by its ability to ferment lactose but also by its failure to produce an IgA protease[5], the latter characteristic perhaps contributing to its lack of pathogenicity[86].

Exposure to *N. lactamica* is probably of great importance in the development of immunity to meningococcal disease since children colonised with these organisms develop antibodies reactive with strains of meningococci of serogroups A, B and/or C[39]; the antibody induced is not directed against capsular polysaccharide, as *N. lactamica* does not appear to possess a capsule[85]. Common lipo-oligosaccharide epitopes shared by meningococci and *N. lactamica* may well be important[87].

Studies in the USA[39], England[18], the Faroes[27] and Nigeria[41] all show that *Neisseria lactamica* is carried predominantly by infants and young children, with up to 50% colonisation rates at any one time, thus substantially outnumbering meningococcal carriers in this population (Figure 5.1). Turnover of strains is rapid by comparison with meningococci, with relatively short duration of carriage (3–4 months or less) and a high acquisition rate, particularly in infants. Males outnumber female carriers in children under 14, but this ratio is reversed in older carriers, perhaps due to mothers acquiring strains from close contact with their young children.

RISK FACTORS FOR MENINGOCOCCAL DISEASE

Introduction

Invasive disease can be produced by a pathogenic organism, a susceptible host, by the influence of extrinsic environmental factors, or perhaps most frequently by a combination of all three. Although there can be sudden and large changes in rates of meningococcal acquisitions and carriage, there is in general very much less variation in rates of carriage than in rates of disease. Increased rates of acquisition probably account in part for the fact that the increased risk of meningococcal disease in the military is largely limited to the period immediately after enlistment[34,38].

The annual incidence of meningococcal disease throughout the world remains remarkably capricious[89]. In the 'meningitis belt' of sub-Saharan Africa outbreaks of disease occur at intervals of 5–10 years[90,91]. Elsewhere, sudden, brief but unpredictable upsurges of disease activity interspersed with long periods of quiescence have been a common pattern in many European and American countries. England, Germany and the USA all experienced severe outbreaks at or around the time of mobilisation in World War II. Recently, some countries such as Norway have experienced increased levels of disease activity over prolonged periods (more than 15 years)[19]. When the incidence of disease rises suddenly an upward shift in the age distribution of cases is often observed[92–94], consistent with the hypothesis that a cohort of individuals susceptible to a particular, perhaps new meningococcal strain, has accumulated within the population over a period of years.

Meningococcal serogroup, serotype and serosubtype

There are clear differences in the pathogenic potential of different meningococcal serogroups. Although 12 serogroups are recognised currently, most disease worldwide is caused by organisms of only three serogroups—A, B or C[89]. When meningococcal disease is caused by strains of other serogroups there is a strong possibility that the affected individual will be found to have increased immunological susceptibility such as a terminal complement component deficiency. Strains of serogroup Y appear to have a predilection for causing pneumonia and are the commonest serogroup to be isolated in this rarely diagnosed condition. Most large outbreaks between 1914 and 1945 are thought to have been caused by serogroup A organisms. Since then serogroup A disease has persisted in Africa whereas Europe and North America have increasingly experienced outbreaks and endemic disease due to strains of serogroups B and C. Though there have been introductions of virulent serogroup A strains into Europe from the Middle East[95] these have not given rise to outbreaks of serogroup A disease[1], suggesting that levels of immunity are sufficiently high in European (and American) populations to prevent spread of these strains. The reasons why serogroup A strains predominated, and why they were later supplanted by serogroup B and C strains in some countries during the last 30 years, remain obscure.

Meningococci can be isolated from the nasopharynx of about half of all cases of meningococcal disease. (As the nasopharynx is thought to be the portal of entry in most cases, the failure to isolate them in the remainder is perhaps surprising, and may reflect insensitivity of swabbing techniques.) When nasopharyngeal strains are compared with deep isolates, i.e. from blood or cerebrospinal fluid, the deep isolate is always well endowed with capsular polysaccharide, confirming the importance of a capsule as a virulence factor. Strains from the nasopharynx are more variably capsulated—some are well endowed whereas others have little or no capsular material. From mixed populations such as these, it would appear that only strains with abundant capsular polysaccharide are capable of invading.

Bactericidal antibodies are directed not only against capsular polysaccharide but also against a variety of surface-expressed antigens including outer membrane proteins. Strains of particular serotypes and serosubtypes may predominate for long periods of time, although variation in the genes controlling the class 2, class 3 and class 1 outer membrane proteins gives rise to a constant process of minor variation in the surface antigenicity of organisms which are otherwise genetically closely related (clones). This continuing antigenic evolution probably confers increased colonisation potential on meningococci.

Meningococcal lipo-oligosaccharide (LOS) immunotype

A number of variants of LOS have been described, giving rise to a typing system[96]. A recent discovery is that there appears to be an association between a particular LOS immunotype and invasive disease. In a study of 36 case and 76 carrier isolates, all of the ET-5 clone, 97% of case isolates expressed the L3,7,9 immunotype, whereas the LOS immunotypes of the carrier strains were much more heterogeneous; only 24% expressed the L3,7,9 immunotype alone[97]. The combination of capsule expression and LOS immunotype appears to be related to virulence. Investigation of four family clusters of ET-5 strains suggested that the L3,7,9 immunotype might be 'switched on' during the colonisation of a new host, or during the process of invasion itself.

Age and sex

In northern Europe and in the USA the age and sex distribution of cases tends to be remarkably similar[93,98,99]. There is usually a modest excess of male cases which may be explained by the higher meningococcal acquisition rate in males; age-specific incidence peaks in the first year of life at about six months, declining subsequently. This pattern is related to immunological susceptibility (see below). A smaller secondary peak of disease in teenagers and young adults is sometimes observed, particularly in association with periods of high disease incidence. The reasons for teenagers and adults developing meningococcal disease are almost certainly more complex; they are discussed later.

Season

In the African meningitis belt outbreaks of disease start during the dry season (the 'harmattan') and come to an end with the arrival of the rains. Humidity, rainfall, wind and airborne dust all undergo marked changes at the time of this climatic transition, as do social behaviour patterns, making it very difficult to identify which, if any of these environmental factors might be important in precipitating disease and bringing outbreaks to an end. For example during the harmattan, individuals in rural communities spend more time inside their huts (Robinson P, personal communication) in order to avoid the dusty winds; in their huts they are exposed to smoke from cooking fires, which may increase the chances of meningococcal acquisition.

In temperate climates, season has a strong influence on the rate of meningococcal disease, in contrast to its lack of effect on carriage rates. In northern Europe and the North American continent meningococcal disease peaks in the first quarter of the year, declining to low levels by late summer[98,100]. A winter peak followed by a summer decline was also observed in relation to invasive haemophilus disease in England and Wales prior to the introduction of conjugated Hib vaccines[101]. Attempts to associate particular weather patterns and humidity levels with localised outbreaks of meningococcal disease in England have given inconclusive results[102].

Exposure to smoking and smokers

Case—control studies in Norway and England have shown that exposure to passive smoking is an important risk factor for meningococcal disease[60,103,104]. In the Norwegian study exposure to passive smoking was analysed in children under 12 years; in the first English study an increased risk was found for all age groups except teenagers. Active smoking was not found to be a risk factor in any of the studies, although numbers of adult cases in each study were relatively small. The observation that smokers are more likely to be meningococcal carriers[46] provides a plausible explanation for the increased risk. Those exposed to passive smoking also experience greater exposure to meningococcal carriers.

However, other factors may also be operating. It also seems likely that smokers may disseminate oropharyngeal bacteria, including meningococci, more efficiently through increased coughing. Smokers are more likely to associate socially with other smokers. Exposure to smoke causes direct damage to the nasopharyngeal mucosa; passive smoking is associated with an increased risk of respiratory disease in young children[105,106], and children in particular, with more delicate mucous membranes, may be more liable to acquire meningococci if living in a smoky atmosphere.

In the later English case—control study[60] it was hypothesised that children brought up in smoking families might be less susceptible to meningococcal disease in later life as a consequence of greater exposure to meningococci in their early years. The data supported this hypothesis; cases of meningococcal disease aged over 5 when they developed their illness were less likely than controls to have been brought up in households with smokers.

Socio-economic factors

Low socio-economic status did not increase susceptibility to meningococcal disease in The Gambia[107] but meningococcal disease cases were more likely than controls to come from lower-income households in an English study[104] and outbreaks have been described in homeless men in the USA[108]. Low socio-economic status could increase risk through a number of different mechanisms. High rates of smoking and respiratory infections, poor diet, damp, poor quality housing and overcrowding at home and at school could all contribute to increased risk.

Glover thought overcrowded sleeping accommodation contributed to the risk of meningococcal disease in the military outbreaks of 1916–17[72] and this association has also been found in civilian populations[60], though not consistently[109]. Overcrowding probably has to be severe before it affects the rate of disease[76]. There was no association between overcrowding and meningococcal disease in a Gambian study[107].

Contact with a case

Close contacts of cases run a substantially increased risk of disease. De Wals found a relative risk of 1245 amongst household contacts of cases when compared with the same age groups in the community[110], while Cooke found a relative risk of 144[111], though some secondary cases may have been missed in this study. High attack rates amongst close contacts of cases have also been recorded by other groups[78,112].

When chemoprophylaxis is not used, the interval between primary and secondary cases is short—usually no more than 2 weeks. However, when chemoprophylaxis is given the mean interval between primary and secondary cases extends to several months[113]. Chemoprophylaxis is highly effective in eradicating nasopharyngeal meningococcal carriage and may also abort some co-primary infections; subsequent recolonisation of contacts from the wider community (with its attendant risk of disease) is difficult or impossible to prevent, but because meningococci are not highly transmissible such recolonisation occurs only slowly. Recolonisation may explain some apparent failures of chemoprophylaxis. Chemoprophylaxis is more likely to be successful when it can be used in conjunction with vaccination, i.e. for contacts of cases infected with serogroup A or C meningococci. There is some doubt as to whether it has any effect on reducing the rate of secondary disease when the causative organism is of serogroup B[113].

It is unusual to be able to demonstrate any clear-cut evidence of immune deficiency even in families where more than one case of disease has occurred and it is normally suggested that secondary cases within families occur because of the presence of a known pathogenic meningococcus. An alternative explanation is that more subtle immune defects are present which cannot be detected by the more routine tests of immunological competence. The numerous reports of failure of chemoprophylaxis to prevent secondary cases are consistent with this hypothesis as is the occurrence of families in which cases of meningococcal disease occur over periods of years without any obvious evidence of immune deficiency.

De Wals noted an increased risk of disease amongst school contacts of cases, though the risk was lower than for household contacts (relative risks of

76 and 23 respectively for day-care nursery contacts and for contacts at pre-primary school)[110], and outbreaks in schools are well documented[47,114–116]. A few investigators have not found any evidence of increased risk among school contacts of cases[117,118], though whether these negative findings are broadly applicable has been questioned[119]. When school outbreaks occur, serogroup C meningococci appear to have a greater capacity to spread rapidly than most strains of serogroup B, which are more likely to cause smouldering endemic disease with cases occurring over many months[120], (Cartwright K, unpublished observations). Whether transmission of meningococci is occurring in the classroom or within the wider community is extremely difficult to determine[42]. The failure to isolate meningococci from the household contacts of the majority of cases of meningococcal disease is persuasive evidence that at least a proportion of these cases are acquiring their infecting strains from settings outside the immediate family.

Host immunity

Bactericidal antibody protects against meningococcal disease; conversely, lack of bactericidal antibody is associated with an increased risk of disease[84]. Infants are protected from meningococcal disease for the first few months of life by passively transferred maternal antibodies and by an extremely low meningococcal acquisition rate. As maternal antibody is lost, susceptibility rises, peaking at about 6 months, then falling progressively as bactericidal antibodies are acquired through exposure to *Neisseria lactamica*, non-pathogenic meningococci and other bacteria expressing surface antigens in common with meningococci[85].

Complement

The roles of complement and complement deficiency in meningococcal infection have been comprehensively reviewed recently[121]. The complement system plays a critical role in the host's defences against invasive meningococcal disease. Complement can be activated via the classical pathway by antigen–antibody complexes, or via the alternative pathway by bacteria which express one of a number of repeating chemical structures such as lipo-oligosaccharides or teichoic acid on their surfaces. Activated complement brings about bacterial cell death by opsonisation and lysis[122].

Immunity to meningococcal disease is associated with the presence of complement-fixing bactericidal antibodies. Serogroup A meningococci can activate complement by either the classical or alternative pathways, whereas meningococci of serogroup B, whose capsular polysaccharide is heavily sialylated, only activate the cascade via the classical pathway[123]. Occasional individuals who experience multiple attacks of meningococcal disease have a high prevalence of complement component deficiency[124], usually a terminal component (C7–C9), i.e. part of the membrane attack complex. Terminal complement component deficiencies are rare, with a population prevalence of about 0.03%, but approximately 50% of affected individuals will experience an attack of meningococcal disease during their lifetime. The risk of meningococcal disease is close to 10 000 fold higher than in immunocompetent individuals. Interestingly, meningococcal disease is the commonest serious bacterial infection in complement deficiency states.

There are a number of unusual characteristics of meningococcal disease in complement-deficient individuals which are worth exploring briefly. Firstly, meningococcal disease in complement-deficient individuals tends to occur in late teenage or early adulthood rather than in early childhood. This suggests that additional factors come into play after the first decade of life to further increase susceptibility to infection. Secondly, although these individuals run a considerably greater risk of meningococcal disease, the course of the infection is usually milder, and mortality is lower[125]. Since meningococcal endotoxin acts as a potent activator of complement *in vivo*[126] the milder illness may be due to a reduction in the release of endotoxin from invading organisms as a consequence of the host's inability to kill the bacteria by formation of membrane attack complexes[127]. Thirdly, relapses are up to ten times commoner, suggesting that complement plays an important role in promoting efficient intracellular killing of meningococci. Fourthly, meningococcal disease in complement-deficient individuals is more likely to be due to unusual serogroups[125,128].

Properdin

Properdin, a protein whose gene is located on the X chromosome, up-regulates the alternative complement pathway by stabilising C3 and C5 convertases[129]. Individuals with properdin deficiency have an intact classical pathway but impaired alternative pathway activation. Such functional deficiency may be partial or complete. More than half of the affected individuals will experience meningococcal disease, usually at a later age than the average. Meningococcal disease in properdin deficiency is frequently fulminant, with a case fatality rate approaching 75%[130]. Vaccination of properdin-deficient individuals is likely to abolish the risk of meningococcal disease caused by serogroups represented in the vaccine, as IgG complement-fixing antibodies are generated, enabling activation of complement (and thus bacterial killing) via the classical pathway.

Immune deficiency

Patients with gross defects of immune function such as those receiving chemotherapy for leukaemia or lymphoma do not appear to run significantly increased risks of meningococcal disease. Many such patients may possess some prior immunity to meningococcal infection. However, meningococcal infection occurs more frequently than would be expected in postsplenectomy patients[131,132], and vaccination has been recommended for this group[131,133], although the additional risk of meningococcal disease is much lower than that of pneumococcal infection[134].

The possibility of an increased risk of meningococcal disease in patients infected with HIV has caused considerable concern because of the high rates of both diseases in sub-Saharan Africa, but the evidence to date suggests that there is no association between the two[135,136]. Heavy alcohol consumption, a potent suppressor of T and B cell function[137], was associated with an increased risk of meningococcal disease in skid row communities in the western USA during an outbreak in 1975[108]. Stress appears to influence the risk of many infectious diseases, sometimes increasing, and sometimes reducing it[138]. Such effects may be mediated by changes in catecholamine levels or by a variety of immunosuppressive mechanisms. Though 'stress' is difficult to measure accurately, Haneberg and his colleagues found significantly reduced case fatality rates in patients who had been exposed to stressful events prior to developing meningococcal disease[103]. Stanwell-Smith found no association between overall stress levels and subsequent risk of meningococcal disease, but particular life events including changes in residence, marital arguments and recent legal disputes were associated with an increased risk of disease[60].

Subversion of pre-existing immunity—the rôle of IgA antibodies

Infants and young children have a high risk of meningococcal disease because they lack protective (bactericidal) antibodies. The reasons why older children and adults, who should mostly possess such antibodies, sometimes develop invasive disease are more puzzling. It is necessary to postulate a mechanism involving subversion of pre-existing immunity to explain disease in some of these older cases.

IgA antibodies are less efficient activators of the complement pathway than IgG and IgM immunoglobulin isotypes, and IgA antibodies are not bactericidal for meningococci when bound to capsular polysaccharide. Convalescent sera from some patients with meningococcal disease can be shown to contain circulating IgA antibodies capable of blocking IgG and IgM mediated serum bactericidal activity[139,140], and high levels of circulating IgA antibodies have been noted in cases in African outbreaks[107]. Such blocking is serogroup specific[139], suggesting that the blocking IgA antibody may bind to capsular polysaccharide.

Griffiss has further proposed that secretory (rather than circulating) IgA antibodies generated by exposure to cross-reacting organisms in the gastrointestinal tract could bind to meningococci in the oropharynx. Such bacteria, with immunoglobulin binding sites blocked by non-lethal IgA antibody, would, on invasion, be protected from the lethal effects of circulating bactericidal IgG and IgM antibodies[141]. Colonisation of the affected population with enteric organisms expressing surface antigens cross-reacting with disease-producing meningococci has been documented in two serogroup A meningococcal outbreaks[55,142]. *E. coli* K100 strains, which induce antibodies cross-reacting with *H. influenzae* type b (Hib)[143], were found in the stools of 20% of cases of invasive Hib disease compared with 2.5% of healthy infants and 0.9% of newborn babies[144].

The proposed mechanism has been further refined by Griffiss and by Kilian and colleagues[86] who suggest that the timing of prior exposure to the cross-reacting enteric organism may be crucial, allowing the development of secretory and serum IgA_1 antibodies reactive with meningococcal surface epitopes but without the simultaneous development of IgA_1 protease-neutralising antibodies. If a meningococcus then colonises the nasopharynx in the next few days, its immunoglobulin binding sites are blocked not by whole IgA molecules (which may still be able to initiate meningococcal killing[145]) but by harmless FAb-α fragments generated by the unimpeded action of IgA_1 protease on secretory IgA_1.

There is circumstantial evidence for the importance of IgA_1 proteases as bacterial virulence factors. Enzymes with this specificity are produced by pathogenic, but not non-pathogenic, members of the genera *Neisseria*, *Haemophilus*, *Streptococcus*, *Bacteroides* and *Capnocytophaga*. Though *N. meningitidis* IgA_1 protease can cleave IgA at one of two sites in the hinge region of the molecule, almost all epidemic clones of meningococci produce an enzyme with type 1 specificity, whereas non-epidemic meningococcal clones produce IgA proteases divided equally between type 1 and type 2 specificity[146].

In view of the evidence above, it might be expected that selective IgA deficiency, which occurs in about one in 700 of the Western population, might influence susceptibility to meningococcal disease. In practice, it does not do so. The explanation may lie in the fact that in such individuals, IgM-producing cells expand greatly in number in the intestinal mucosa to make up for the lack of IgA secretion[147].

The rôle of viruses and mycoplasmas

A possible association between virus infections and increased susceptibility to bacterial meningitis has been postulated since the last century. The relationship between influenza (and other respiratory infections) and meningococcal disease was considered at some length by Sir Humphrey Rolleston in his first Lumleian lecture to the Members and Fellows of the Royal College of Physicians, London in 1919[148]. He concluded that impaired resistance to infection, together with the presence of chronic meningococcal carriers with influenzal coughs, may have facilitated the spread of meningococcal infection after influenza outbreaks.

The similar patterns of seasonal variation in the incidence of meningococcal disease and of respiratory virus activity[45] in the northern hemisphere, with a pronounced winter peak and summer trough, suggest that there might be a relationship between the two. Interactions between bacteria and viruses in the respiratory tract have been recognised and investigated for many years[149,150]. Early studies of the influence of viruses on meningococcal disease in US military recruits led to conflicting opinions; Artenstein and colleagues thought that any effect of respiratory viral infection on invasive meningococcal disease was probably small[67], while Edwards *et al.* thought that acute respiratory infection may have contributed to meningococcal disease[151].

Viruses might influence the risk of meningococcal disease in a number of ways. The possibility of increased dissemination of meningococci or of increased susceptibility to meningococcal colonisation induced by viruses have both been discussed above in the section on meningococcal carriage. Neither hypothesis is supported by the lack of seasonal variation in meningococcal nasopharyngeal carriage. When invasive meningococcal disease occurs, it is thought to follow shortly after nasopharyngeal colonisation[151]. By damaging the nasopharyngeal mucosa viruses might facilitate the meningococcal invasion process. If this were a common event, it should be possible to isolate viruses frequently from the nasopharynx of acute cases of meningococcal disease.

Krasinski *et al.* attempted virus isolation and serology in a group of 160 children with bacterial meningitis (though only 16 of these had meningococcal meningitis). The specificity of the serological data is difficult to interpret, but viruses were isolated from 23 patients[152]. Unfortunately a control population was not sampled at the same time. Moore *et al.* redressed this deficiency in a study of viral and mycoplasma infection in children with meningococcal disease during an outbreak of serogroup A infections in Chad in 1988[153]. They isolated viruses from 15/62 cases compared with 6/62 controls, a difference which borders on statistical significance. They also isolated *Mycoplasma* species (predominantly *M. hominis*) from 14/62 cases but from only 1/62 controls. Attempts to confirm the latter finding in cases of meningococcal disease in the USA have been unsuccessful (Broome CV, personal communication), and in an English multicentre case–control study of meningococcal disease *M. hominis* was not isolated from the throat swabs of any of 25 case–control pairs (Cartwright K, unpublished findings). It appears, therefore, that the *M. hominis* strains isolated in Moore's study may have been laboratory contaminants (or possibly, that *M. hominis* is only found in African serogroup A disease).

The failure, despite careful attempts over many years, to isolate viruses more than occasionally from acute cases of meningococcal disease during an outbreak in Gloucestershire, England, suggests that viruses cultivable by routine methods are only infrequently present in the nasopharynx in such cases.

Influenza A

A third possibility is that viruses might reduce the host's resistance to infection by an effect on the immune system. There is now a large body of direct and indirect evidence to support this mechanism, at least in the specific case of infection with influenza A virus. There have been several anecdotal reports of an association between influenza virus infection and subsequent meningococcal disease[65,154–156]. In each case influenza virus infection preceded meningococcal disease, usually by about two weeks. Serological and epidemiological investigations in England and Wales in the aftermath of the 1989 influenza A outbreak showed that cases of meningococcal disease aged 10 or more who became ill in the month after the influenza outbreak were three times more likely to have had recent influenza A infection than matched controls[157]. There was also a shift in the age distribution of meningococcal disease cases in the month after the influenza outbreak, with a significantly greater proportion of teenage and adult cases than the average for the preceding 5 years (52.7% versus 40.4%, $p < 0.01$). There was a clear interval of 2 weeks separating the rise in numbers of cases of influenzal illness and the subsequent rise in the numbers of meningococcal disease cases. The early December rise in meningococcal disease incidence in 1989 was observed neither in the 2 preceding years, nor in the following winter (Figure 5.2).

The epidemiological findings of the UK study have since been confirmed by a detailed analysis of national data on influenza-like illness and meningococcal disease in France[158]. The French workers also noted a marked increase in the severity of meningococcal disease for 2 months after epidemic influenza, with more cases developing a purpuric rash, and a 25% increase in the meningococcal disease mortality rate. Recent anecdotal evidence in the UK supports the finding of increased disease severity after influenza, and a substantial increase in numbers of cases of meningococcal disease was again noted at the UK Meningococcal Reference Unit in November 1993 after a relatively modest increase in influenza activity in the community in the preceding few weeks[159]. Wang et al. also speculated on an association between epidemic influenza A and epidemic meningococcal disease in China throughout most of this century[160].

All the above evidence supports the hypothesis that influenza A infection increases susceptibility to meningococcal disease primarily by subversion of pre-existing immunity, rather than through one of the other possible

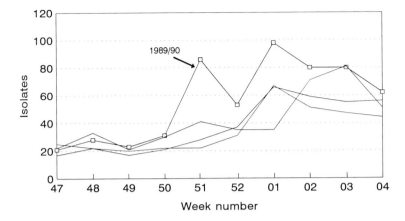

Figure 5.2 *Meningococcal isolates received at the UK Reference Laboratory, winter seasons 1987/88 to 1990/91. A large outbreak of influenza A occurred in weeks 47–49 of 1989, but not in any of the other three winters. The sharp rise in influenza activity preceded the rise in meningococcal cases by about 2 weeks, suggesting that influenza A infection does not precipitate meningococcal disease by directly facilitating the passage of meningococci from nasopharynx by bloodstream*[157]. Reproduced with permission from The Lancet. © *Cartwright KAV et al. Influenza A and meningococcal disease. Lancet 1991; 338: 554–7*

mechanisms discussed above. The failure (in general) to isolate influenza A viruses from acute cases of meningococcal disease, and the finding that influenza antibodies are already raised when patients are acutely unwell with meningococcal disease, support the theory that influenza A infection precedes, rather than accompanies, meningococcal disease. An increase in meningococcal transmission during influenza outbreaks cannot be ruled out, because no large-scale studies of meningococcal acquisition and carriage during influenza A outbreaks have yet been undertaken. However, the 2 week interval between influenza A infection and meningococcal disease, the upward shift in the age distribution of meningococcal disease cases in the month after the influenza outbreak, the increase in meningococcal disease severity, and the documented immunosuppressive capacity of influenza A are all consistent with influenza-induced immune suppression.

Young children are already susceptible to invasive meningococcal disease; the rate of disease may be at a level where it cannot be further increased by exposure to influenza (though disease may perhaps become more severe), whereas older children and adults, most of whom should have protective antibodies, may be made temporarily susceptible to meningococcal invasion by influenza A infection. Influenza A is known to damp down many aspects of immune function[161–163]; it is also known to predispose to other bacterial infections such as pneumococcal and staphylococcal pneumonia[164].

While the case for influenza A infection precipitating meningococcal disease is now overwhelmingly strong, the same cannot yet be said for other viral infections. For example, though meningococci bind in increased numbers to Hep-2 cells infected with respiratory synctial virus (RSV)[165], the sharp peak of RSV infection which causes widespread infection of infants each winter, usually in November or December, does not coincide regularly with any upsurge in meningococcal disease; nor is there a shift in the age distribution of meningococcal disease in those months to the infant population in whom RSV infection is most prevalent. More detailed work will be needed to discover whether other viruses predispose to meningococcal infection, and if they do, to elucidate the pathogenic mechanism.

REFERENCES

1. Schwartz B, Moore P, Broome CV. Global epidemiology of meningococcal disease. Clin Microbiol Rev 1989; 2: S118–24.
2. Salit IE, Morton G. Adherence of Neisseria meningitidis to human epithelial cells. Infect Immun 1981; 31: 430–5.
3. Stephens DS, Hoffman LH, McGee ZA. Interaction of Neisseria meningitidis with human nasopharyngeal mucosa—attachment and entry into columnar epithelial cells. J Infect Dis 1983; 148: 369–76.
4. Nassif X, Lowy J, Stenberg P, O'Gaora P, Ganji A, So M. Antigenic variation of pilin regulates adhesion of Neisseria meningitidis to human epithelial cells. Mol Microbiol 1993; 8: 719–25.
5. Mulks MH, Plaut AG. IgA protease production as a characteristic distinguishing pathogenic from harmless Neisseriaceae. N Engl J Med 1978; 299: 973–6.
6. Delacroix DL, Dive C, Rambaud JC, Vaerman JP, IgA subclasses in various secretions and in serum. Immunology 1982; 47: 383–5.
7. Schryvers AB, Morris LJ. Identification and characterisation of the transferrin receptor from Neisseria meningitidis. Mol Microbiol 1988; 2: 281–8.
8. Schryvers AB, Morris LJ. Identification and characterisation of the human lactoferrin-binding protein from Neisseria meningitidis. Infect Immun 1988; 56: 1144–9.
9. Schryvers AB, Gonzalez GC. Receptors for transferrin in pathogenic bacteria are specific for the host's protein. Can J Microbiol 1990; 36: 145–7.
10. Stephens DS, McGee ZA. Attachment of Neisseria meningitidis to human mucosal surfaces: influence of pili and type of receptor cell. J Infect Dis 1981; 143: 525–32.
11. Janda WM, Bohnhoff M, Morello JA, Lerner SA. Prevalence and site-pathogen studies of Neisseria meningitidis and N gonorrhoeae in homosexual men. JAMA 1980; 244: 2060–4.
12. Condé-Glez CJ, Calderon E. Urogenital infection due to meningococcus in men and women. Sex Transm Dis 1991; 18: 72–5.
13. Maini M, French P, Prince M, Bingham JS. Urethritis due to Neisseria meningitidis in a London genitourinary medicine clinic population. Int J STD & AIDS 1992; 3: 423–5.
14. Broome CV. The carrier state: Neisseria meningitidis. J Antimicrob Chemother 1986; 18: (Suppl A) 25–34.

15. De Wals P, Gilquin C, De Maeyer S, Bouckaert A, Noel A, Lechat MF, Lafontaine A. Longitudinal study of asymptomatic meningococcal carriage in two Belgian populations of schoolchildren. J Infect 1983; *6*: 147–56.

16. Greenfield S, Sheehe PR, Feldman HA. Meningococcal carriage in a population of 'normal' families. J Infect Dis 1971; *123*: 67–73.

17. Cartwright KAV, Stuart JM, Robinson PM. Meningococcal carriage in close contacts of cases. Epidemiol Infect 1991; *106*: 133–41.

18. Cartwright KAV, Stuart JM, Jones DM, Noah ND. The Stonehouse survey: nasopharyngeal carriage of meningococci and *Neisseria lactamica*. Epidemiol Infect 1987; *99*: 591–601.

19. Lystad A, Aasen S. The epidemiology of meningococcal disease in Norway 1975–91. NIPH Annals 1991; *14*: 57–65.

20. Poolman JT, Lind I, Jonsdottir K, Frøholm LO, Jones DM, Zanen HC. Meningococcal serotypes and serogroup B disease in North-West Europe. Lancet 1986; *ii*: 555–8.

21. Moore PS, Reeves MW, Schwartz B, Gellin BG, Broome CV. Intercontinental spread of an epidemic group A *Neisseria meningitidis* strain. Lancet 1989; *ii*: 260–3.

22. Caugant DA, Høiby EA, Rosenqvist E, Frøholm LO, Selander RK. Transmission of *Neisseria meningitidis* among asymptomatic military recruits and antibody analysis. Epidemiol Infect 1992; *109*: 241–53.

23. Dudley SF, Brennan JR. High and persistent carrier rates of *Neisseria meningitidis* unaccompanied by cases of meningitis. J Hyg 1934; *34*: 525–41.

24. Wenzel RP, Davies JA, Mitzel JR, Beam WE. Non-usefulness of meningococcal carriage rates. Lancet 1973; *ii*: 205.

25. Hollis DG, Wiggins GL, Weaver RE. *Neisseria lactamicus* sp. n., a lactose-fermenting species resembling *Neisseria meningitidis*. Appl Microbiol 1969; *17*: 71–7.

26. Branham SE. Serological relationships among meningococci. Bact Rev 1953; *17*: 175–88.

27. Olsen SF, Djurhuus B, Rasmussen K, Joensen HD, Larsen SO, Zoffman H et al. Pharyngeal carriage of *Neisseria meningitidis* and *Neisseria lactamica* in households with infants within areas with high and low incidences of meningococcal disease. Epidemiol Infect 1991; *106*: 445–57.

28. Olcén P, Kjellander J, Danielsson D, Lingquist BL. Culture diagnosis of meningococcal carriers: yield from different sites and influence of storage in transport medium. J Clin Pathol 1979; *32*: 1222–5.

29. Norton JF, Baisley IE. Meningococcus meningitis in Detroit in 1928–1929 IV. Meningococcus carriers. J Prevent Med 1931; *5*: 357–67.

30. Schoenbach EB, Phair JJ. Appraisal of the techniques employed for the detection of subclinical (inapparent) meningococcal infections. Am J Hyg 1948; *47*: 271–81.

31. van Peenen PPD, Suiter LE, Mandel AD, Mitchell MS. Field evaluation of Thayer-Martin medium for identification of meningococcus carriers. Am J Epidemiol 1965; *82*: 329–33.

32. Pether JVS, Lightfoot NF, Scott RJD, Morgan J, Steele-Perkins AP, Sheard SC. Carriage of *Neisseria meningitidis*: investigations in a military establishment. Epidemiol Infect 1988; *101*: 21–42.

33. Phair JJ, Schoenbach EB. The dynamics of meningococcal infections and the effect of chemotherapy. Am J Hyg 1944; *39–40*: 318–44.

34. Aycock WL, Mueller JH. Meningococcus carrier rates and meningitis incidence. Bact Rev 1950; *14*: 115–60.

35. Caugant DA, Høiby EA, Magnus P, Scheel O, Hoel T, Bjune G et al.

Asymptomatic carriage of *Neisseria meningitidis* in a randomly sampled population. J Clin Microbiol 1994; *32*: 323–30.

36. Craven DE, Peppler MS, Frasch CE, Mocca LF, McGrath PP, Washington G. Adherence of *Neisseria meningitidis* from patients and carriers to human buccal epithelial cells. J Infect Dis 1980; *142*: 556–68.

37. Reller LB, MacGregory RR, Beaty HN. Bactericidal antibody after colonization with *Neisseria meningitidis*. J Infect Dis 1973; *127*: 56–62.

38. Fraser PK, Bailey GK, Abbott JD, Gill JB, Walker DJC. The meningococcal carrier rate. Lancet 1973; *i*: 1235–7.

39. Gold R, Goldschneider I, Lepow ML, Draper TF, Randolph M. Carriage of *Neisseria meningitidis* and *Neisseria lactamica* in infants and children. J Infect Dis 1978; *137*: 112–21.

40. Marks MI, Frasch CE, Shapera RM. Meningococcal colonisation and infection in children and their household contacts. Am J Epidemiol 1979; *109*: 563–71.

41. Blakebrough IS, Greenwood BM, Whittle HC, Bradley AK, Gilles HM. The epidemiology of infections due to *Neisseria meningitidis* and *Neisseria lactamica* in a northern Nigerian community. J Infect Dis 1982; *146*: 626–37.

42. Rønne T, Berthelsen L, Buhl LH, Lind I. Comparative studies on pharyngeal carriage of *Neisseria meningitidis* during a localised outbreak of serogroup C meningococcal disease. Scand J Infect Dis 1993; *25*: 331–9.

43. Njoku-Obi AN, Agbo JAC. Meningococcal carrier rates in parts of Eastern Nigeria. Bull WHO 1976; *54*: 271–3.

44. Ichhpujani RL, Mohan R, Grover SS, Joshi PR, Kumari S. Nasopharyngeal carriage of *Neisseria meningitidis* in general population and meningococcal disease. J Com Dis 1990; *4*: 264–8.

45. Fleming DM, Crombie DL. The incidence of common infectious diseases: the weekly returns service of the Royal College of General Practitioners. Health Trends 1985; *17*: 13–16.

46. Stuart JM, Cartwright KAV, Robinson PM, Noah ND. Effect of smoking on meningococcal carriage. Lancet 1989; *ii*: 723–5.

47. Blackwell CC, Weir DM, James VS, Todd WTA, Banatvala N, Chaudhuri AKR et al. Secretor status, smoking and carriage of *Neisseria meningitidis*. Epidemiol Infect 1990; *104*: 203–9.

48. Thomas JC, Bendana NS, Waterman SH, Rathbun M, Arakere G, Frasch CE et al. Risk factors for carriage of meningococcus in the Los Angeles County Men's jail system. Am J Epidemiol 1991; *133*: 286–95.

49. Blackwell CC, Tzanakaki G, Kremastinou J, Weir DM, Vakalis N, Elton RA et al. Factors affecting carriage of *Neisseria meningitidis* among Greek military recruits. Epidemiol Infect 1992; *108*: 441–8.

50. Cope GF, Heatley RV. Cigarette smoking and intestinal defences. Gut 1992; *33*: 721–3.

51. Barton JR, Riad MA, Gaze MN, Maran AGD, Ferguson A. Mucosal immunodeficiency in smokers, and patients with epithelial head and neck tumours. Gut 1990; *31*: 378–82.

52. Ertel A, Eng R, Smith SM. The differential effect of cigarette smoke on the growth of bacteria found in humans. Chest 1991; *100*: 628–30.

53. Colebrook L. Bacterial antagonism, with particular reference to meningococcus. Lancet 1915; *ii*: 1136–8.

54. Gordon MH. Great Britain Medical Research Committee, Special Report Series No 3, 1917; 106–11.

55. Filice GA, Hayes PS, Counts GW, Griffiss JM, Fraser DW. Risk of group A

meningococcal disease: bacterial interference and cross-reactive bacteria among mucosal flora. J Clin Microbiol 1985; 22: 152–6.

56. Blackwell CC, Jonsdottir K, Hanson M, Todd WTA, Chaudhuri AKR, Mathews B *et al*. Non-secretion of ABO antigens predisposing to infection by *Neisseria meningitidis* and *Streptococcus pneumoniae*. Lancet 1986; ii: 284–5.

57. Blackwell CC, Weir DM, James VS, Cartwright KAV, Stuart JM, Jones DM. The Stonehouse study: secretor status and carriage of *Neisseria* species. Epidemiol Infect 1989; 102: 1–10.

58. Kristiansen B-E, Elverland H, Hannestad K. Increased meningococcal carrier rate after tonsillectomy. Br Med J 1984; 288: 974.

59. Jeschke R, Stroder J. Continual observation of clinical and immunological parameters, in particular of salivary IgA, in tonsillectomised children. Arch Otorhinolaryngol 1980; 226: 73–84.

60. Stanwell-Smith RE, Stuart JM, Hughes AO, Robinson P, Griffin MB, Cartwright K. Smoking, the environment and meningococcal disease: a case control study. Epidemiol Infect 1994; 112: 315–28.

61. Smith CB, Golden C, Klauber MR, Kanner R, Renzetti A. Interactions between viruses and bacteria in patients with chronic bronchitis. J Infect Dis 1976; 134: 552–61.

62. Ramírez-Ronda CH, Fuxench-López Z, Nevárez M. Increased pharyngeal bacterial colonisation during viral illness. Arch Intern Med 1981; 141: 1599–603.

63. Gwaltney JM, Sande MA, Austrian R, Hendley JO. Spread of *Streptococcus pneumoniae* in families. II. Relation of transfer of *S. pneumoniae* to incidence of colds and serum antibody. J Infect Dis 1975; 132: 62–8.

64. Kostyukova NN, Alexeev AB, Gorlina MK *et al*. A study on meningococcal colonization of epithelium. In: Achtman M, Kohl P, Marchal C, Morelli G, Seiler A, Thiesen B, eds. *Neisseriae 1990*. Berlin: Walter de Gruyter, 1991; 609–14.

65. Young LS, LaForce FM, Head JJ, Feeley JC, Bennett JV. A simultaneous outbreak of meningococcal and influenza infections. N Engl J Med 1972; 287: 5–9.

66. Olcén P, Kjellander J, Danielsson D, Lindquist BL. Epidemiology of *Neisseria meningitidis*: prevalence and symptoms from the upper respiratory tract in family members to patients with meningococcal disease. Scand J Infect Dis 1981; 13: 105–9.

67. Artenstein MS, Rust JH, Hunter DH, Lamson TH, Buescher EL. Acute respiratory disease and meningococcal infection in army recruits. JAMA 1967; 201: 1004–8.

68. Gotschlich EC, Goldschneider I, Artenstein MS. Human immunity to the meningococcus V. The effect of immunization with meningococcal group C polysaccharide on the carrier state. J Exp Med 1969; 129: 1385–95.

69. Stroffolini T, Angelini L, Galanti I, Occhionero M, Congiu ME, Mastrantonio P. The effect of meningococcal group A and C polysaccharide vaccine on nasopharyngeal carrier state. Microbiologica 1990; 13: 225–9.

70. Blakebrough IS, Greenwood BM, Whittle HC, Bradley AK. Failure of meningococcal vaccination to stop the transmission of meningococci in Nigerian schoolboys. Ann Trop Med Parasitol 1983; 77: 175–8.

71. Hassan-King MKA, Wall RA, Greenwood BM. Meningococcal carriage, meningococcal disease and vaccination. J Infect 1988; 16: 55–9.

72. Glover JA. Observations on the meningococcal carrier rate and their application to the prevention of cerebrospinal fever. Special report series of the Medical Research Council (London) 1920; 50: 133–65.

73. Farrell DG, Dahl EV. Nasopharyngeal carriers of *Neisseria meningitidis*. Studies

among Air Force recruits. JAMA 1966; *198*: 1189–92.
74. Phair JJ. Meningococcal meningitis. In: Coates JB, Hoff EC, Hoff PM, eds. *Preventive Medicine In World War II. Volume IV: Communicable diseases transmitted chiefly through respiratory and alimentary tracts.* 1958. Washington DC. Office of the Surgeon General, Department of the Army.
75. Anon. A factor in the spread of cerebrospinal meningitis. JAMA 1931; *96*: 1634.
76. Kaiser AB, Hennekens CH, Saslaw MS, Hayes PS, Bennett JV. Sero-epidemiology and chemoprophylaxis of disease due to sulphonamide-resistant *Neisseria meningitidis* in a civilian population. J Infect Dis 1974; *130*: 217–24.
77. Greenfield S, Feldman HA. Familial carriers and meningococcal meningitis. N Engl J Med 1967; *277*: 498–502.
78. Munford RS, Taunay AE, de Morais JS, Fraser DW, Feldman RA. Spread of meningococcal infection within households. Lancet 1974; *i*: 1275–8.
79. Blakebrough IS, Gilles HM. The effect of rifampicin on meningococcal carriage in family contacts in northern Nigeria. J Infect 1980; *2*: 137–43.
80. Sáez-Nieto JA, Campos J, Latorre C, Juncosa T, Sierra M, Garcia-Tornell T, Garcia-Barrenzo B, Lopez-Galindez C, Casal J. Prevalence of *Neisseria meningitidis* in family members of patients with meningococcal infection. J Hyg (Camb) 1982; *89*: 139–48.
81. Frasch CE, Mocca LF. Strains of *Neisseria meningitidis* isolated from patients and their close contacts. Infect Immun 1982; *37*: 155–9.
82. Rake G. Studies of meningococcus infection VI. The carrier problem. J Exp Med 1934; *59*: 553–76.
83. Altmann G, Egoz N, Bogokovsky B. Observations on asymptomatic infections with *Neisseria meningitidis*. Am J Epidemiol 1973; *98*: 446–52.
84. Goldschneider I, Gotschlich EC, Artenstein MS. Human immunity to the meningococcus. II. Development of natural immunity. J Exp Med 1969; *129*: 1327–48.
85. Griffiss JM, Brandt BL, Jarvis GA. Natural immunity to *Neisseria meningitidis*. In: Vedros NA, ed. *Evolution of meningococcal disease.* Vol II. Boca Raton, Florida: CRC Press Inc, 1987; 99–119.
86. Kilian M, Mestecky J, Russell MW. Defense mechanisms involving Fc-dependent functions of immunoglobulin A and their subversion by bacterial immunoglobulin A proteases. Microbiol Rev 1988; *52*: 296–303.
87. Kim JJ, Mandrell RE, Griffiss JM. *Neisseria lactamica* and *Neisseria meningitidis* share lipooligosaccharide epitopes but lack common capsular and class 1, 2, and 3 protein epitopes. Infect Immun 1989; *57*: 602–8.
88. Gauld JR, Nitz RE, Hunter DH, Rust JH, Gauld RL. Epidemiology of meningococcal meningitis at Ford Ord. Am J Epidemiol 1965; *82*: 56–72.
89. Peltola H. Meningococcal disease: still with us. Rev Infect Dis 1983; *5*: 71–90.
90. Lapeyssonnie L. La méningite cérébro-spinale en Afrique. Bull WHO 1963; *28*: 3–114.
91. Tikhomirov E. Meningococcal meningitis: global situation and control measures. World Health Stat Q 1987; *40*: 98–109.
92. Mihalcu F, Pasolescu O, Coban V, Cuciureanu G, Dumitrescu S. Aspects actuels de la meningite cerebro-spinale epidemique en Roumanie. Arch Roum Path Exp Microbiol 1972; *31*: 125–34.
93. Peltola H, Kataja JM, Mäkelä PH. Shift in the age-distribution of meningococcal disease as predictor of an epidemic? Lancet 1982; *ii*: 595–7.
94. Cartwright KAV, Stuart JM, Noah ND. An outbreak of meningococcal disease in Gloucestershire. Lancet 1986; *ii*: 558–61.

95. Jones DM, Sutcliffe EM. Group A meningococcal disease in England associated with the Haj. J Infect 1990; *21*: 21–5.

96. Zollinger WD, Mandrell RE. Outer membrane protein and lipopolysaccharide serotyping of *Neisseria meningitidis* by inhibition of a solid-phase radio-immunoassay. Infect Immun 1977; *18*: 424–33.

97. Jones DM, Borrow R, Fox A, Gray S, Cartwright KA, Poolman JT. The lipooligosaccharide immunotype as a virulence determinant in *Neisseria meningitidis*. Microb Pathogen 1992; *13*: 219–24.

98. Band JD, Chamberland ME, Platt T, Weaver RE, Thornberry C, Fraser DW. Trends in meningococcal disease in the United States, 1975–1980. J Infect Dis 1983; *148*: 754–8.

99. Abbott JD, Jones DM, Painter MJ, Young SEJ. The epidemiology of meningococcal infections in England and Wales, 1912–1983. J Infect 1985; *11*: 241–57.

100. Jones DM, Kaczmarski EB. Meningococcal infections in England and Wales: 1991. Commun Dis Rep Rev 1992; *2*: R61–3.

101. Nazareth B, Slack MPE, Howard AJ, Waight PA, Begg NT. A survey of invasive *Haemophilus influenzae* infections. Communicable Disease Report 1992; *2*: R13–16.

102. Collier CG. Weather conditions prior to major outbreaks of meningococcal meningitis in the United Kingdom. Int J Biometeorol 1992; *36*: 18–29.

103. Haneberg B, Tønjum T, Rodahl K, Gedde-Dahl T. Factors preceding the onset of meningococcal disease with special emphasis on passive smoking, stressful events, physical fitness and general symptoms of ill-health. NIPH Ann 1983; *6*: 169–73.

104. Stuart JM, Cartwright KAV, Dawson JA, Rickard J, Noah ND. Risk factors for meningococcal disease: a case control study in south west England. Commun Med 1988; *10*: 139–46.

105. Colley JRT, Holland WW, Corkhill RT. Influence of passive smoking and parental phlegm on pneumonia and bronchitis in early childhood. Lancet 1974; *ii*: 1031–4.

106. Bonham GS, Wilson RW. Children's health in families with cigarette smokers. Am J Public Health 1981; *71*: 290–3.

107. Greenwood BM, Greenwood AM, Bradley AK, Williams K, Hassan-King M, Shenton FC *et al*. Factors influencing susceptibility to meningococcal disease during an epidemic in The Gambia, West Africa. J Infect 1987; *14*: 167–84.

108. Filice GA, Englender SJ, Jacobsen JA, Jourden JL, Burns DA, Gregoy D *et al*. Group A meningococcal disease in skid rows: epidemiology and implications for control. Am J Public Health 1984; *74*: 253–4.

109. Norton JF, Gordon JE. Meningococcus meningitis in Detroit in 1928–1929. J Prev Med 1930; *4*: 207–14.

110. De Wals P, Hertoghe L, Borlée-Grimée I, De Maeyer-Cleempoel S, Reginster-Haneuse G, Dachy A *et al*. Meningococcal disease in Belgium. Secondary attack rate among household, day-care nursery and pre-elementary school contacts. J Infect 1981; *3* (Suppl. 1): S53–61.

111. Cooke RPD, Riordan T, Jones DM, Painter MJ. Secondary cases of meningococcal infection among close family and household contacts in England and Wales, 1984–7. Br Med J 1989; *298*: 555–8.

112. Meningococcal Disease Surveillance Group. Analysis of endemic meningococcal disease by serogroup and evaluation of chemoprophylaxis. J Infect Dis 1976; *134*: 201–4.

113. Stuart JM, Cartwright KAV, Robinson PM, Noah ND. Does eradication of meningococcal carriage in household contacts prevent secondary meningococcal disease? Br Med J 1989; 298: 569–70.

114. Feigin RD, Baker CJ, Herwaldt LA, Lampe RM, Mason EO, Whitney SE. Epidemic meningococcal disease in an elementary school classroom. N Engl J Med 1982; 307: 1255–7.

115. Hudson PJ, Vogt RL, Heun EM, Brondum J, Coffin RR, Plikaytis BD et al. Evidence for school transmission of Neisseria meningitidis during a Vermont outbreak. Pediatr Infect Dis J 1986; 5: 213–17.

116. Morrow HW, Slaten DD, Reingold AL, Werner SB, Fenstersheib MD. Risk factors associated with a school-related outbreak of serogroup C meningococcal disease. Pediatr Infect Dis J 1990; 9: 394–8.

117. French MR. Epidemiological study of 383 cases of meningococcus meningitis in the city of Milwaukee 1927–28 and 1929. Am J Public Health 1931; 21: 130–8.

118. Jacobsen JA, Camargos PAM, Ferreira JT, McCormick JB. The risk of meningitis among classroom contacts during an epidemic of meningococcal disease. Am J Epidemiol 1976; 104: 552–5.

119. Wall R, Wilson J, MacArdle B, Vellani Z. Meningococcal infection: evidence for school transmission. J Infect 1991; 23: 155–9.

120. Cann KJ, Rogers TR, Jones DM, Noah ND, Burns C. Neisseria meningitidis in a primary school. Arch Dis Child 1987; 62: 1113–17.

121. Figueroa JE, Densen P. Infectious diseases associated with complement deficiencies. Clin Microbiol Rev 1991; 4: 359–95.

122. Ross SC, Rosenthal PJ, Berberich HM, Densen P. Killing of Neisseria meningitidis by human neutrophils: implications for normal and complement-deficient individuals. J Infect Dis 1987; 155: 1266–75.

123. Di Ninno VL, Chenier VK. Activation of complement by Neisseria meningitidis. FEMS Microbiol Lett 1981; 12: 55–60.

124. Merino J, Rodriguez-Valverde V, Lamelas JA, Riestra JL, Casanueva B. Prevalence of deficits of complement components in patients with recurrent meningococcal infections. J Infect Dis 1983; 148: 331.

125. Ross SC, Densen P. Complement deficiency states and infection: epidemiology, pathogenesis and consequences of neisserial and other infections in an immune deficiency. Medicine (Baltimore) 1984; 63: 243–73.

126. Brandtzaeg P, Mølnnes TE, Kierulf P. Complement activation and endotoxin levels in systemic meningococcal disease. J Infect Dis 1989; 160: 58–65.

127. Lehner PJ, Davies KA, Walport MJ, Cope AP, Wurzner R, Orren A et al. Meningococcal septicaemia in a C6-deficient patient and effects of plasma transfusion on lipopolysaccharide release. Lancet 1992; 340: 1379–81.

128. Fijen CA, Kuijper EJ, Hannema AJ, Sjøholm AG, van Putten JP. Complement deficiencies in patients over ten years old with meningococcal disease due to uncommon serogroups. Lancet 1989; ii: 585–8.

129. Fearon DT, Austen KF. Properdin; binding to C3b and stabilisation of the C3B-dependent C3 convertase. J Exp Med 1975; 142: 856–63.

130. Densen P, Weiler JM, Griffiss JM, Hoffmann LG. Familial properdin deficiency and fatal meningococcaemia. Correction of the bactericidal defect by vaccination. N Engl J Med 1987; 316: 922–6.

131. Francke EL, Neu HC. Postsplenectomy infection. Surg Clin N Am 1981; 61: 135–55.

132. Ellison EC, Fabri PJ. Complications of splenectomy. Etiology, prevention and management. Surg Clin North Am 1983; 63: 1313–30.

133. Shaw JHF, Print CG. Postsplenectomy sepsis. Br J Surg 1989; *76*: 1074–81.
134. Brigden ML. Postsplenectomy sepsis syndrome. How to identify and manage patients at risk. Postgrad Med J 1985; *77*: 215–26.
135. Brindle R, Simani P, Newnham R, Waiyaki P, Gilks C. No association between meningococcal disease and human immunodeficiency virus in adults in Nairobi, Kenya. Trans Roy Soc Trop Med Hyg 1991; *85*: 651.
136. Kipp W, Kamugisha J, Rehle T. Meningococcal meningitis and HIV infection: results from a case-control study in Western Uganda. AIDS 1992; *6*: 1557–8.
137. Dunne FJ. Alcohol and the immune system. Br Med J 1989; *298*: 543–4.
138. Peterson PK, Chao CC, Molitor T, Murtaugh M, Strgar F, Sharp BM. Stress and pathogenesis of infectious disease. Rev Infect Dis 1991; *13*: 710–20.
139. Griffiss JM. Bactericidal activity of meningococcal antisera. Blocking by IgA of lytic antibody in human convalescent sera. J Immunol 1975; *114*: 1779–84.
140. Griffiss JM, Bertram MA. Immunoepidemiology of meningococcal disease in military recruits. II. Blocking of serum bactericidal activity by circulating IgA early in the course of invasive disease. J Infect Dis 1977; *136*: 733–9.
141. Griffiss JM. Epidemic meningococcal diseases: synthesis of a hypothetical immuno-epidemiological model. Rev Infect Dis 1982; *4*: 159–72.
142. Guirguis N, Schneerson R, Bax AD, Egan W, Robbins JB, Shiloach J *et al*. *Escherichia coli* K51 and K93 capsular polysaccharides are cross-reactive with the group A capsular polysaccharide of *Neisseria meningitidis*. J Exp Med 1986; *162*: 1837–51.
143. Handzel ZT, Argaman M, Parke JC, Schneerson R, Robbins JB. Heteroimmunization to the capsular polysaccharide of *Haemophilus influenzae* type b induced by enteric cross-reacting bacteria. Infect Immun 1975; *11*: 1045–52.
144. Ginsburg CM, McCracken GH, Schneerson R, Robbins JB, Parke JC. Association between cross-reacting *Escherichia coli* K100 and disease caused by *Haemophilus influenzae* type b. Infect Immun 1978; *22*: 339–42.
145. Lowell GH, Smith LF, Griffiss JM, Brandt BL. IgA-dependent, monocyte-mediated, antibacterial activity. J Exp Med 1980; *152*: 452–7.
146. Lomholt H, Poulsen K, Caugant DA, Kilian M. Molecular polymorphism and epidemiology of *Neisseria meningitidis* immunoglobulin A1 proteases. Proc Natl Acad Sci USA 1992; *89*: 2120–4.
147. Crabbé PA, Heremans JF. Selective IgA deficiency with steatorrhoea. A new syndrome. Am J Med 1967; *42*: 319–26.
148. Rolleston H. Lumleian lectures on cerebro-spinal fever. Lecture 1. Lancet 1919; *i*: 541–9.
149. Nichol KP, Cherry JD. Bacterial–viral interrelations in respiratory infections of children. N Engl J Med 1967; *277*: 667–72.
150. Loosli CG. Influenza and the interaction of viruses and bacteria in respiratory infections. Medicine 1973; *52*: 369–84.
151. Edwards EA, Devine LF, Sengbusch CH, Ward HW. Immunological investigations of meningococcal disease. III. Brevity of group C acquisition prior to disease occurrence. Scand J Infect Dis 1977; *9*: 105–10.
152. Krasinski K, Nelson JD, Butler S, Luby JP, Kusmiesz H. Possible association of mycoplasma and viral respiratory infections with bacterial meningitis. Am J Epidemiol 1987; *125*: 499–508.
153. Moore PS, Hierholzer J, DeWitt W, Gouan K, Djoré D, Lippeveld T *et al*. Respiratory viruses and Mycoplasma as cofactors for epidemic group A meningococcal meningitis. JAMA 1990; *264*: 1271–5.
154. Lal HB, Narayan TK, Kalra SL, Lal R. Simultaneous outbreaks of influenza and

meningitis. J Ind Med Assoc 1963; 40: 113–15.

155. Pether JVS. Bacterial meningitis after influenza. Lancet 1982; i: 804.

156. Schübiger G, Munzinger J, Dudli C, Wipfli U. Meningokokken-Epidemie in einer Internats-schule: Sekundarerkrankung mit rifampicin-resistentem Erreger unter Chemoprophylaxe. Schweiz Med Wschr 1986; 116: 1172–5.

157. Cartwright KAV, Jones DM, Smith AJ, Stuart JM, Kaczmarski EB, Palmer SR. Influenza A and meningococcal disease. Lancet 1991; 338: 554–7.

158. Hubert B, Watier L, Garnerin P, Richardson S. Meningococcal disease and influenza-like syndrome: a new approach to an old question. J Infect Dis 1992; 166: 542–5.

159. Jones DM. Influenza and meningococcal disease. Lancet 1994; 343: 119.

160. Wang J-F, Caugant DA, Li X, Hu X, Poolman JT, Crowe BA, Achtman M. Clonal and antigenic analysis of serogroup A Neisseria meningitidis with particular reference to epidemiological features of epidemic meningitis in the People's Republic of China. Infect Immun 1992; 60: 5267–82.

161. Kleinerman ES, Snyderman R, Daniels CA. Depressed monocyte chemotaxis during acute influenza infection. Lancet 1975; ii: 1063–6.

162. Larson HE, Blades R. Impairment of human polymorphonuclear leucocyte function by influenza virus. Lancet 1976; i: 283.

163. Cambridge G, MacKenzie J, Keast D. Cell-mediated immune response to influenza virus infections in mice. Infect Immun 1976; 13: 36–43.

164. Parker MT. Necropsy studies of the bacterial complications of influenza. J Infect 1979; 1 (suppl 2): 9–16.

165. Raza MW, Ogilvie MM, Blackwell CC, Stewart J, Elton RA, Weir DM. Effect of respiratory syncytial virus infection on binding of Neisseria meningitidis and Haemophilus influenzae type b to a human epithelial cell line (HEp-2). Epidemiol Infect 1993; 110: 339–47.

6
Epidemiology of Meningococcal Disease in Europe and the USA

DENNIS JONES

Meningococcal Reference Unit, Public Health Laboratory, Manchester, UK

INFLUENCE OF SEASON ON MENINGOCOCCAL INFECTION

In the 'meningitis belts' of Africa the incidence of meningococcal infection rises sharply towards the end of the dry and dusty season (the 'harmattan') and falls with the onset of the rains. It is postulated that the presence of dust interferes with local IgA secretion in the nasopharynx, altering the balance of immunity.

In temperate climates meningococcal infection due to both serogroup B and serogroup C strains has a seasonal peak with most cases regularly occurring in the first quarter of the year (Figure 6.1). Although the reasons for this seasonality are not clear it is postulated that in the winter there is closer personal contact, lack of ventilation and catarrhal infections that may facilitate transmission of meningococci. The seasonal pattern is seen irrespective of age[1]. It is likely that virus infections that affect the upper respiratory tract play some part in the seasonality of meningococcal infection. The advent of a nationwide outbreak of influenza A in England and Wales in November/December 1989 provided the opportunity to collect serological data and observe the pattern of meningococcal infection during that winter[2]. The results indicated that there had been an excess of cases of meningococcal infection related to the occurrence of influenza, and the seasonal peak that year occurred earlier than usual having a temporal

Meningococcal Disease. Edited by Keith Cartwright © 1995 John Wiley & Sons Ltd

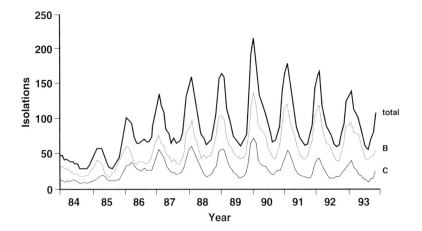

Figure 6.1 *Meningococci from clinical cases received at the Meningococcal Reference Unit 1984–93 (four weekly moving averages). B: serogroup B; C: serogroup C*

relationship to the influenza outbreak, occurring in its wake. A temporal relationship between influenza and meningococcal infection was also observed in France[3]. Other organisms may also exert an influence. We have observed an outbreak in military personnel to follow closely on an outbreak of rubella, and it has been postulated that mycoplasmas may have a similar role[4].

INFLUENCE OF AGE AND GENDER

In general the incidence of meningococcal infection is related to the degree of immunity prevailing in the population so that it is common amongst the young, although the age profile of cases varies according to the serogroup causing disease. In developed countries serogroup B infections are relatively more common in the very young, serogroup A in older children with serogroup C strains holding an intermediate position. In Norway, where B15:P1.16 strains of the ET-5 clone have been responsible for the majority of recent infections, the relative age distribution of cases was 40% in children under 5 years, with a peak in the under ones, and 30% in the age group 13–20; amongst older children the peak incidence was seen in those aged 16–17 years[5]. In England and Wales in recent years, where serogroup B and C strains have been prevalent, the peak age-specific attack rate occurs at 6 months, at a time when maternal (passive) immunity has largely disappeared and active immunity has yet to be developed.

Based on cases whose isolates were submitted in recent years to the Meningococcal Reference Laboratory, the meningococcal disease annual attack rate in the first month of life was 5.9 per 100 000, rising to over 50 per 100 000 at 6 months. The annual attack rate then fell subsequently to 10 per 100 000 at age 2, continuing to fall still further in children of primary school age. The rate then rose again, albeit slowly, to a smaller second peak amongst 17–18 year olds (Figure 6.2). The overall adult rate of infection is 0.4 per 100 000 per annum.

The relatively high rates in neonates when compared with adults is probably the result of incomplete transmission of maternal immunity coupled with the immaturity of the neonatal immune system. Neonates have a late complement factor deficiency which would interfere with the efficiency of the serum bactericidal system[6]. The reasons for the second peak in teenagers are not clear but may be related to the social activities of the age group increasing the likelihood of transmission of pathogenic meningococci. It is interesting to note that there is a relative excess of ET-5 complex strains in older children and young adults and that these meningococci, irrespective of phenotype, all exhibit this property. This predilection for older age groups is also shared by some sulphonamide sensitive serogroup C2a and serogroup C non-typable strains belonging to other genotypic groups.

Although it has long been recognised that slightly more males than females get invasive infections, the ratio of males to females varies with age. In England and Wales the male to female ratio is highest in infants and becomes gradually reduced with increasing age. At 17–18 years more girls than boys become infected, but thereafter males predominate once more; the reasons for this variation are obscure.

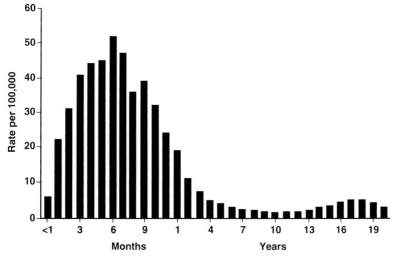

Figure 6.2 *Age-specific rates for meningococcal infection, England and Wales, 1984–91*

EUROPEAN EPIDEMIOLOGY

The annual incidence of meningococcal infection is generally in the range of 1–3 per 100 000 in European countries although this fluctuates. Many countries have shown an increase during the 1980s and are now showing decreases in the 1990s, but the fluctuations are not usually in synchrony. In Europe, the disease commonly follows a seasonal pattern with most cases in the first quarter of the year. Once again, this pattern is not invariable, and particularly in smaller population groups, autumn or even occasionally summer peaks of incidence may be recorded.

Even within closely adjacent European countries with apparently similar socio-economic structures there are very wide (and unexplained) differences in patterns of meningococcal disease incidence. For example, in the Scandinavian countries in the period 1970 to 1985 the highest rates of infection were observed in Denmark and Finland in 1974, in Sweden in 1975, in Iceland in 1976, in the Faroes in 1981 and in Norway in 1983[7,8]. The maximum incidence attained during this period in each of the different countries varied from 2.8 per 100 000 in Sweden (a rate barely higher than background levels) to 95 cases per 100 000 in the Faroes.

Across Europe the disease is most prevalent in children under five, and nearly half of infections in this age group occur in the under 1 year olds—a finding of very great importance for the development and subsequent targeting of vaccines. Minor variations in the age distribution of cases, particularly in teenagers, are often related to the relative proportions of serogroup B and serogroup C infections in particular countries, although serogroup B remains predominant in Europe as a whole.

MENINGOCOCCAL DISEASE IN ENGLAND AND WALES

Sources of data on meningococcal disease in England and Wales are statutory notifications (returned to the Office of Population Censuses and Surveys, OPCS), case reports to the Public Health Laboratory Service *Communicable Disease Surveillance Centre* and case reports with isolates to the *Meningococcal Reference Unit* (MRU), located at the Public Health Laboratory, Manchester. Although each set of data is slightly different, the trends are internally consistent and, in practice, follow each other closely. Under-notification, a well-recognised problem, may mean that only about 65% of cases are reported, so the true incidence of disease is probably considerably higher than any of the sources quoted[9]. More efficient notification of fatal cases means that estimates of the proportion of fatal cases that are based on notifications will be falsely high. Both these sources of bias are important when cost–benefit analyses of potential vaccines are being undertaken.

The trends in meningococcal disease are illustrated by the notifications (Figure 6.3) which provide a record since 1912. The large peaks in incidence that coincided with the two World Wars were caused by serogroup A strains, as was the peak in the 1930s. As the incidence fell during the 1950s the basic endemic level of disease of some 400–500 cases per year remained, and was caused mainly by serogroup B strains with 20–30% of infections due to serogroup C strains.

In 1972 there began a 3–4 year period when the incidence rose and then fell again quite sharply. The excess of cases above the basic level was almost entirely due to serogroup B serotype 2a strains, which were perhaps new to the community. This increase in infections appeared and disappeared quite sharply, and B2a strains have occurred only in small numbers since then. In 1985 another hyperendemic period began. At this time B15:P1.16 strains of the ET-5 complex were responsible for nearly 50% of serogroup B infections. This state of affairs did not persist, for as the total number of cases went up, those due to B15:P1.16 strains did not increase proportionately. The overall increased incidence of cases was due to a composite of various serotypes of serogroup B strains and an increase in serogroup C strains such that no single serotype predominated.

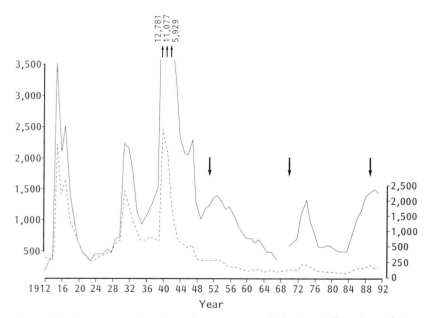

Figure 6.3   Statutory notifications of meningococcal infection (Office of Population Censuses and Surveys) 1912–92. The solid line denotes the number of cases and the dashed line the number of deaths

The B15:P1.16 strains were epidemiologically important because of their property of persisting year after year in the same locality and they were responsible for several localised and persisting outbreaks notably in Gloucestershire[10], Plymouth and Merseyside. These local outbreaks were characterised by proportionately higher attack rates in teenagers than in young children and by their causing increased numbers of cases over several years. In the first year of the Gloucestershire outbreak the disease was almost completely restricted to the age group 15–25, but over the next 10 years a bimodal age distribution developed gradually, with equal numbers of teenagers and much younger cases. B15:P1.16 strains were first encountered in Norway in the 1970s and have been responsible there for a hyperendemic period which has only recently shown some signs of declining. In England and Wales these strains were responsible for approximately 15–20% of serogroup B infections during the present hyperendemic period (Figure 6.4).

The overall incidence of disease as reflected by isolates received at the MRU in the period 1984–92 is shown in Figure 6.1. This demonstrates a steady rise and fall in the total number of cases but also that rise and fall of serogroup C infections does not coincide with that of serogroup B strains. These actual trends obscure much regional variation both in incidence and prevalence of particular serogroups[11].

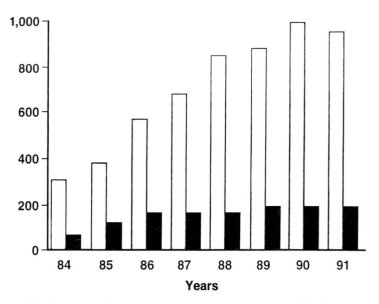

Figure 6.4   Serogroup B serotype 15 P1.16 infections compared with total group B infections 1984–91. □, total Serogroup B; ■, B15: P1.16

Distribution of serotypes

Serotypes and serosubtypes are very useful markers for localised epidemiology but are also of interest on a national or continental scale. Determination depends on the availability and specificity of monoclonal antibodies, but these are not available for all the possible antigens. Indeed there are changes that occur that are presently masked by our inability to serotype a significant proportion of strains..

In England and Wales serogroup B meningococcal disease is currently caused by a variety of serotypes, but certain phenotypes are more important than others. Strains of B15:P1.16 phenotype remain the most numerous (18%), closely followed by B2b:P1.10 (13%). The former are ET-5 strains and the latter belong to the A4 cluster and each has a different age range. Some strains of the phenotype B4:P1.15 also belong to the ET-5 complex and these are under-represented in the figure because the monoclonal antibody in use currently does not detect all serotype 4 strains so that many appear as Bnt P1.15. Strains of the phenotype B4:P1.10 (another ET-5 phenotype) have been localised to one area in England for several years and are rarely detected outside Worcestershire. Although the overall pattern has not changed, the proportion of the various phenotypes varies from year to year[11].

This general pattern of the prevalence of various phenotypes is repeated in other European countries. For example, a period of increasing incidence of meningococcal disease in The Netherlands during the 1980s was also associated with a complex variety of serogroup B meningococcal phenotypes[12].

Serotyping and serosubtyping monoclonal antibodies applied to serogroup C strains detect far less variation than with the serogroup B strains; 80% of serogroup C strains are either serotype 2a or 2b, with the remainder untypable. In addition, 40% of serogroup C strains were not serosubtypable. New DNA-based typing systems[13] will mean that the full extent of the genetic variation involved in the expression of the serotyping and serosubtyping outer membrane proteins will be discernible in the future and may therefore clarify some of the obscurities that occur with the present (serologically based) phenotyping system.

DNA probes

Another molecular method, using a random fragment of DNA, has thrown new light on the epidemiology of the B15 strains. Using both the probe and a monoclonal antibody that detected a point mutation in the class 1 outer membrane protein in combination[14], four variants of P1.16 were defined. The geographical distribution of these variants shows them to be widely disseminated through England and Wales (Figure 6.5). However, each variant has remained in its respective locality, as shown, for a number of years.

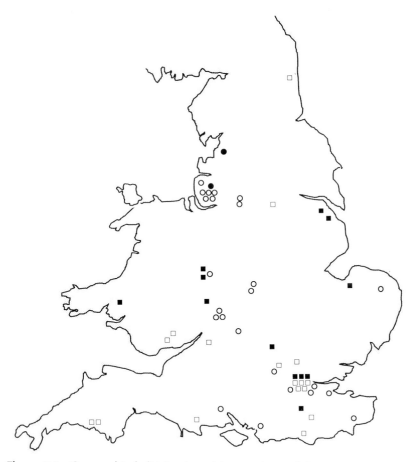

Figure 6.5   *Geographical distribution of four variants of B15: P1.16 strains in England and Wales, January 1991. Defined by molecular variations of class 1 protein P1.16 and RFLP (restriction fragment length polymorphism) typing. □, P1.16a-21; ■, P1.16a-1; ●, P1.16b-21; ○, P1.16b-1*

For example, in Gloucestershire all the isolates over a decade have been B15:P1.16b-1 and in Plymouth, another area with a prolonged upsurge of B15 infections over the same period of time, all the isolates have been B15:P1.16a-21. Only the large cosmopolitan conglomerate of the London area shows a mixture of P1.16 variants. This molecular approach to the epidemiology demonstrates that individual meningococcal strains are not particularly mobile in terms of spreading from one town to another as the same strain can be found causing disease in a locality over a number of years. This is perhaps consistent with the long duration of nasopharyngeal carriage (e.g. of the B15:P1.16 phenotype) and with the known slow movement of such meningococcal strains through populations.

We can no longer consider the country-wide upsurge of B15 strains across England in the 1980s as being due to a single strain, though the variants detected appear to be so closely related that they probably originated as a single bacterial clone. These variants appear to be very stable and have been detected amongst a sample of strains from Norway, where B15 infections were first encountered in Europe[8,15]. The variants of the class 1 protein P1.16a and P1.16b are detectable by appropriate monoclonal antibodies that differ in their respective specific bactericidal activities. On the other hand, convalescent human sera from patients infected with either variant show no difference in the specificity of the bactericidal response, giving similar bactericidal titres with either variant. The stability of these variants, in terms of a particular strain remaining localised in a particular community, may reflect the absence of selection pressure in the human immune response to these epitopes in natural infection. Another example of the lack of mobility of individual meningococcal strains is the restriction of B4:P1.10 isolates to Worcester and the neighbouring village of Malvern over several years. Outside this small area, this phenotype is not being encountered elsewhere in the Midlands of England.

EPIDEMIOLOGY IN THE USA

In a laboratory-based study of four selected areas of the USA, the annual incidence of meningococcal infection has recently been estimated at about 1/100 000 with age-specific rates probably very similar to those in Europe[16]. The seasonal pattern is also generally similar to that in Europe[17,18]. An important difference is that a significantly higher incidence of infection was observed in the black population (1.5 compared to 1.1/100 000). Overall, 46% of isolates were serogroup B and 45% were serogroup C with, interestingly, a much higher rate of serogroup C infection in blacks. The differences between the races were thought to reflect differences in the presence of various risk factors for meningococcal disease such as poor housing, overcrowding, socio-economic factors and exposure to tobacco smoke. Just as in Europe, serogroup C strains caused proportionately more infections in older age groups and serogroup B strains were especially common in very young children.

MORTALITY AND MORBIDITY

Meningococcal disease is traditionally divided clinically into syndromes of meningitis and septicaemia. The differentiation is not at all clear. Patients with meningococci in the bloodstream may have innocuous and benign bacteraemia, or fulminant overwhelming septicaemia, fatal within a few hours. A haemorrhagic rash is observed in more than 50% of patients with symptoms of meningitis and from whom a meningococcus is isolated from the cerebrospinal fluid. Do these patients have meningitis or septicaemia, or both[19]? The mortality in septicaemic illness is much higher than in the meningitic form of disease, but there are some difficulties in arriving at accurate case fatality ratios.

As noted earlier, notification figures may be low due to under-reporting whereas certification of deaths is likely to be much more accurate. Only since 1989 has meningococcal septicaemia as well as meningitis been notifiable in England and Wales, and in other countries meningitis only may be notifiable. However, based on notifications, in each of the last three years in England and Wales the case fatality rate has been 12%. This case fatality rate is an average of the rate for meningitis (about 7%) and septicaemia (about 20%). Age-specific death rates are highest in infants and the elderly; teenagers have the lowest mortality[20,21]. In the American laboratory-based study the overall case fatality rate was also 12%. Case fatality rates have declined marginally over the last twenty years. The recent slight decline could reflect higher awareness of meningococcal disease amongst the general public and family doctors (with recognition and treatment of the disease at an earlier stage), more efficient treatment of severe cases in hospital, more complete ascertainment and/or notification of surviving cases, or a combination of the three effects.

As well as mortality, long-term morbidity rates are also dependent on the severity of the acute illness. The development of new forms of treatment, such as the use of a variety of immunomodulators may produce some improvements, but use early enough in a fulminating infection will always remain a difficulty. The long-term solution to the problem lies in the development and deployment of effective vaccines. Accurate ascertainment of disease incidence is a prerequisite for determining vaccine efficacy.

REFERENCES

1. Jones DM, Mallard RH. Age incidence of meningococcal infection, England and Wales 1984–1991. J Infect 1993; 27: 83–8.
2. Cartwright KAV, Jones DM, Smith AJ, Stuart JM, Kaczmarski EB, Palmer SR. Influenza A and meningococcal disease. Lancet 1991; 338: 554–7.
3. Hubert B, Watier L, Garnerin P, Richardson S. Meningococcal disease and influenza-like syndrome; a new approach to an old question. J Infect Dis 1992; 166: 542–5.
4. Moore PS, Hierholzer J, Dewitt W. Respiratory viruses and mycoplasma as co-factors for epidemic group A meningococcal meningitis. JAMA 1990; 264: 1271–5.

5. Lystad A, Asen S. Epidemiology of meningococcal disease in Norway 1975–91. NIPH Ann 1991; *14*: 57–64.
6. Lassiter HA, Watson SW, Seifring ML, Tanner JE. Complement factor 9 deficiency in serum of neonates. J. Infect Dis 1992; *166*: 53–7.
7. Peltola H. Meningococcal disease: an old enemy in Scandinavia. In: Vedros NA ed. *Evolution of Mengingococcal Disease*. Volume I. Boca Raton; CRC Press Inc, 1987; 91–102.
8. Poolman JT, Lind I, Jonsdottir K, Frøholm LO, Jones DM, Zanen HC. Meningococcal serotypes and serogroup B disease in north-west Europe. Lancet 1986; *ii*: 555–8.
9. Davies LA. Assessing the value of different sources of information of meningococcal diseases. Community Med 1989; *11*: 239–46.
10. Cartwright KAV, Stuart JM, Noah ND. An outbreak of meningococcal disease in Gloucestershire. Lancet 1986; *ii*: 558–61.
11. Jones DM, Kaczmarski EB. Meningococcal infections in England and Wales (1992). Commun Dis Rep Rev 1993; *9*: R129–31.
12. Scholten RJPM, Bijlmer HA, Poolman JT. Kuifers B, Caugant DA, Alphen L, Dankert J, Valkenberg HA. Meningococcal disease in the Netherlands 1958–1990. A study increase in the incidence since 1982 potentially caused by new serotypes and subtypes of *Neisseria meningitidis*. Clin Infect Dis 1993; *16*: 237–46.
13. Maiden MCJ, Bygraves JA, McCarvil J, Feavers IM. Identification of meningococcal serosubtypes by the polymerase chain reaction. J Clin Microbiol 1992; *6*: 489–95.
14. McGuinness BT, Clarke IN, Lambden PR, Barlow AK, Poolman JT, Jones DM, Heckels JE. Point mutation in meningococcal *por A* gene associated with increased endemic disease. Lancet 1991; *337*: 514–17.
15. Holten E. Serotypes of *Neisseria meningitidis* isolated from patients in Norway during the first six months of 1978. J Clin Microbiol 1979; *9*: 186–8.
16. Jackson LA, Wenger JD. Laboratory-based surveillance of meningococcal disease in selected areas, United States 1989–91. MMWR 1993; *42*: 21–30.
17. Schlech WF, Ward JI, Band JD, Hightower A, Fraser DW, Broome CV. Bacterial meningitis in the United States, 1978 through 1981: the national bacterial meningitis surveillance study. JAMA 1985; *253*: 1749–54.
18. Pinner RW, Gellin BG, Bibb WF, Baker CN, Weaver R, Hunter SB *et al.* Meningococcal disease in the United States—1986. J Infect Dis 1991; *164*: 368–74.
19. Tarlow MJ, Geddes AM. Meningococcal meningitis or septicaemia: a plea for diagnostic clarity. Lancet 1992; *340*: 1481.
20. Beeson PB, Westerman E. Cerebro-spinal fever. Analysis of 3575 case reports, with special reference to sulphonamide therapy. Br Med J 1943; *i*: 497–500.
21. Banks HS. Meningococcosis. A protean disease. Lancet 1948; *ii*: 635–40.

7
Global Epidemiology of Meningococcal Disease

MARK ACHTMAN
Max-Planck Institut für molekulare Genetik, Berlin, Germany

PREAMBLE

All countries suffer from endemic meningococcal disease, primarily in children under the age of 5, at an annual rate of at least 1/100 000 population. In addition, some countries, predominantly but not exclusively in the developing world, suffer from occasional or even regular epidemics of meningitis. The underlying mechanisms leading to spread of meningococci and to epidemic outbreaks of meningococcal disease remain unknown. For example, amongst the Scandinavian countries Norway experienced a small outbreak of serogroup A disease in the late 1960s[1] followed by relatively high levels of serogroup B disease (approx. 10/100 000) which only began to decline slowly after 1988[2]. Finland was affected by a fairly large serogroup A epidemic in the mid-1970s (maximal annual incidence 15/100 000)[3]. In contrast, meningococcal epidemics were last registered in Sweden during World War I[3]. There is no obvious explanation why the epidemiology of the disease in these neighbouring countries should differ so much in modern times when travel and population movement are so widespread.

Documenting the spread of particular meningococcal strains through the world requires that we should be able to recognise them and differentiate them from other pathogenic (and non-pathogenic) meningococci. Traditionally this has been done by serological methods, but more powerful analytical tools are now available.

Meningococcal Disease. Edited by Keith Cartwright © 1995 John Wiley & Sons Ltd

Multi-locus enzyme electrophoresis (MLEE)

Multi-locus enzyme electrophoresis (MLEE) is a technique which uses the natural variation in electrophoretic mobility of diverse cytoplasmic allozymes (enzyme variants), and in some cases outer membrane proteins (OMPs), as markers for different genetic alleles on the bacterial chromosome. Indistinguishable bacteria are assigned to a common electrophoretic type (ET). MLEE analysis of thousands of individual meningococci has defined numerous ETs that differ from each other by at least one allozyme or OMP. Depending on the laboratory, groups of related ETs (as defined by cluster analysis) have been designated *subgroup* (serogroup A), *cluster* or *complex* (for serogroups B and C).

Each such genetic grouping (whether called subgroup, cluster or complex) is postulated to consist of bacteria descended from a single ancestral cell and which have undergone only minor genetic changes subsequently. Whereas numerous genetic groupings are detected among endemic isolates, most isolates from any one outbreak or epidemic belong to a common grouping. Furthermore, only a few genetic groupings of meningococci have been associated with epidemic disease[4–10]. Most epidemics since World War II, regardless of geographical location, have been caused by serogroup A bacteria of subgroups I, III, IV-1 and V[5], serogroup B bacteria of the ET-5 complex[9] or the A4 cluster[7,8], or by serogroup C bacteria of the ET-37 complex[4]. The epidemic spread of some of these groupings between countries and even continents has been demonstrated. The bacterial population genetics underlying this fairly consistent pattern of spread will be described in some detail.

However, even these 'epidemic' strains can cause endemic disease, as illustrated once again by the experience of the Scandinavian countries. Serogroup A subgroup III meningococci from an outbreak in Norway in 1969 were indistinguishable[1] from strains associated with an epidemic in Finland in the mid-1970s[11]. These two epidemics represent stages in the global spread of these bacteria (see below) from China via Russia to Brazil[12]. During the 1970s, a large proportion of the small number of cases of meningococcal disease in Sweden were also caused by subgroup III serogroup A bacteria[13]. Thus, at about the same time, subgroup III bacteria spread to three Scandinavian countries where they caused respectively a limited outbreak, an epidemic and no detectable increase in meningococcal disease incidence.

There have been attempts to define epidemic-specific 'clones' within serogroup A subgroups[11] but more recent data indicate that even though most isolates from any one epidemic usually belong to a single ET, meningococci are subject to sufficient genetic variation[14] that MLEE cannot resolve any collection of strains smaller than a subgroup, which is associated with epidemic spread[5].

Serological classification systems

Serological classification schemes were developed prior to and independently of MLEE[15]. Serogrouping is performed with polyclonal sera while serotype (based on the class 2 or 3 OMP) and the serosubtype (class 1 OMP) are determined using murine monoclonal antibodies (MAbs)[16,17]. Many serotyping MAbs appear to recognise epitopes which exist only in conformational form in nature, as these MAbs bind poorly to fully denatured class 2 or 3 OMPs in immunoblots. By contrast, many serosubtyping MAbs recognise linear epitopes within the two variable regions (VR1 and VR2) of the class 1 OMP[18,19]. A full serological description would therefore consist of serogroup, serotype and dual serosubtype, e.g. B15:P1.16,7. Unfortunately, MAbs for many serosubtypes present in nature are still lacking[19-22] and comprehensive serological typing is therefore not yet possible.

Though in special cases certain serological variants are characteristic of individual genetic groupings, recent DNA sequence data has confirmed that there is sufficient genetic variation amongst meningococcal strains such that it will be impossible to develop serotyping and serosubtyping schemes which are as reliable as MLEE for recognising the genetic groupings (Figure 7.1)[20]. Because this interpretation is not whole-heartedly accepted by all scientists, and because of the time-consuming nature of MLEE, numerous publications continue to appear containing serological data not supported by assignment of meningococcal strains to groupings defined by MLEE. Inconsistency of designations to genetic groupings in the past also renders it difficult to interpret some of the recent epidemiological literature. Re-evaluation of outbreaks and epidemics in the more distant past is hampered by the lack of surviving meningococcal strains.

This chapter focuses on epidemiology from the perspective of genetic groupings of meningococci. Interested readers wishing a more traditional presentation are referred to the superb older summaries by Peltola[3] or Vedros[23,24] and to recent reviews[25,26]. The molecular epidemiology of serogroup A disease has also been recently reviewed[27,28].

EPIDEMIC PATTERNS

Subgroup I

The data presented by Olyhoek *et al.*[11] has been subjected to a reinterpretation imposed by recognition of the fact that the subgroup is the basic unit of

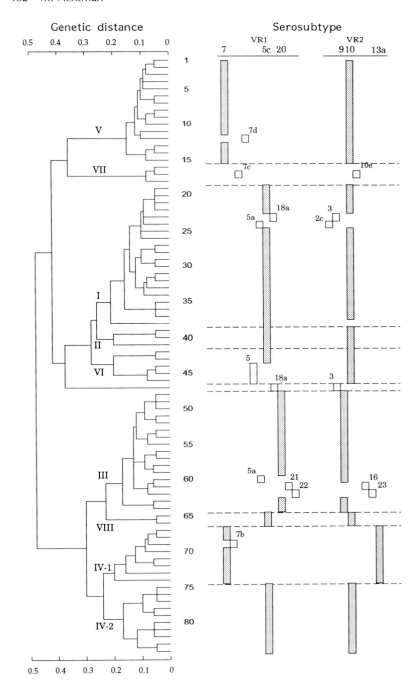

epidemic spread for serogroup A organisms[5]. The oldest identified strain of subgroup I was isolated in the UK in 1941. In the early 1960s, subgroup I bacteria were isolated during an epidemic in Niger, from cases of endemic disease in Algeria and Chad, and from US army personnel stationed in West Germany. In 1967, epidemic disease caused by subgroup I flared up in North Africa and the Mediterranean region and spread throughout West Africa by 1968–72. Subgroup I strains caused outbreaks among native Americans in Canada in the early 1970s, followed by outbreaks among 'skid row' inhabitants of the Pacific Northwest of the USA[11,29]. Epidemics in Nigeria and Rwanda in the late 1970s were caused by subgroup I[11], as were outbreaks amongst Maoris and Pacific Islanders in New Zealand in 1985[25], and in aboriginals in central Australia in the late 1980s[30] (Caugant DA, personal communication). During the 1970s subgroup I meningococci were isolated globally from cases of endemic disease[11].

Although most isolates from individual epidemics caused by subgroup I were of the ET-19 clone[5], other ETs were encountered commonly in particular outbreaks[5,11]. Bacteria from England (1941) and West Germany (1964) were ET-28, those from Niger and Chad in the early 1960s were clone I-3[11] (now ET-32[5]), and those from Canada and the Pacific Northwest were ET-23. Whereas most subgroup I isolates express the serosubtype epitopes P1.5c,10, ET-23 bacteria were P1.18a,3,6 and rare bacteria expressing the epitopes P1.5a,2c or having a deletion of the P1.10 epitope were also found (Figure 7.1)[5,20].

Subgroup III

Figure 7.2 summarises current knowledge of the patterns of epidemic spread of these bacteria. The oldest isolates are from a large epidemic in China in the

Figure 7.1 (*opposite*)   *Cluster analysis and serosubtypes of 84 electrophoretic types (ETs) of serogroup A meningococci. Left: dendrogam derived by cluster analysis showing the 84 ETs and the subgroups I to VIII[5]. Right: a composite diagram based on reactivities of individual isolates with MAbs to serosubtypes[4] and on DNA sequences[20]. The VR1 and VR2 regions of the porA gene determining the serosubtype have been sequenced from most but not all of the representatives of the 84 ETs[20]. Common VR serosubtypes are shown by shaded rectangles and with designations at the top while exceptional serosubtypes are indicated by open rectangles. No sequence data are available for ETs 16 and 18 and these are left blank. The blank space for VR2 of ET-38 reflects a deletion of that region. No MAbs are available which distinguish serosubtypes with the P1.5, P1.7 and P1.10 families and MAbs have not yet been isolated which react with P1.5c, P1.18a, P1.21 or P1.23. Within a subgroup, the PorA proteins were indicated as being the same when an identical porA gene had been sequenced from several ETs and the PorA protein from other bacteria migrated identically upon SDS PAGE and was indistinguishable with the available MAbs*

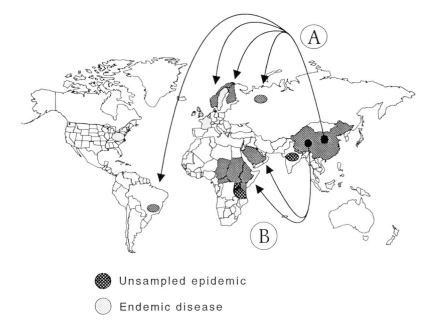

⬤ Unsampled epidemic

◯ Endemic disease

Figure 7.2   *Spread of serogroup A, subgroup III bacteria during two pandemic waves. A: first pandemic beginning in China in the mid-1960s and extending to Moscow and Norway in 1969 followed by Finland and Brazil in the mid-1970s. B: second pandemic beginning in China and Nepal in the early 1980s, followed by Saudi Arabia in 1987 and East Africa as of 1988. Epidemics occurred in India (1985) and Tanzania (1989) which have not been sampled but which fit into the same pattern of spread. In addition, the few cases of disease caused by bacteria imported from Mecca to the USA, England and France have been summarised, together with cases from Sweden, as 'endemic disease'*

mid-1960s[5]. In 1969 these organisms caused an epidemic in Moscow[5] and an outbreak in western Norway[1]. There were no bacteria available for testing from a serogroup A epidemic which broke out in the same year in Romania[31]. In the mid-1970s subgroup III bacteria caused epidemics in Finland and Brazil[11] and were the most common meningococcal strains to be isolated from cases of endemic disease in Sweden[13]. In the early 1980s subgroup III bacteria caused an epidemic in Nepal[11] and an increase in disease in China[5]. No bacteria have been tested from cases occurring during an epidemic in northern India in 1985.

In 1987 subgroup III bacteria caused an outbreak during the annual Haj (pilgrimage to Mecca, Saudi Arabia) which is attended by Muslim pilgrims from most countries[32]. Approximately 10% of the estimated 1000 pilgrims from the USA carried subgroup III bacteria in the nasopharynx on their return[33]. Isolated cases of disease caused by subgroup III were reported shortly thereafter from England[5,34], France[35,36], Israel[5,37], and The Gambia[38,39]. Serogroup A disease was also noted in Qatar[40] and Egypt[32]. Subgroup III epidemics broke out in 1988 in Sudan[13], Chad[32] and Ethiopia[38], followed by epidemics in 1989 in Kenya, Tanzania[41] and in 1992 in the Central African Republic[42]. Although it has been claimed that subgroup III bacteria had been isolated (once) in Africa prior to the epidemic in the Haj[39], this has since been disputed[43].

Subgroup III is very homogeneous and most reported isolates have been assigned to ET-48 and serosubtype P1.20,9 (formerly called P1.x,9), expressing pili with both class I and IIa epitopes[5,12,20]. Subgroup III bacteria have also been fairly homogenous when examined by pulse-field gel electrophoresis[44] and by DNA fingerprinting[39,45]. Lipopolysaccharide (LPS) immunotyping has disclosed more variation and isolates expressing L9, L10, L11, L12 or L13 immunotypes have all been found[12]. Two genetic changes have been documented during spread from Asia to Mecca, namely in an *opa* gene and in the IgA_1 protease[46].

Subgroup IV-1

Subgroup IV-1 is associated with different epidemiological patterns than are subgroups I and III. Almost all endemic isolates from West Africa since the early 1960s belong to subgroup IV-1[11] despite two waves of epidemic disease caused by subgroup I in the 1960s and 1970s. In addition, some isolates from an epidemic in Niger in the early 1960s and all isolates from epidemics in West Africa in the early 1980s belonged to subgroup IV-1[11]. All subgroup IV-1 bacteria thus far isolated have come from West Africa[5,11], with the exception of four Indian strains[39].

Many meningococci were isolated from patients and healthy carriers in The Gambia during the epidemic of 1982–3 and thereafter. All serogroup A meningococci from patients and carriers which were tested were of subgroup IV-1, and essentially all meningococci isolated from diseased patients were of serogroup A[47]. These bacteria resemble other subgroup IV-1 isolates in that they are largely homogeneous both in serosubtype, P1.7,13a[5,20,47] (Figure 7.1), and in LOS immunotype (L9); when piliated, they react with MAb to pilin epitope I[5,47].

Subgroup V

Subgroup V bacteria have only been isolated in China, where they caused an epidemic during the 1970s[5]. They express P1.7,10 and their pili react with MAb to epitope IIb[5]. As with subgroup IV-1 strains, it still remains unclear why these bacteria have not spread from China, and conversely, why subgroup I and IV-1 bacteria have never been isolated in China.

ET-5 complex

Serogroup B bacteria of the ET-5 complex seem to have been rare prior to 1970. Since then they have been responsible for elevated disease levels in a number of countries[9,48]. Retrospective analyses show that these bacteria were common as causes of meningococcal disease in Norway and Spain from the early 1970s through to the early 1990s[48]. ET-5 complex bacteria caused an epidemic in Cuba in the early 1980s[9] and in Iquique, Chile[49] followed by an epidemic in Brazil in the late 1980s[50]. ET-5 strains have been isolated from diverse sites within Europe and the Americas[9,51] and in a number of countries their presence has been documented several years prior to the occurrence of outbreaks[48,50]. The ET-5 complex has been associated with different serological markers: bacteria from Norway tend to be 15:P1.16, those from Spain and Brazil 4:P1.15 and those from Iquique 15:P1.3. In the UK, many of these bacteria have been 15:P1.16 and have been sulphonamide-resistant; such bacteria have been responsible for localised outbreaks[52]. Due to the variability in serological markers and the proven existence of these bacteria in several countries prior to elevation of disease rates, it is impossible to reconstruct their patterns of spread.

A4 cluster

Though there has been no analysis dedicated exclusively to the epidemiology of disease caused by the A4 cluster, comparison of different sources of epidemiological data indicate that these bacteria caused numerous cases of disease in the 1970s and 1980s. The A4 cluster describes a group of meningococci, often serogroup B and type 2b, isolated between 1974 and 1984 in the USA and between 1978 and 1980 in South Africa[7]. Strains of the same clone were also isolated in Canada and in several European countries at about the same time. Most B2b meningococci belong to the A4 cluster[7,8]. Recently, serogroup C bacteria of the A4 cluster have caused elevated disease levels in Brazil[53]. The serological distinction between serotypes 2a, 2b and 2c was ignored in earlier analyses and it is not possible now to reconstruct just how widespread B2b bacteria were. The available data suggests that they may also have been common in the 1970s in Canada[54] and England and Wales[55].

ET-37 complex

Bacteria of the ET-37 complex caused numerous cases of disease in US military recruits in the late 1960s[4,56] and have been isolated frequently from cases of endemic disease in the USA, Europe and Mali, West Africa[4,7,8,57]. Epidemics in Burkina Faso, West Africa, in the early 1980s and recent outbreaks in Canada[58] and Mali[4] have also been caused by strains of this complex. Many of these bacteria are 2a:P1.5,2 or C:2a:P1.5,y and almost all express pili which react with MAb to the class IIb epitope only[4]. In some countries, including the UK and Italy, almost all C2a bacteria belong to the ET-37 complex[4,59].

GENETIC VARIABILITY IN MENINGOCOCCI

As is evident from the above, the correlation between genetic grouping and serological properties is incomplete. Serotypes and serosubtypes of bacterial strains belonging to the ET-5 complex, A4 cluster and the ET-37 complex are somewhat variable. Whereas most ET-5 complex and A4 cluster meningococci tested to date have been serogroup B, some have been assigned to serogroup C or to other serogroups. Similarly, although most ET-37 complex bacteria are serogroup C, some have been assigned to serogroup B or other serogroups. Serogroup A meningococci seem to be much more homogeneous than serogroup B or C strains, but subgroup VI bacteria from East Germany may be serogroup A, B or C[4,51]. A serogroup B strain of subgroup III (which is otherwise exclusively associated with serogroup A) has been isolated in Brazil[4]. The genetic basis for changes in capsular polysaccharide and serotype remain unknown but analyses of serosubtype variants have shown that the class 1 protein *porA* gene is a mosaic, reflecting the results of genetic recombination[20,22]. Meningococci are naturally transformable and recombinational events have also been implicated to explain the variability of the Opa proteins[14,60] and IgA$_1$ protease[46,61].

Long-term studies of meningococci isolated from particular regions have shown changes with time. In China, sequential epidemics and periods of increased disease incidence between the mid-1960s and the mid-1980s were associated respectively with serogroup A bacteria of serogroups III, V and III[5]. In Africa, successive epidemic waves from the early 1960s to the early 1990s were associated with serogroup A bacteria of subgroups I (in the early 1960s), I (again, in the late 1960s), IV-1 and III[5,11], although occasional cases of disease and even local outbreaks have been caused by unrelated meningococcal strains, especially in West Africa (see ET-37 complex above).

In Norway, a serogroup A subgroup III outbreak in the late 1960s was followed in the early 1970s by a protracted period of high disease incidence caused by ET-5 complex (and to a minor extent ET-37 complex) strains[48]. B2b (A4 cluster?) meningococci were isolated frequently in The Netherlands between the 1960s and the late 1970s but the bacteria isolated at various times differed in electrophoretotype[62]. For some serogroup A bacteria, these patterns can be explained by epidemic spread but in other cases they seem to reflect the influence of unknown factors leading to clonal expansion of pre-existing strains which are then reflected in increased disease levels. The slow sequential replacement of clonal groupings has been attributed to herd immunity[26] but the available evidence suggests that natural immunity triggered by exposure to meningococci or by immunisation with OMP vaccines is effective against unrelated bacteria, despite antigenic diversity[12,46,63].

Local and even extensive spread of recombinant and mutant bacteria has been observed. Meningococci with single nucleotide changes in the P1.16 VR2 epitope of the serosubtype class 1 protein have been found in England, and mutants with a small deletion in P1.16 have been found in Norway[64,65]. Whereas serogroup A, subgroup I bacteria are normally P1.5c,10, a P1.18a, 3 recombinant variant was common in The Netherlands and caused outbreaks in North America[5,20]. Subgroup III bacteria underwent at least two independent changes, one in an *opa* gene and another in the *iga* gene, in spreading from Asia in the early 1980s to Saudi Arabia in 1987[46]. Such variants may be selected by immunological pressures[26,64,65], but it has also been argued that variants may be selected randomly[14].

SECONDARY FACTORS

Carriage of meningococci does not necessarily lead to disease. Classical studies in US army recruits showed that five of 13 recruits (38%) whose sera lacked bactericidal antibodies and who became carriers of serogroup C, ET-37 complex meningococci manifested clinical disease[66]. Carriage of meningococci is rare in inter-epidemic periods in West Africa[67], suggesting that population-wide acquired immunity may be rare at the beginning of an epidemic, if nasopharyngeal carriage of meningococci is an important factor in the development of a protective immune response.

During the (subgroup IV-1 serogroup A) epidemic of 1982–3 in The Gambia, the carriage rate was approximately 15% in spot surveys and the cumulative disease rate was slightly over 1% in the region investigated most intensively[67,68]. Children who developed meningococcal disease were shown to have possessed bactericidal antibodies prior to the outbreak of disease[68]. Acute phase sera from patients and also sera from non-carriers who subsequently became healthy carriers lacked antibodies to IgA_1 protease[69] as well as bactericidal antibodies[12]. Most sera from persistent carriers possessed both types of antibodies. Given the higher frequency of carriers than of diseased patients, these observations indicate that during an epidemic, acquisition of bacteria by immunologically naive individuals results in carriage and production of protective antibodies while only a small proportion of the colonised individuals go on to develop disease. In the African environment, carriage of all meningococci, even non-pathogenic serogroups, is rare in inter-epidemic periods whereas during an outbreak carriage of both pathogenic and non-pathogenic serogroups is common[67]. Serogroup B bacteria are very rare in the African Meningitis Belt, even during an epidemic.

Carriage rates during periods of epidemic disease

These observations raise two questions.

1. Why does the carriage rate increase so dramatically during an epidemic?
2. Why do some individuals become sick rather than becoming healthy carriers?

Several different mechanisms have indeed been proposed to explain why epidemic disease happens during periods of elevated carriage. Increased carriage rates of pathogenic meningococci are probably a prerequisite for epidemic disease. After the outbreak of serogroup A, subgroup III meningococcal disease in Haj pilgrims in 1987, the same bacteria were imported to numerous countries (see above) where they caused only a few cases of disease. Similarly, most cases of meningococcal meningitis in Sweden during the 1970s were caused by subgroup III bacteria, but the incidence of meningococcal disease remained low. These observations may reflect carriage of subgroup III bacteria by only a small proportion of the healthy populations of those countries. Had a higher rate of carriage occurred, then more cases might have resulted. However, no mechanisms have yet been suggested to account for differences in carriage rates of the same bacterial clones in different countries.

Carriage or disease?

Based on data obtained in a subgroup I outbreak, Griffiss hypothesised that disease arises from co-infection with a pathogenic meningococcus and an enteric organism which stimulates cross-reacting IgA[70,71]. IgA blocks binding of IgG and IgM and thus prevents complement activation. In support of this hypothesis, bacteria with cell surface antigens cross-reactive with meningococcal capsular polysaccharide and lipopolysaccharide have been isolated from contacts of diseased individuals[29], and elevated IgA levels have been recorded in patients suffering from epidemic disease[70].

In a case–control study during a subgroup III epidemic in Chad, Moore implicated upper respiratory infection (possibly associated with mucosal *Mycoplasma* infection) as a potential factor contributing to disease rather than oropharyngeal carriage[72]. Other analyses have implicated antecedent infection with influenza A virus based on elevated antibody levels to influenza among meningococcal disease patients[73] and on epidemiological associations[5,73,74]. Infection with influenza A virus has numerous effects on the human immune system[75] and *in vitro*, direct adhesion of meningococci to influenza virus-infected Hep-2 cells has been shown[76]. All three mechanisms implicate antecedent or concurrent infection with a virus or another bacterium as being of importance in the development of disease, rather than simply a lack of bactericidal antibodies. The relative importance of these three mechanisms for inducing immunosusceptibility in previously immunocompetent individuals remains to be determined. Possibly these secondary factors contribute individually or jointly towards the development of outbreaks.

Though deficiency of terminal complement components is a well-documented contributory factor to endemic meningococcal disease[77], complement deficiencies are too rare to account for epidemic disease.

SUMMARY

The availability of MLEE has led to a recognition that epidemic meningococcal disease is caused by only a few 'epidemic' clonal groupings, which are somewhat variable in their serological properties. Availability of standard reference strains in laboratories undertaking MLEE (and serological characterisation) will lead to the use of consistent and uniform designations for these epidemic clonal groupings. Outbreaks caused by an epidemic clonal grouping are a cause for alarm whereas simple import of these bacteria to a new locale need not necessarily result in elevated disease levels.

Endemic disease is associated with a greater diversity of meningococcal strains and the endemic disease rate will probably remain fairly low while most cases of disease are caused by non-epidemic clones. Our understanding of the mechanisms which cause epidemic disease is still fragmentary and it is still not yet possible to predict future disease rates reliably.

REFERENCES

1. Hjetland R, Caugant DA, Hofstad T, Frøholm LO, Selander RK. Serogroup A *Neisseria meningitidis* of clone III-1 in Western Norway, 1969–73. Scand J Infect Dis 1990; 22: 241–2.
2. Lystad A, Aasen S. The epidemiology of meningococcal disease in Norway 1975–91. NIPH Annals 1991; 14: 57–66.
3. Peltola H. Meningococcal disease: still with us. Rev Infect Dis 1983; 5: 71–91.
4. Wang J-F, Caugant DA, Morelli G, Koumaré B, Achtman M. Antigenic and epidemiological properties of the ET-37 complex of *Neisseria meningitidis*. J Infect Dis 1993; 167: 1320–9.
5. Wang J-F, Caugant DA, Li X, Hu X, Poolman JT, Crowe BA *et al*. Clonal and antigenic analysis of serogroup A *Neisseria meningitidis* with particular

reference to epidemiological features of epidemic meningitis in China. Infect Immun 1992; *60*: 5267–82.

6. Caugant DA, Kristiansen B-E, Frøholm LO, Bøvre K, Selander RK. Clonal diversity of *Neisseria meningitidis* from a population of asymptomatic carriers. Infect Immun 1988; *56*: 2060–8.

7. Caugant DA, Mocca LF, Frasch CE, Frøholm LO, Zollinger WD, Selander RK. Genetic structure of *Neisseria meningitidis* populations in relation to serogroup, serotype, and outer membrane protein pattern. J Bacteriol 1987; *169*: 2781–92.

8. Caugant DA, Zollinger WD, Mocca LF, Frasch CE, Whittam TS, Frøholm LO *et al.* Genetic relationships and clonal population structure of serotype 2 strains of *Neisseria meningitidis*. Infect Immun 1987; *55*: 1503–13.

9. Caugant DA, Frøholm LO, Bøvre K, Holten E, Frasch CE, Mocca LF *et al.* Intercontinental spread of a genetically distinctive complex of clones of *Neisseria meningitidis* causing epidemic disease. Proc Natl Acad Sci USA 1986; *83*: 4927–31.

10. Caugant DA, Bøvre K, Gaustad P, Bryn K, Holten E, Høiby EA *et al.* Multilocus genotypes determined by enzyme electrophoresis of *Neisseria meningitidis* isolated from patients with systemic disease and from healthy carriers. J Gen Microbiol 1986; *132*: 641–52.

11. Olyhoek T, Crowe BA, Achtman M. Clonal population structure of *Neisseria meningitidis* serogroup A isolated from epidemics and pandemics between 1915 and 1983. Rev Infect Dis 1987; *9*: 665–92.

12. Achtman M, Kusecek B, Morelli G, Eickmann K, Wang J, Crowe B *et al.* A comparison of the variable antigens expressed by clone IV-1 and subgroup III of *Neisseria meningitidis* serogroup A. J Infect Dis 1992; *165*: 53–68.

13. Salih MAM, Danielsson D, Bäckman A, Caugant DA, Achtman M, Olcén P. Characterization of epidemic and non-epidemic *Neisseria meningitidis* serogroup A strains from Sudan and Sweden. J Clin Microbiol 1990; *28*: 1711–19.

14. Achtman M. Clonal spread of serogroup A meningococci. A paradigm for the analysis of microevolution in bacteria. Mol Microbiol 1994; *11*: 15–22.

15. Frasch CE, Zollinger WD, Poolman JT. Serotype antigens of *Neisseria meningitidis* and a proposed scheme for designation of serotypes. Rev Infect Dis 1985; *7*: 504–10.

16. Abdillahi H, Poolman JT. Whole-cell ELISA for typing *Neisseria meningitidis* with monoclonal antibodies. FEMS Microbiol Lett 1987; *48*: 367–71.

17. Abdillahi H, Poolman JT. *Neisseria meningitidis* group B serosubtyping using monoclonal antibodies in whole-cell ELISA. Microb Pathog 1988; *4*: 27–32.

18. McGuinness B, Barlow AK, Clarke IN, Farley JE, Anilionis A, Poolman JT *et al.* Deduced amino acid sequences of class 1 protein (PorA) from three strains of *Neisseria meningitidis*. Synthetic peptides define the epitopes responsible for serosubtyping specificity. J Exp Med 1990; *171*: 1871–82.

19. McGuinness BT, Lambden PR, Heckels JE. Class 1 outer membrane protein of *Neisseria meningitidis*: epitope analysis of the antigenic diversity between strains, implications for subtype definition and molecular epidemiology. Mol Microbiol 1993; *7*: 505–14.

20. Suker J, Feavers IM, Achtman M, Morelli G, Wang J-F, Maiden MCJ. The *porA* gene in serogroup A meningococci: evolutionary stability and mechanism of genetic variation. Mol Microbiol 1994; *12*: 253–65.

21. Maiden MCJ, Bygraves JA, McCarvil J, Feavers IM. Identification of meningococcal serosubtypes by the polymerase chain reaction. J Clin Microbiol 1992; *30*: 2835–41.

22. Feavers IM, Heath AB, Bygraves JA, Maiden MCJ. Role of horizontal genetic exchange in the antigenic variation of the class 1 outer membrane protein of *Neisseria meningitidis*. Mol Microbiol 1992; *6*: 489–95.

23. Vedros NA, ed. *Evolution of Meningococcal Disease*. Vol I. Boca Raton, FL: CRC Press Inc, 1987; 1–142.

24. Vedros NA, ed. *Evolution of Meningococcal Disease*. Vol II. Boca Raton, FL: CRC Press Inc, 1987; 1–149.

25. Schwartz B, Moore PS, Broome CV. Global epidemiology of meningococcal disease. Clin Microbiol Rev 1989; *2* Suppl: S118–24.

26. Moore PS. Meningococcal meningitis in sub-Saharan Africa: A model for the epidemic process. Clin Infect Dis 1992; *14*: 515–25.

27. Achtman M. Molecular epidemiology of epidemic bacterial meningitis. Rev Med Microbiol 1990; *1*: 29–38.

28. Achtman M. Clonal properties of meningococci from epidemic meningitis. Trans R Soc Trop Med Hyg 1991; *85*, Suppl 1: 24–31.

29. Counts GW, Gregory DF, Spearman JG, Barrett AL, Filice GA, Holmes KK *et al*. Group A meningococcal disease in the US Pacific Northwest: epidemiology, clinical features, and effect of a vaccine control program. Rev Infect Dis 1984; *6*: 640–8.

30. Patel MS, Merianos A, Hanna JN, Vartto K, Tait P, Morey F *et al*. Epidemic meningococcal meningitis in central Australia, 1987–1991. Med J Aust 1993; *158*: 336–40.

31. Kuzemenska P, Kriz B. Epidemiology of meningococcal disease in central and eastern Europe. In: Vedros NA, ed. *Evolution of Meningococcal Disease*. Volume I. Boca Raton, FL: CRC Press Inc, 1987; 103–37.

32. Moore PS, Reeves MW, Schwartz B, Gellin BG, Broome CV. Intercontinental spread of an epidemic group A *Neisseria meningitidis* strain. Lancet 1989; *ii*: 260–3.

33. Moore PS, Harrison LH, Talzak EE, Ajello GW, Broome CV. Group A meningococcal carriage in travelers returning from Saudi Arabia. JAMA 1988; *260*: 2686–9.

34. Jones DM, Sutcliffe EM. Group A meningococcal disease in England associated with the Haj. J Infect 1990; *21*: 21–5.

35. Denamur E, Pautard JC, Ducroix JP, Masmoudi K, Eb F, Riou JY *et al*. Meningococcal disease due to group A *Neisseria meningitidis* in contacts of Mecca pilgrims. Lancet 1987; *ii*: 1211.

36. Riou JY, Caugant DA, Selander RK, Poolman JT, Guibourdenche M, Collatz E. Characterization of *Neisseria meningitidis* serogroup A strains from an outbreak in France by serotype, serosubtype, multilocus enzyme genotype and outer membrane protein pattern. Eur J Clin Microbiol Infect Dis 1991; *10*: 405–9.

37. Slater PE, Roitman M, Costin C. Meningitis in Israel: an imported outbreak. Israel J Med Sci 1989; *25*: 41–2.

38. Haimanot RT, Caugant DA, Fekadu D, Bjune G, Belete B, Frøholm LO *et al*. Characteristics of serogroup A *Neisseria meningitidis* responsible for an epidemic in Ethiopia, 1988–89. Scand J Infect Dis 1990; *22*: 171–4.

39. Bjorvatn B, Hassan-King M, Greenwood B, Haimanot RT, Fekade D, Sperber G. DNA fingerprinting in the epidemiology of African serogroup A *Neisseria meningitidis*. Scand J Infect Dis 1992; *24*: 323–32.

40. Novelli VM, Lewis RG, Dawood ST. Epidemic group A meningococcal disease in pilgrims. Lancet 1987; *ii*: 863.

41. Anon. Epidemic meningococcal disease – Kenya and Tanzania: Recommendations for travellers, 1990. MMWR 1990; *39*: 13–14.

42. Guibourdenche M, Caugant DA, Herve V *et al.* Characteristics of serogroup A *Neisseria meningitidis* strains isolated in Central African Republic in February 1992. Eur J Clin Microbiol Infect Dis 1994; *13*: 174–7

43. Achtman M, Wang J-F. DNA fingerprinting of serogroup A meningococci. Scand J Infect Dis 1993; *25*: 161–2.

44. Bygraves JA, Maiden MCJ. Analyses of the clonal relationships between strains of *Neisseria meningitidis* by pulsed field gel electrophoresis. J Gen Microbiol 1992; *138*: 523–31.

45. Olyhoek T, Crowe BA, Wall RA, Achtman M. Comparison of clonal analysis and DNA restriction analysis for typing of *Neisseria meningitidis*. Microb Pathog 1988; *4*: 45–51.

46. Morelli G, del Valle J, Lammel CJ, Pohlner J, Müller K, Blake M *et al.* Immunogenicity and evolutionary variability of epitopes within IgA$_1$ protease from serogroup A *Neisseria meningitidis*. Mol Microbiol 1994; *11*: 175–87.

47. Crowe BA, Wall RA, Kusecek B, Neumann B, Olyhoek T, Abdillahi H *et al.* Clonal and variable properties of *Neisseria meningitidis* isolated from cases and carriers during and after an epidemic in the Gambia, West Africa. J Infect Dis 1989; *159*: 686–700.

48. Caugant DA, Frøholm LO, Sacchi CT, Selander RK. Genetic structure and epidemiology of serogroup B *Neisseria meningitidis*. In: Achtman M, Kohl P, Marchal C, Morelli G, Seiler A, Thiesen B, eds. *Neisseriae 1990*. Berlin: Walter de Gruyter, 1991; 37–42.

49. Cruz C, Pavez G, Aguilar E, Grawe L, Cam J, Mendez F *et al.* Serotype-specific outbreak of group B meningococcal disease in Iquique, Chile. Epidemiol Infect 1990; *105*: 119–26.

50. Sacchi CT, Pessoa LL, Ramos SR, Milagres LG, Camargo MCC, Hidalgo NTR *et al.* Ongoing group B *Neisseria meningitidis* epidemic in Sao Paulo, Brazil, due to increased prevalence of a single clone of the ET-5 complex. J Clin Microbiol 1992; *30*: 1734–8.

51. Grahlow W-D, Caugant DA, Høiby EA, Selander RK. Occurrence of clones of the ET-5 complex of *Neisseria meningitidis* in the German Democratic Republic. Z Klin Med 1990; *45*: 947–50.

52. Poolman JT, Lind I, Jónsdóttir K, Frøholm LO, Jones DM, Zanen HC. Meningococcal serotypes and serogroup B disease in North-west Europe. Lancet 1986; *ii*: 555–8.

53. Sacchi CT, Zanella RC, Caugant DA, Frasch CE, Hidalgo NT, Milagres LG *et al.* Emergence of a new clone of serogroup C *Neisseria meningitidis* in Sao Paulo, Brazil. J Clin Microbiol 1992; *30*: 1282–6.

54. Ashton FE, Ryan JA, Diena BB. Serotypes and major outer membrane proteins of *Neisseria meningitidis* strains isolated in Canada. In: Vedros NA, ed. *Evolution of Meningococcal Disease*. Volume I. Boca Raton, FL: CRC Press Inc, 1987; 57–63.

55. Jones DM, Abbott JD. Meningococcal diseases in England and Wales. In: Vedros NA, ed. *Evolution of Meningococcal Disease*. Volume I. Boca Raton, FL: CRC Press Inc, 1987; 65–90.

56. Brundage JF, Zollinger WD. Evolution of meningococcal disease epidemiology in the U.S. Army. In: Vedros NA, ed. *Evolution of meningococcal disease*. Volume I. Boca Raton, FL: CRC Press Inc, 1987; 5–25.

57. Pinner RW, Gellin BG, Bibb WF, Baker CN, Weaver R, Hunter SB *et al.* Meningococcal disease in the United States – 1986. J Infect Dis 1991; *164*: 368–74.

58. Ashton FE, Ryan JA, Borczyk A, Caugant DA, Mancino L, Huang D. Emergence of a virulent clone of *Neisseria meningitidis* serotype 2a that is

associated with meningococcal group A disease in Canada. J Clin Microbiol 1991; *29*: 2489–93.

59. Mastrantonio P, Congiu ME, Selander RK, Caugant DA. Genetic relationships among strains of *Neisseria meningitidis* causing disease in Italy, 1984–7. Epidemiol Infect 1991; *106*: 143–50.

60. Hobbs MM, Seiler A, Achtman M, Cannon JG. Microevolution within a clonal population of pathogenic bacteria: recombination, gene duplication and horizontal genetic exchange in the *opa* gene family of *Neisseria meningitidis*. Mol Microbiol 1994; *12*: 171–80.

61. Lomholt H, Poulsen K, Caugant DA, Kilian M. Molecular polymorphism and epidemiology of *Neisseria meningitidis* immunoglobulin A1 proteases. Proc Natl Acad Sci USA 1992; *89*: 2120–4.

62. Caugant DA, Bol P, Høiby EA, Zanen HC, Frøholm LO. Clones of serogroup B *Neisseria meningitidis* causing systemic disease in the Netherlands, 1958–1986. J Infect Dis 1990; *162*: 867–74.

63. Rosenqvist E, Høiby EA, Wedege E, Kusecek B, Achtman M. The 5C protein of *Neisseria meningitidis* is highly immunogenic in humans and stimulates bactericidal antibodies. J Infect Dis 1993; *167*: 1065–73.

64. Rosenqvist E, Høiby, EA, Wedege E, Caugant DA, Frøholm LO, McGuiness BT *et al.* A new variant of serosubtype P1.16 in serogroup B *Neisseria meningitidis* associated with increased resistance to bactericidal antibodies. Microb Pathog 1993; *15*: 197–205.

65. McGuinness BT, Clarke IN, Lambden PR, Barlow AK, Poolman JT, Jones DM *et al.* Point mutation in meningococcal *porA* gene associated with increased endemic disease. Lancet 1991; *337*: 514–17.

66. Goldschneider I, Gotschlich EC, Artenstein MS. Human immunity to the meningococcus I. The role of humoral antibodies. J Exp Med 1969; *129*: 1307–26.

67. Hassan-King MKA, Wall RA, Greenwood BM. Meningococcal carriage, meningococcal disease and vaccination. J Infect 1988; *16*: 55–9.

68. Greenwood BM, Greenwood AM, Bradley AK, Williams K, Hassan-King M, Shenton FC *et al.* Factors influencing susceptibility to meningococcal disease during an epidemic in the Gambia, West Africa. J Infect 1987; *14*: 167–84.

69. Brooks GF, Lammel CJ, Blake MS, Kusecek B, Achtman M. Antibodies against IgA$_1$ protease are stimulated both by clinical disease and by asymptomatic carriage of serogroup A *Neisseria meningitidis*. J Infect Dis 1992; *166*: 1316–21.

70. Griffiss JM, Brandt BL, Jarvis GA. Natural immunity to *Neisseria meningitidis*. In: Vedros NA, ed. *Evolution of Meningococcal Disease*, Volume II. Boca Raton, FL: CRC Press Inc, 1987; 99–119.

71. Griffiss JM. Epidemic meningococcal disease: synthesis of a hypothetical immunoepidemiologic model. Rev Infect Dis 1982; *4*: 159–72.

72. Moore PS, Hierholzer J, DeWitt W, Gouan K, Djoré D, Lippeveld T *et al.* Respiratory viruses and *Mycoplasma* as cofactors for epidemic group A meningococcal meningitis. JAMA. 1990; *264*: 1271–5.

73. Cartwright KAV, Jones DM, Smith AJ, Stuart JM, Kaczmarski EB, Palmer SR. Influenza A and meningococcal disease. Lancet 1991; *338*: 554–7.

74. Hubert B, Watier L, Garnerin P, Richardson S. Meningococcal disease and influenza-like syndrome: a new approach to an old question. J Infect Dis 1992; *166*: 542–5.

75. Shaw MW, Arden NH, Maassab HF. New aspects of influenza viruses. Clin Microbiol Rev 1992; *5*: 74–92.

76. Kostyuukova NN, Alexeev AB, Gorlina MK *et al.* A study on meningococcal

colonization of epithelium. In: Achtman M, Kohl P, Marchal C, Morelli G, Seiler A, Thiesen B, eds. *Neisseriae 1990*. Berlin: Walter de Gruyter, 1991; 609–14.
77. Figueroa JE, Densen P. Infectious diseases associated with complement deficiencies. Clin Microbiol Rev 1991; 4: 359–95.

8
The Clinical Spectrum of Meningococcal Disease

NEIL STEVEN and MARTIN WOOD
Department of Infection and Tropical Medicine, Birmingham
Heartlands Hospital, Birmingham, UK

INTRODUCTION

Neisseria meningitidis typically causes an acute infective illness. By far the most common presentation is with acute purulent meningitis but less commonly, patients present with meningococcal septicaemia, a catastrophic constellation of fever, fulminant haemorrhagic rash and shock of frighteningly rapid onset. The clinical syndromes of meningitis, meningococcaemia and meningococcal septicaemia overlap, as illustrated by a paediatric series[1]. Most children (93%) had meningitis; this included 37% who had both meningitis and bacteraemia but 7% had bacteraemia without evidence of meningitis. A tenth were shocked.

Benign and chronic meningococcaemia

The terms 'benign' and 'chronic' meningococcaemia have been used interchangeably by some authors. However, they are best used to describe quite different, albeit overlapping, clinical patterns. Each is confirmed by a blood culture positive for *N. meningitidis*. Benign or occult meningococcaemia describes an acute febrile illness, often with an exanthem, indistinguishable from many, much more common, nondescript viral illnesses, but without features of meningitis or septicaemia. It may progress to more serious disease but spontaneous resolution is known. The symptoms of chronic

Meningococcal Disease. Edited by Keith Cartwright © 1995 John Wiley & Sons Ltd

meningococcaemia are intermittent or persistent fever, arthralgia and rash, which, by convention, last longer than one week. It is a rare cause of pyrexia of unknown origin. Organisms may localise to cause meningitis or carditis, but the chronic symptoms respond rapidly to appropriate antibiotic therapy.

Less common manifestations

Other organs may be involved in patients with acute meningococcal meningitis, septicaemia or meningococcaemia, either at presentation or later as complications. These include the joints, the pericardium, the skin and the eye. Symptoms can arise either through direct metastatic infection or as a result of immune mechanisms. In one series[1], 27% of children with *N. meningitidis* infections had one or more extra-meningeal complication. Occasionally, acute meningococcal infection may be localised solely to an extra-meningeal site, and present as septic arthritis, conjunctivitis, pericarditis, pneumonia or pelvic infection.

ACUTE MENINGOCOCCAL DISEASE

Presentation

The common presenting symptoms are listed in Table 8.1[2–5]. They are generally non-specific, particularly in children under 5 years who make up the majority of cases. The most frequent symptoms are fever and chills, vomiting, lethargy and drowsiness, or irritability. Infants stop feeding. Confusion or coma may be the presenting symptoms in the context of an otherwise nondescript febrile illness. Older children and adults frequently complain of headache, even when meningococcaemia occurs without meningitis. The headache of meningitis is very severe and may be 'bursting' in nature. Photophobia and neck stiffness are less frequent complaints. A rash may have been noticed. Myalgia is described by a quarter of patients, and painful joints in about 8%. Abdominal symptoms—pain and diarrhoea—may occur. Rarely they are sufficiently prominent to suggest erroneously a diagnosis of gastroenteritis[6,7].

Seizures, either before or shortly after admission, are reported in up to 20% of cases. In most instances these appear to be simple febrile convulsions, that is generalised fits lasting less than 15 minutes occurring during periods of high fever in children under the age of 4 years. However, Voss et al.[5] described 19 children presenting with convulsions of whom two had focal fits and in another series[3], 29% of cases presenting with convulsions were children more than 4 years old. Kilpi et al.[8] noted an association between rapid onset of symptoms in bacterial meningitis and the occurrence of convulsions, at least in children older than one year.

Table 8.1   *Presenting symptoms of acute meningococcal disease*

Study	Olcén et al. 1979[2]	Donald et al. 1981[3]	Wong et al. 1989[4]	Voss et al. 1989[5]
Number of patients	69	298	100	122
Age range	5/12–65 y	3/52–69 y	6/52–13 y	under 14 y
Fever	96%	100%	71%	98%
Vomiting	61%	44%	34%	69%
Somnolence/lethargy/ drowsiness/irritability	57%			Majority
Headache	51%			34%
Skin rash	49%			
Photophobia				18%
Painful/stiff neck	23%			
Myalgia	23%			
Diarrhoea	13%		6%	
Abdominal pain	12%			
Joint pain	7%		8%	
Convulsions	1%	21%	8%	16%
Cough		27%	8%	
Rhinorrhoea			10%	
Onset <1 day	62%	59%		
<2 days		20%		82%
>2 days		19%		

Acute meningococcal infection is typically an illness of rapid onset. On presentation, about 60% of cases have had their symptoms for less than 24 hours. However, between 12% and 20% have had symptoms for more than 2 days, and durations of a week or more are described. An association between the duration of symptoms prior to presentation and the presence of a rash has been noted[3]; of those with symptoms for less than a day, 56% had a purpuric rash, compared with 30% of those with a 3 day history and none of those with a 4 day history. Kilpi *et al.*[9] prospectively investigated the pattern of onset in 286 children with bacterial meningitis, of whom 23% were infected with *Neisseria meningitidis*. Those with only a 1 day history were more likely to be comatose on admission and to have seizures than were those with longer histories, irrespective of the causative organism. A more prolonged onset of illness was found particularly in infants. Children with a long duration of symptoms were more likely to have symptoms of an upper respiratory tract infection and to have received pre-admission oral antibiotics than were those with a rapidly developing illness. This may reflect the mild and non-specific onset in these cases, rather than any effect of oral antibiotics on the clinical course.

About half of all patients with acute meningococcal infection describe prodromal symptoms in the week prior to hospital admission[2]. In most cases, symptoms suggest an upper respiratory tract infection, and include sore throat, coryza, cough, painful ears and conjunctivitis. A few describe fever only. The common presenting signs on admission are summarised in Table 8.2. Most patients look ill and are distressed. Oral herpes simplex re-activation may occur. Fever, usually between 38 °C and 41 °C, is almost universal among patients with acute meningococcal disease, although a few may be afebrile or even hypothermic, particularly in septicaemia.

The findings on examination and results of investigations may be grouped into three main areas: meningitis, the presence and appearance of a skin rash, and evidence of sepsis syndrome. Also noteworthy are those patients with occult meningococcaemia, in whom there is a remarkable dearth of features of serious disease.

Meningitis

The signs of meningeal irritation are neck stiffness and positive Kernig and Brudzinski signs[9]. Neck stiffness is detected as resistance to passive flexion or gentle lateral rolling of the head with the patient supine. It is caused by spasm of the paraspinal muscles and in extreme forms may produce opisthotonos. It is usually possible to be confident about the presence of neck stiffness but confusion may be caused by cervical spondylitis, cervical osteomyelitis and soft tissue inflammation—of which painful cervical lymphadenopathy is by far the most common. Kernig's sign is elicited by extension of the knee while the hip is flexed and the patient is supine. It is positive if knee extension causes pain in the back or neck. Brudzinski's sign is

Table 8.2   Signs of acute meningococcal disease

Study	Olcén et al. 1979[2]	Wong et al. 1989[4]
Number of patients	69	100
Age range	5/12–65 years	6/52–13 years
Fever	96%	71%
Stiff neck	76%	
Focal neurological deficit	3%	
Rash	75%	71%
Petechiae		49%
Purpura fulminans	71%	16%
Maculopapular rash		10%
Pustules		1%
Fully alert	9%	
Fatigued/somnolent	87%	
Unresponsive	4%	
Hypotension	23%	42%
Anuria	4%	

a reflex flexion of the hips and knees on neck flexion, with the patient sitting with legs outstretched.

Signs of meningeal irritation are present in most, but not all, cases of meningitis. Infants, who form a large proportion of the cases of meningococcal meningitis, frequently present with non-specific symptoms and without localising signs, although they may have a tense, bulging fontanelle. Meningitis may also occur without specific signs in patients with overwhelming meningococcal sepsis, and in elderly or immunocompromised individuals.

Though patients with meningococcal meningitis may be fully alert, most are lethargic, drowsy or confused. However, coma, or a marked reduction in the level of consciousness, occurs in a minority. By contrast Carpenter and Petersdorf[10] reported that 58% of patients with pneumococcal meningitis were unresponsive on admission, or responded only to pain.

The cerebrospinal fluid

In meningococcal meningitis cerebrospinal fluid (CSF) is usually under pressure and appears cloudy if there are more than about $500 \times 10^6/l$ leucocytes present. In a typical series[2], the CSF leucocyte count ranged from 0 to $55\,000 \times 10^6/l$, with a mean of $3800 \times 10^6/l$. The mean was higher in patients with evidence only of meningitis ($6450 \times 10^6/l$) than in patients who also had a rash or positive blood cultures ($2850 \times 10^6/l$). The proportion of polymorphonuclear leucocytes ranged between 49% and 98%, with a mean of 86%. CSF glucose was usually reduced to below 1.5 mmol/l or less than 40% of the value of a plasma glucose sample taken simultaneously. Protein was typically raised, ranging from 0.19 to 9.54 g/l, with a mean of 2.59 g/l. Direct microscopy was positive for gram-negative diplococci in 72% of cases.

If a Gram stained smear does not demonstrate organisms, other CSF abnormalities can assist in making a diagnosis of bacterial meningitis. The most useful feature is the CSF leucocyte differential count. A polymorphonuclear picture is strongly suggestive of a bacterial aetiology. Rarely it may be found in early viral meningitis, but then the total cell count is usually less than $100 \times 10^6/l$. A lymphocytic pleocytosis, which can lead to confusion with viral or even tuberculous meningitis, is unusual in meningococcal meningitis, although it has been reported[11-13]. A CSF glucose of less than 40% of the plasma value and/or a protein exceeding 2 g/l are not features of viral meningitis, but are found in more than 80% of cases of bacterial meningitis[14].

Meningitis with apparently normal CSF findings

Bacterial meningitis is sometimes confirmed by isolation of an organism from a CSF specimen whose initial direct examination was normal. Polk and

Steele[15] found that 2.7% of culture-positive CSF specimens from one children's hospital had normal glucose and protein levels and less than $9 \times 10^6/l$ leucocytes.

Meningococcal meningitis with apparently normal CSF may occur in two clinical settings[3,5,16]. In the more frequent, patients have clinical evidence of meningococcaemia, often of fulminating septicaemia, and the need for treatment is clear. Confusion may occur in patients who have a nondescript fever complicated at most by non-specific features such as meningism or a febrile convulsion. Donald *et al.*[3] describe five such children, aged from 7 months to 9 years, who had a lumbar puncture as part of the investigation of a seizure and fever. Two had lower respiratory tract infections. None had evidence of meningitis or a rash. CSF examination was completely normal (except for one child who had $4 \times 10^6/l$ lymphocytes) but *N. meningitidis* was subsequently isolated from all five specimens. Three patients received oral antibiotics—one recovered with these alone, one was recalled, found to be still unwell and given more intensive therapy, and the third died at home the following day. The two children not given antibiotics both progressed to a typical picture of purulent meningitis by the following day.

The acute meningococcal rash

Most patients with acute meningococcal infection have a skin rash. The appearances of the rash have been described extensively, in both adults and children[11,17,18]. Three patterns may be seen: a maculopapular rash, a petechial rash, and an ecchymotic haemorrhagic or necrotic rash. A mixed pattern may occur, or there may be progression over time to a more haemorrhagic type. In a prospective study of 69 children with acute meningococcal disease a maculopapular rash was noted in 13%, a mixed maculopapular/purpuric rash in 25%, and a purpuric rash in 55%. There was no difference in age distribution between the three groups. However, five children who had no rash were significantly younger than others[17].

The lesions of the maculopapular rash are pink, raised toward the centre, 2–15 mm in diameter, and have indistinct borders. They are not confluent and they blanch completely on pressure. They are usually distributed on the trunk alone or on the trunk and the extremities. Less often they involve the limbs only, including the palms and soles. Lesions are non-pruritic, transient, and may last for less than a day after treatment. Careful examination may reveal inconspicuous petechiae in the centre of a few macules. A maculopapular rash may progress within hours to a haemorrhagic rash, with general deterioration and a worsening prognosis[19].

The lesions of the petechial rash are small, about 1–2 mm in diameter, non-blanching and found mainly on the trunk and lower limbs. They may also occur on the face, the palate and the conjunctivae. Petechiae may be found with, or progress to, larger purpuric lesions, which may be raised and which may have black, necrotic centres. Petechiae may become confluent, and may develop into haemorrhagic bullae. Extensive areas of cyanosis may develop, particulaly involving the extremities. Cyanotic areas are well demarcated, often symmetrical and do not blanch on pressure. Peripheral pulses in affected limbs are usually still palpable. Digits or whole limbs may become necrotic. The appearances may evolve in hours, and are described as purpura fulminans. Haemorrhagic bullae and easy bleeding from puncture sites are features associated with depleted coagulation factors and fibrinolysis.

A fulminant purpuric rash is more commonly found in patients with a short history of illness. Such patients are much more likely to be hypotensive, and to have evidence of disseminated intravascular coagulation (DIC), than are patients with a maculopapular or petechial rash. Mortality is higher in purpura fulminans than in other forms of meningococcal disease—44% compared with 3%[18]. Survivors of purpura fulminans may suffer considerable morbidity; one of our patients required amputation of three limbs for peripheral necrosis; Seyfer and Kiefer[20] described a case in which 35% of the total body skin surface was lost, requiring extensive grafting.

Clotting abnormalities

Acute meningococcal disease is the most common infective cause of DIC[21] and mild prolongation of clotting times is frequently found in patients with a petechial rash. Patients with purpura fulminans have prothrombin times and activated partial thromboplastin times of between 1.5 and 2 times normal, associated with diminished plasma fibrinogen levels and elevated fibrinogen degradation product titre. The platelet count may be markedly reduced. In one paediatric series, a platelet count below $100 \times 10^9/l$ was found in 14% of cases, of whom more than half died[4].

Septicaemia

Most patients with meningococcal disease have meningococcaemia, i.e. blood cultures positive for N. meningitidis, or a typical meningococcal rash with N. meningitidis isolated from another usually sterile site such as CSF. A minority of these patients meet the criteria for the definition of sepsis syndrome. The most important additional features are related to impaired tissue perfusion—hypoxaemia, acidosis, an elevated plasma lactate level and oliguria. Hypotension (systolic blood pressure less than 90 mmHg in an adult or less than 70 mmHg in a child) without other cause, leads to this condition being described as septic shock[22].

When present, shock dominates the clinical picture. The patient is ill, with cool, cyanosed peripheries. The conscious state is variable. Patients may remain alert despite systemic hypotension, although complete unresponsiveness is not unusual. Oliguria occurs, although it is usually transient in survivors. A cardiac gallop rhythm is sometimes heard. Evidence for some degree of myocardial depression contributing to shock comes from haemodynamic studies within 6 hours of presentation in 19 patients (mean age 20 years), with meningococcaemia, hypotension, acidosis and oliguria, who were compared with 20 patients (mean age 47 years) with septic shock from other organisms[23]. The group with meningococcaemia had a significantly higher mean wedge pressure and lower cardiac index. Furthermore, fluid challenge led to a greater increase in wedge pressure for a smaller increase in cardiac index in the meningococcal group. Peripheral vascular resistance was significantly higher in the meningococcal group. In this study, electrocardiography (ECG), echocardiography and serial creatinine phosphokinase (CK) measurements were undertaken in 49 patients with meningococcal infection. Seventeen had echocardiographic evidence of impaired myocardial contractility (septal systolic amplitude motion less than 5 mm and/or posterior endocardial systolic motion less than 10 mm and fractional shortening less than 28%). Of these, 12 (71%) developed shock and five died. Autopsy on three showed an acute interstitial myocarditis and myocardial histology of one showed gram-negative diplococci. Of the other 32 patients with no echocardiographic evidence of impaired myocardial function, two were hypotensive. Both were successfully treated with plasma volume expansion without inotropic support. There was a correlation between a raised CK level, abnormal ECG and echocardiographic evidence of impaired myocardial contractility.

Low-grade uraemia is not uncommmon in meningococcaemia. Transient proteinuria, microscopic haematuria, pyuria and the presence of granular casts in the urine have often also been noted[11]. Patients with septic shock may develop more severe uraemia, sometimes necessitating dialysis. Renal failure is usually transient if the patient survives, although permanent impairment does occur. Metabolic acidosis is a further feature of sepsis syndrome. There may be a negative base excess of 8–10 mmol/l, associated with a raised plasma lactate.

Most patients with meningococcal septicaemia have meningitis as well, even though signs of meningeal irritation may be absent; a few patients have normal CSF which subsequently yields a meningococcus on culture.

Occult meningococcaemia

Patients with meningococcal infection may present with fever, sometimes accompanied by a maculopapular rash, but without petechiae, purpura or signs of septicaemia. Meningeal irritation may be absent and CSF examination may be normal. There is often evidence of upper respiratory tract infection, usually otitis media. Children may present with a febrile convulsion. Peripheral blood leucocytosis is usual. By definition, *N. meningitidis* is isolated from blood culture.

This pattern of presentation is very difficult to differentiate from the more frequent, mild, self-limiting febrile illnesses thought to be caused by viruses. It occurs mainly in children and young adults, particularly in infants. The age distribution is similar to that of other forms of acute meningococcal infection[13,24]. No evidence for reduced virulence or correlation with serotype of the infecting organism has been shown.

There is an overlap between this syndrome and the prodromal illness frequently reported by patients with meningococcal meningitis or obvious meningococcaemia. However, in many patients with what turns out to have been occult meningococcaemia the infection resolves with oral antibiotics only, or with no therapy at all. Sullivan and La Scolea[24] described 13 cases with nondescript febrile illnesses, six with otitis media. All were recalled after blood cultures were reported positive for *N. meningitidis*. Seven were well and two had persisting fever; all of these had sterile repeat blood cultures. Four others developed meningitis and two of these had had normal CSF at their first visit. All 13 received further antibiotic therapy. Edwards *et al.*[13] reported seven more such cases, of whom five had otitis and two a macular rash. When recalled, five had recovered on oral antibiotics and one on no therapy at all. One case still had low-grade fever and a rash and improved on parenteral antibiotics.

The most common cause of occult bacteraemia in children is *Streptococcus pneumoniae*. However, children with occult meningococcaemia have a much higher risk of developing meningitis than those with occult pneumococcaemia[25]. There is a correlation between the presence of clinical features of meningococcaemia and the intensity of bacteraemia[24], but no other clear risk factors for disease progression have been identified. Shapiro *et al.*[25], who studied 310 children with occult bacteraemia due to *S. pneumoniae*, *N. meningitidis* and *Haemophilus influenzae*, found that 22 (7%) progressed to meningitis. Importantly, there was no evidence that having a lumbar puncture on presentation caused meningitis. These children did not have evidence of serious infection such as a petechial rash or an abnormal CSF examination, or their bacteraemia would not have been classed as occult. Other clinical features such as lethargy, irritability, toxicity, neck stiffness, a bulging fontanelle or very high fever did not predict progression to meningitis.

Other investigations in acute meningococcal infection

The peripheral blood white cell count varies widely, ranging from 0.9 to 46.2 × 10^9/l (mean 14.2 × 10^9/l) in a recent series[4]. Most patients have a polymorphonuclear leucocytosis. However, low white cell counts are not uncommon, especially in overwhelming sepsis. In the same series, 21% of children, including all the fatal cases in which the blood count was measured, had a white count below $5 \times 10^9/l$. A low serum sodium is common in meningitis. With fluid restriction, it usually returns to normal within 48 hours. Transient hyperglycaemia has also been observed.

MORTALITY IN ACUTE MENINGOCOCCAL DISEASE

Systemic meningococcal disease carries a significant risk of death. Based on data from a large study of notifications of infections and deaths, and smaller hospital-based studies, the crude mortality rate in technologically advanced countries is about 7% to 10% (Table 8.3). However, deaths are notified more efficiently than cases. Most deaths occur early in the illness, within the first 24–48 hours.

The mortality rate has not changed significantly over the past three decades despite changes in antibiotic prescribing and improvements in intensive care facilities. Havens et al.[26] reviewed mortality rates in meningococcal infection in children in one hospital over thirty years. The crude mortality rate was 10.3% (27/261). There was no significant trend in the case fatality ratio over time. There was an increase in the proportion of cases assessed retrospectively as having severe disease, from 14% in 1957 to 1963, to 38% in 1980 to 1987. This assessment was based on data such as heart rate, leucocyte count in peripheral blood and in the CSF, and the mental state. Over the whole period, those assessed as having severe disease had a mortality rate of 29.7%, compared with 2.7% for the others. The fatality rate stratified for disease severity showed no significant trend over time.

Clinical features associated with a fatal outcome

There are three aspects of the clinical presentation which have a strong association with a fatal outcome: the presence of shock, the appearance of the skin rash, and the level of consciousness. Death from acute meningococcal

Table 8.3 *Case fatality ratios for acute meningococcal disease*

Study	Patient group	No. of patients	Mortality
Wolf and Birbara 1968[11]	Military recruits	112	7.1%
Voss et al. 1989[5]	Children	122	7%
Olcén et al. 1979[2]	All ages	69	7.2%
Wong et al. 1989[4]	Children	100	10%
Fallon et al. 1984[30]	Notifications in Scotland 1972–82	1912	7.5%

disease is consistently associated with hypotension at or soon after presentation. Failure of hypotension to improve with aggressive fluid resuscitation is also an adverse prognostic indicator. Tesoro and Selbst[27] studied 73 children with meningococcal infection and found that of 19 who were shocked, six died (32%). Twelve were given pressor agents in addition to fluids, including the six who later died. Only one of the other patients died (from cerebral oedema), a 2% mortality in those who were not shocked.

Patients with a purpuric or ecchymotic rash are significantly more likely to be hypotensive, to have evidence of consumption coagulopathy, and to die. In a population consisting mostly of military recruits, Toews and Bass[18] found a mortality rate of 44% in such patients, compared with a case fatality rate of 3% in those who had no purpura. Similar results have been found in children[1,4,28].

Patients without a rash, or with maculopapular lesions only, have a very good prognosis if adequately treated[17]. However, deaths have been recorded. It is very important to consider the diagnosis of meningococcal infection in children with fever and a non-petechial rash, and to review the rash regularly. The development of petechiae within macules may be a pointer to the need for more aggressive therapy, and a worsening prognosis.

Patients who are comatose or obtunded have a relatively poor outlook. Tesoro and Selbst[27] recorded a mortality of 41% in such children, whereas there were no deaths in those described as being normal, lethargic or irritable.

Fatal cases usually have a short duration of illness prior to presentation, although a short history is common in meningococcal disease in any case. There is an apparent paradox in that those patients in whom treatment is delayed have a better outcome than those treated early. This reflects the better outcome in those with a slow and non-specific onset to their illness[8,10]. Stiehm and Damrosch's[28] observation that a history of petechial rash not exceeding 12 hours was indicative of a more fulminant infection and a poorer outcome has not been confirmed in other studies.

Laboratory features associated with a fatal outcome

Several of the easily available laboratory investigations are significantly associated with a fatal outcome—a blood leucocyte count of less than 5×10^9/l, a platelet count of less than 100×10^9/l, a prolonged prothrombin and activated partial thromboplastin time, and an elevated serum creatinine[4,27]. Leclerc et al.[29] found that the C-reactive protein (CRP) level predicted survival in children who were shocked and who had purpura caused by bacterial infection. 17/18 children whose CRP level exceeded 0.1 g/l survived, a positive predictive value of 94%, whereas 12/17 children with a CRP level below 0.1 g/l died, a negative predictive value of 71%. Stiehm and Damrosch[28] found that children with a normal or near-normal erythrocyte sedimentation rate (ESR) had a worse prognosis than those with a raised ESR. In general, laboratory features pointing to a failure of the acute phase response to infection, the presence of DIC, or to poor tissue perfusion, are associated with a higher mortality.

Other factors, such as the serogroup of the infecting organism[30], are less clearly associated with poor outcome. Wong et al.[4] noted that seizures occurred in 6% of non-fatal cases compared with 30% of those who later died. In the same study fever occurred with similar frequency in surviving and fatal cases, but hypothermia on presentation occurred exclusively in those who died. Though Stiehm and Damrosch[28] found that a CSF white cell count of less than $20 \times 10^6/l$ was associated with fatal outcome in meningococcal disease, others have not confirmed this observation.

Scoring systems

The use of scoring systems, combining data of prognostic significance in the assessment of patients with acute meningococcal disease, has attracted much interest. Scores can be applied to patients with obvious or suspected meningococcal infection, both on presentation and on review. The use of a prognostic score obliges clinicians to make observations in each of the areas of prognostic significance and to come to a conclusion as to the seriousness of the case. This can be readily applied to management protocols, in which the indications for invasive monitoring and aggressive therapy can more clearly be defined. Medical management and the patient's outcome can be compared with that anticipated from the prognostic score, as part of clinical audit. Scores may also be used to stratify trials of new therapies by case severity.

Several systems have been devised. The Glasgow Meningococcal Septicaemia Prognostic Score (GMSPS) (Table 8.4) has the advantage of being based on bedside examination and results of readily available tests[31]. It gives emphasis to measurements reflecting shock and poor tissue perfusion, combining these with assessments of rash, conscious state and rapidity of deterioration. It has been tested in a retrospective study of 120 paediatric cases[32]. All 104 children with scores of seven or less survived (a negative predictive value of 100%). Of 19 children who scored eight or above on, or soon after admission, 14 died, giving a positive predictive value of 73.7%. Two survivors were post-ictal at assessment, and their scores reverted to less than eight soon after admission.

If the system is used solely to predict mortality from observations on admission, a cut-off value of 10 provides the best discrimination. However, if the system is used to identify the iller patients needing an intensive care environment, then a lower cut-off value is more useful. The score is not designed to identify patients whose prognosis is so poor that intervention is not attempted; patients with scores as high as 14 have survived.

Table 8.4 *The Glasgow Meningococcal Septicaemia Prognostic Score*[31]

Criterion	Score
Hypotension:	
Systolic blood pressure <75 mmHg if less than 4 years age	
<85 mmHg if older	3
Skin–rectal temperature difference >3 °C	3
Base deficit (capillary sample) <8 mmol/l	1
Coma score* <8 at any one time or deterioration >3 in an hour	3
Lack of meningism	2
Parental opinion that child's condition has worsened in past hour	2
Widespread ecchymoses, or lesions extending on review	1
	15

* Modified paediatric coma scale:
Eyes open spontaneously 4, to speech 3, to pain 3, none 1.
Best verbal response oriented 6, words 4, vocal sounds 3, cries 2, none 1.
Best motor response obeys commands 6, localise pain 4, flexion to pain 1, extension to pain 1, none 0.

FOCAL MANIFESTATIONS OF MENINGOCOCCAL DISEASE

Neurological complications

Focal cerebral deficits are uncommon presenting features or sequelae of meningococcal meningitis. Hemiparesis in an alcoholic has been described[33] and two children have been reported in whom hemiparesis, homonymous hemianopia and dysphasia developed following convulsions which themselves occurred after several days of otherwise uncomplicated recovery[34]. Subdural empyema (leading to a relapse of meningitis), and subdural effusions are rare complications[1]. General psycho-neurological sequelae are also uncommon though headaches and lassitude commonly persist for some months after meningococcal meningitis. In Olcén's series[2] one patient developed hydrocephalus and dementia, and two were found to have poor concentration and emotional lability which persisted one year after the illness.

Bacterial meningitis is an important cause of acquired sensorineural deafness in childhood. It occurs more frequently in pneumococcal meningitis than in meningitis caused by *N. meningitidis* or *H. influenzae*[35]. In one prospective study in children with meningococcal infection 9% of survivors had impaired hearing[1]. Other studies suggest an incidence of 4 to 6%[2,5,34]. This may be an underestimate as follow-up audiometry is not always undertaken. Hearing loss may be bilateral and severe, potentially impairing language acquisition in young children.

Prospective studies on children with bacterial meningitis caused by any of the three commonest organisms have helped to clarify the relationship between the pattern of onset of hearing loss and its outcome[35–37]. On admission with meningitis patients commonly have otitis media, which may cause some reversible conductive hearing loss. When it occurs, impairment of auditory nerve function, as assessed by brainstem auditory evoked potentials (BAEP), is detectable within 48 hours of admission. In some children, damage to the auditory nerve is severe and irreversible. The two weeks after admission form a crucial period during which hearing may deteriorate further, or during which some recovery may occur. Children whose hearing is assessed as normal at 48 hours do not develop hearing loss later in the illness. The interpretation of these studies should be qualified by the fact that none of those whose hearing impairment proved permanent had meningitis caused by *N. meningitidis*. In bacterial meningitis[35,36] and specifically in meningococcal meningitis[5], a very low CSF glucose level has been found to be associated with deafness. However, in another study of meningococcal infections, deafness was associated with a peripheral blood leucocytosis or leucopenia, with a CSF pleocytosis exceeding $10\,000 \times 10^6/l$, but not with hypoglycorrhachia[1]. Farmer reported in 1945[34] that about two-thirds of patients with complete deafness following meningococcal disease also had an unsteady gait and evidence of vestibular damage. This association has not been reported in other series[1,2,5]. Survivors of bacterial meningitis left with other severe neurological deficits frequently have hearing damage as well[35].

Though several cases have been reported in which cerebellar ataxia occurred either as a presenting feature or as a later complication of meningitis caused by *H. influenzae*[38], it is a very rare complication of meningococcal meningitis. One case has been described in a 28 month old girl[39]. Recovery was complete.

Other cranial nerve deficits occur uncommonly in the acute phase of meningococcal meningitis. A unilateral or, occasionally, bilateral sixth nerve lesion, presenting with diplopia on admission, was the most commonly reported in a large series in the 1940s, with an incidence of about 10%[34]. Very occasionally diplopia can be the main presenting symptom. It occurs in all age groups, and the prognosis is good. Third nerve palsy with ptosis, divergent strabismus and a dilated pupil, and fourth nerve palsy are occasionally seen. Fifth and ninth nerve palsies have also been reported[2,34].

Seventh nerve palsy causing paralysis of the muscles of facial expression, and sometimes also ipsilateral loss of taste sensation on the anterior two-thirds of the tongue occurs infrequently; Farmer[34] reported an incidence of 1% to 5% in an early series, and cases continue to be reported[40]. Facial palsy typically occurs between the 5th and 14th day of the patient's illness. Occasionally it is bilateral, and in these cases paralysis on the second side develops 1–4 days after the first.

Peripheral nerve lesions are rare, and apparently transient. Wolf and

Birbara[11] reported two cases, each involving more than one nerve in the upper limb. Olcén[2] also noted a case with paresis of the brachial plexus, and another with a peroneal nerve lesion. Engber *et al.*[41] reported a patient in whom paresis of the median and ulnar nerves on opposite sides occurred during severe meningococcal sepsis. Recovery was slow and still incomplete at 9 months. Conus medullaris syndrome in a 20 year old man recovering from meningococcaemia and meningitis has been reported[42]. He developed a flaccid paralysis of both legs, extensor Babinski reflexes, hypoaesthesia in a stocking distribution and perianal anaesthesia, urinary retention, erectile failure and faecal incontinence. Myelography demonstrated no spinal lesion, CSF showed a resolving meningitic picture, and electromyelography confirmed denervation of the anal sphincter. Recovery was incomplete.

Arthritis

Arthritis is common in acute meningococcal disease. An excellent review of series published from 1898 to 1979 showed a mean incidence of 10.8% in adults, 4.9% in children and 6.7% overall[43]. It may complicate any of the invasive forms of meningococcal disease and may develop at any stage in the acute illness[44]. Affected joints are red, swollen and painful and an effusion is often present. Tenosynovitis may occur, though this is rare[45,48]. In slightly more than half the cases in which arthritis occurs, a single joint is affected; in the remainder it is polyarthritic[43]. Large joints are most commonly affected, particularly the knee (40%), followed by the elbow, wrist, ankle, small joints of the hands and feet, shoulder and hip. Case reports[45-48] suggest that arthritis occurring around the time of presentation typically affects several joints, often symmetrically. Arthritis developing after several days treatment more often affects a single joint. However, this distinction is not clear-cut. Resolution of arthritis is usually rapid but some cases take 2–4 weeks to settle[47,48].

Synovial fluid from affected joints is usually turbid and contains polymorphs. In a minority of cases, *N. meningitidis* may be demonstrated by Gram stain or culture. A few patients have been studied in sufficient detail to conclude that arthritis in acute meningococcal disease is sometimes immunologically mediated. Globular deposits of meningococcal antigen, meningococcal antibody and the C3 component of complement have been found in white cells from the synovial fluid and in synovial biopsy specimens. These patients also had a fall in the level of meningococcal antigen and a rise in meningococcal antibody titres in the serum, and a fall in serum C3 at the same time as the arthritis. In these cases arthritis may result either from the deposition of circulating immune complexes in the synovium, or from an Arthus reaction to meningococcal antigens fixed in the synovium[49]. It would be reasonable to expect arthritis on presentation to be septic, and that occurring later to be caused by hypersensitivity, but this has yet to be confirmed[43].

Radiological changes other than soft tissue swelling are rare. Erosion of the distal femoral epiphyseal centre was reported in a 13 month old child with arthritis of the knee occurring after meningococcal meningitis[50]. This showed progressive re-calcification over 6 months. Periosteal elevation and demineralisation of the distal humerus was also described in an infant with meningococcaemia and a sterile effusion of the elbow[51]. Longer term sequelae of arthritis are rare. Only seven of 1001 patients treated in the antibiotic era had residual problems; one had ankylosis and six had limited function[43].

Primary meningococcal arthritis and the acute arthritis–dermatitis syndrome

Rarely, *N. meningitidis* may cause arthritis without typical features of acute meningococcal disease such as purpura or meningitis, thus leading to possible confusion with other causes of septic arthritis or with collagen diseases. This primary meningococcal arthritis has been reviewed by Schaad *et al.*[52]. The age distribution was similar to the more common meningococcal illnesses, with peak attack rates in infancy and in military recruits and college students. A male preponderance was noted. Typically, single large joints were affected, usually the knee. However, 30% of cases were polyarthritic, and small joints were also affected. The arthritis was associated with fever, leucocytosis, raised ESR, and in one-third of cases, an erythematous maculopapular rash on the trunk and extremities. In half the cases a preceding upper respiratory tract infection was reported. The synovial fluid was purulent, and yielded meningococci in most cases. Primary meningococcal septic arthritis of the shoulder with culture-proven osteomyelitis of the humerus in a baby has also been described[51].

The constellation of fever, maculopapular rash and flitting polyarthralgia or arthritis in a sexually active young adult may suggest the diagnosis of disseminated gonococcal infection (DGI) or acute arthritis–dermatitis syndrome. In some places DGI is the commonest cause of non-traumatic arthritis in adults aged 15 to 30 years. Meningococcaemia may also present in this way and is an important differential diagnosis. The main distinguishing features are that patients with meningococcaemia usually have many more skin lesions and a higher peripheral blood leucocyte count[53].

Other skin manifestations

Patients with acute meningococcal infection may suffer vasculitic skin lesions late in the course of the disease. This complication occurred in 1.7%

of cases in a Nigerian series[13,44], and in 4.7% of cases in a paediatric series from Texas[1]. The onset is about 5 days after presentation and is often associated with persistence of fever. Vasculitis is more likely in those who suffered shock and purpura at presentation. The lesions start as darkened skin, with a blistered edge, and slightly swollen, warm and tender underlying tissue. They progress over a day to sterile bullae, which after about 3 more days leave a shallow punched out ulcer which soon heals. Lesions may occur on the trunk, lower limbs, over the deltoid and on the dorsum of the hand. They may be single, or occur in crops at irregular intervals over 2 or 3 days. A few cases develop tender, warm nodules similar to Osler's nodes. Seven of 12 patients in the Nigerian series also had arthritis, and three developed signs of heart failure at the same time as the rash. Skin biopsies showed that vasculitis and immune complex mediated damage, or an Arthus reaction, were potential mechanisms for this late-onset cutaneous vasculitis.

Primary meningococcal infection of the skin of the legs with erythema, swelling and pus formation, has been described[54] in an elderly lady with chronic venous statis. A pure growth of *N. meningitidis* was obtained from an aspirate. There were no systemic manifestations and blood cultures were sterile.

Pericarditis

Pericarditis is an unusual feature of acute meningococcal disease. The incidence was reported to vary from zero to 1.6% in several large series between 1942 and 1958[55]. Five of 69 cases in a more recent series had pericarditis[2]. The features described are based on reports of 13 adult cases with pericarditis complicating clinically apparent meningococcal disease[46,55–58]. Eleven had meningitis. All but two developed chest pain, typically anterior and sharp in nature. Lateralisation of the pain was associated with evidence of pulmonary or pleural disease. Three had persistent or recurrent fever associated with the pericarditis. All developed a pericardial friction rub at some time in their illness and one had a pericardial effusion confirmed on echocardiogram. Of the other 12, 11 had enlargement of the cardiac shadow on chest X-ray at some time.

Chest pain started, or a pericardial rub was first found between day 2 and day 20 after admission; in just over half the cases it was within the first 5 days. In three cases increased size of the cardiac silhouette and/or ECG changes suggestive of pericarditis were present on admission, preceding the clinical onset by many days. Most cases resolved within 5–7 days. Three had a prolonged course, with recurrence more than a month after onset. In two cases this appeared to be related to withdrawal of corticosteroid therapy; increasing the corticosteroid dose appeared to aid recovery. Three developed clinical evidence of tamponade. Pericardial aspiration showed sterile purulent fluid with leucocyte counts of $1.2–20 \times 10^9/l$, mostly neutrophils. Seven patients had arthritis and in five cases this occurred several days after the initial presentation and at the same time as pericarditis became apparent. Three patients had pleural effusions (two with arthritis in addition) coincident with the development of pericarditis. Three had evidence of pulmonary infiltrates, two at presentation, and one occurring later with a pleural effusion and pericarditis.

Late, culture-negative pericarditis in an infant with persistent fever, an enlarged cardiac silhouette, pneumonitis and bilateral pleural effusions has been reported[59]. This case contrasts with another infant in whom meningitis and petechial rash were present on admission and pericarditis and tamponade developed later the same day[60]. In the latter case, the pericardial fluid contained gram-negative cocci.

Primary meningococcal pericaditis can occur rarely in the absence of, or before, recognisable meningococcaemia or meningitis. Blaser et al. described only 16 cases in their review[58]. The median age of these patients was 19.5 years; only two were infants. Patients presented in a manner similar to those with purulent pericarditis from other infections. Chest pain, fever and dyspnoea were the commonest initial symptoms. Pleurisy and pneumonia were also sometimes noted. Most patients had experienced a non-specific prodromal illness. Half the patients developed a pericardial rub and tamponade occurred in 11 of the 16 patients. Pericardial fluid was purulent or blood-stained. N. meningitidis was identified in nine of 14 patients who had pericardiocentesis. Blaser found that primary pericarditis was associated with serogroup C infection significantly more often than would have been expected from its overall isolation rate in the United States.

In summary, pericarditis is an uncommon complication of meningococcal disease, and may rarely be the primary focus of infection. Both primary and secondary pericarditis are much more common in adults than children. Primary meningococcal pericarditis is often complicated by tamponade, and N. meningitidis can be cultured from pericardial fluid. By contrast, pericarditis complicating other meningococcal infections typically occurs later in the course of the illness, is complicated less often by tamponade and more often by pleural effusions or arthritis, and, if aspirated, the pericardial fluid is usually sterile. Secondary meningococcal pericarditis is probably the result of hypersensitivity.

Endocarditis

Meningococcal endocarditis is now rare but was described extensively in the earlier part of the century, before antibiotics were widely used[61]. Patients were typically young, and the left sided heart valves were affected. Several patterns were described. Cecil and Soper[62] reported three children with acute purulent meningitis who died after intervals varying from 5 days to 5 weeks and in whom autopsy revealed mitral valve vegetations as well as other focal sites of infection including pneumonia and pericarditis. Cecil and others also described acute endocarditis presenting without evidence of meningitis. In two such cases rheumatic mitral valves were affected[62,63]; another involved a probably normal aortic valve and presented as rapidly progressive heart failure[63]. Endocarditis following a more chronic course has also been described. Gwyn[64] reported a 37 year old woman observed for 8 months with fever, increased heart size, mitral systolic and aortic diastolic murmurs, intermittent petechiae, Osler's nodes and finger clubbing, in whom meningococcal meningitis supervened as the terminal event. Other cases were more typical of chronic meningococcaemia with intermittent fever, rash and migratory polyarthralgia. Signs of cardiac valve lesions, initially absent, became apparent during the course of the illness, which usually, but not always, led to the patients' demise[65-68].

Meningococci have been reported recently as a cause of prosthetic heart valve infection[69,70]. In another recent case the infection involved a native mitral valve in an 88 year old woman who had had rheumatic fever as a child. The diagnosis was proved on blood culture and the patient recovered with penicillin treatment[71].

Ocular complications

The most important meningococcal eye infections are conjunctivitis and endophthalmitis; the first because it may precede invasive disease, and the second because it occurs as a metastatic focus during meningococcaemia. Other ocular manifestations include conjunctival petechiae which may be seen in association with a meningococcal rash, and episcleritis. The latter has been described occurring 6 days after starting therapy for meningitis and resolving after a week[49]. It may result from the reaction of antibody with meningococcal antigen deposited in the sclera during the acute infection. Conjunctivitis caused by herpes simplex spread from a reactivated oral lesion is also not uncommon in acute meningococcal disease.

Conjunctivitis may be one of the presenting features in up to 2% of cases of meningococcaemia or meningitis[72]. Meningococcal conjunctivitis may also occur in isolation, or may precede invasive disease (in a similar way to minor upper respiratory tract infections during the prodromal illness). The incidence of primary meningococcal conjunctivitis is not known.

Meningococcal conjunctivitis has features typical of such bacterial infections with a thick yellow (sometimes mucoid[73]) ocular discharge, hyperaemia of the palpebral conjunctiva, and sometimes injection of the bulbar conjunctiva[74]. Periorbital cellulitis is an uncommon accompaniment[75]. The pupils and anterior chamber are usually normal. Corneal ulcers can occur, but these usually heal well and rarely leave residual opacity. One or both eyes may be affected. Cervical lymphadenopathy and fever may occur, even in cases where CSF and blood cultures have subsequently been found to be sterile. It has been reported in adults and children and occasionally in newborn infants presenting with ophthalmia neonatorum[76]. Primary meningococcal conjunctivitis may progress to severe disease including fulminant septicaemia and death[72]. This happens in only a minority of cases, although an estimate of the frequency of progression is difficult because a specific bacterial aetiology is not usually sought in conjunctivitis. Of 41 reported proven cases, four progressed to meningococcaemia or meningitis[74]. Patients with proven primary meningococcal conjunctivitis have recovered following treatment with topical antibiotics alone. Nonetheless, the rapidity of onset and severity of meningococcal septicaemia mean that systemic therapy is justifiable for meningococcal conjunctivitis when the organism is identified.

Bacterial endophthalmitis is found in two settings—following surgery or trauma, and as a result of haematogenous spread of infection. One case of exogenously acquired post-operative meningococcal endophthalmitis has been described[77]. However, meningococcal endophthalmitis typically occurs as a rare presenting feature of meningococcaemia and meningitis. In a review of 20 cases of bacterial endophthalmitis unrelated to surgery or trauma, N. meningitidis was the cause of 15%[78]. One or both eyes may be affected. Visual acuity is markedly reduced, and the affected eye is painful. Signs of conjunctivitis may be present, but in addition there is ciliary injection, cloudiness of the cornea, keratic precipitates and hypopyon. Posterior synechiae and raised intraocular pressures are also described. Prompt parenteral antibiotic therapy for the systemic infection also leads to complete resolution of the eye infection[55,59,79,80].

Respiratory tract infections

N. meningitidis causes lower and upper respiratory tract infections, both as primary infections, and as part of disseminated meningococcal disease.

Although cough is a common presenting symptom of patients with meningococcaemia or meningitis, the incidence of radiologically confirmed pneumonia in meningococcal disease varies markedly between series. Olcén et al.[2] reported no such cases but Donald et al.[3] noted that 15 of 298 cases of meningococcal disease had evidence of lobar pneumonia or bronchopneumonia. In 10 cases obvious signs of meningococcaemia dominated the presentation. However, five patients had no such distinctive features, and the aetiology was only determined after isolation of N. meningitidis from otherwise normal CSF.

Symptoms of upper respiratory tract infection including rhinitis, otitis media and pharyngitis are common in the prodrome of acute meningococcal infection. Meningococcal otitis media and pharyngitis may occur as isolated infections. Gradon and Lutwick[81] described an 82 year old woman with a retropharyngeal fasciitis, whose blood cultures were positive for *N. meningitidis* W-135. She presented with acute fever, dysphagia, dysphonia and neck swelling. Diffuse prevertebral soft tissue swelling without abscess formation was demonstrated radiologically. Recovery was swift on antibiotic therapy.

Primary meningococcal pneumonia is well recognised particularly in association with serogroup Y strains. In an outbreak in a military camp, of 16 patients with meningococcaemia or meningitis, 10 also had pneumonia. A further 68 patients had primary meningococcal pneumonia, proved by culture of trans-tracheal aspirates in most cases. Ten had positive blood cultures without clinical features typical of meningococcaemia[82]. A recent study of 162 hospital admissions for community-acquired pneumonia found the causative agent to have been *N. meningitidis* in 6% by demonstration of a rising titre of meningococcal antibodies[83].

There are no particular clinical or radiological features of meningococcal pneumonia. Fever, pharyngitis, dyspnoea, pleuritic chest pain, cough productive of purulent and sometimes blood-tinged sputum, and hypoxia are all frequently present. Lobar consolidation or patchy alveolar infiltration may be seen on chest X-ray. Small effusions are often present. Early studies quoted by Galpin *et al.*[84] suggested that meningococcal pneumonia typically followed adenovirus or influenza infections. This has not been confirmed in more recent series[83].

N. meningitidis may also cause acute bronchitis. Davies *et al.*[85] found significant numbers of the organism in 2.2% of positive sputum cultures in one hospital in one year. Most came from patients with acute bronchitis, or exacerbations of chronic bronchitis. Males predominated, with a mean age of 58.6 years in contrast to the age distribution of invasive meningococcal disease. None developed meningitis or evidence of meningococcaemia.

Abdominal and pelvic manifestations

Diarrhoea is a common presenting feature in acute meningococcal infection[2] and is probably due to toxaemia. Occasionally gastrointestinal symptoms can be so severe that they mask the true diagnosis of meningitis or septicaemia. Werne[6] reports four such cases, another was reported by Waldum[7], and we have seen a further two recently. The ages ranged from 14 to 70 years. All had had watery, mostly profuse, diarrhoea from 7 hours to 3 days prior to presentation. Three had prominent abdominal pain. Two were afebrile, six were hypotensive on presentation, and six had meningitis. One was profoundly shocked but did not have meningitis. One survivor required 3 months dialysis following his acute illness, and mild elevations in blood urea and creatinine were noted in five others. All seven developed a petechial rash, but in six cases this was not present when first seen by a doctor. All were resuscitated with fluids when they presented in shock, but in four of the seven definitive treatment of meningococcal infection was delayed because of the unusual symptoms. Two patients died. *N. meningitidis* was cultured from blood or CSF, but not from the stool in any of the cases.

Patients with acute meningococcal disease may have pronounced abdominal pain mimicking peritonitis. This resolves without surgery or antibiotics. We have seen a 20 year old man in whom acute right loin pain and high fever were the sole presenting features of meningococcaemia. He had no features of meningitis or sepsis, and never developed a rash. Liver enzymes, urine microscopy and culture, and abdominal ultrasound examination were normal. His symptoms and fever resolved on treatment with cefotaxime.

Spontaneous bacterial peritonitis is a complication of chronic liver disease, causing abdominal pain, fever and purulent ascites. Occasional cases caused by *N. meningitidis* have been reported in adults with alcoholism or other causes of cirrhosis[86,87], and in an infant with biliary atresia[88]. None developed meningitis. Peritoneal infection is thought to arise from haematogenous spread. Blood cultures are usually positive as well as cultures of the ascitic fluid. One of the above cases had evidence of endocarditis, probably also caused by the meningococcus.

N. meningitidis is a recognised cause of urethritis and endocervicitis in sexually active people. It is particularly associated with oro–genital sex, and cases are described in which the same serotype has been identified from the partner's throat[89]. A study in a Mexico City sexually transmitted disease clinic found that 0.4% of both endocervical and male urethral swabs grew *N. meningitidis* compared to 10% and 37% respectively which were positive for *N. gonorrhoeae*[90]. The meningococcus is not uncommonly cultured from rectal swabs taken from homosexual men, but when present, it appears to cause proctitis less frequently than does the gonococcus[91]. Genital infection is rare in prepubertal patients. Fallon and Robinson, however, described a 3 year old girl with a persistent vaginal discharge since early infancy, from whose high vaginal swab a meningococcus was isolated. The discharge resolved without treatment[92]. None of the above cases progressed to invasive meningococcal disease. A single case of meningococcal peritonitis and salpingitis has been described[89].

CHRONIC MENINGOCOCCAEMIA

This is a rare syndrome of chronic or recurrent fever, vasculitic rash and arthralgia associated with blood cultures positive for *Neisseria meningitidis*. It makes up 1–2% of all cases of meningococcal disease. Benoit[93] reviwed 148 cases up to 1963, and cases continue to be reported. The condition is described predominantly in adults, though paediatric cases are also reported, including that of a 3 month old infant. There is a strong male preponderance in the case reports reviewed by Benoit, although this is probably accounted for by the large proportion which occurred in armed forces personnel. There is no association between any predisposing illness and the development of chronic meningococcaemia. A patient who also had deficiency of the C5 component of complement has been described[94], but cases with normal complement levels are also reported[95]. In the pre-antibiotic era chronic meningococcaemia was a recognised complication of treatment with meningococcal antiserum alone[96].

The typical pattern is of recurrent episodes of fever and chills, starting abruptly and lasting several hours. Daily, tertian and quartan periodicities have been described although the fever does not necessarily occur at the same time each day. When fever occurs much less frequently, such as in the case described by Flaegstad *et al.*[97], it is more difficult to be sure that the episodes prior to the one during which the meningococcal infection was identified were part of the same syndrome, even though other typical features were present. In a third of cases there may be sustained fever[93].

A rash is reported in the vast majority of cases. Characteristically this occurs in crops appearing at the same time as the fevers and fading in the afebrile interludes. The lesions are most commonly maculopapular, between 5 and 15 mm in diameter. Several authors describe a non-blanching bluish-grey centre to some of the lesions[96,98]. Petechiae and nodules are reported less frequently, and a case has been described with target lesions[99]. The rash may be polymorphic. It is distributed on the trunk and limbs, and less commonly on the palms, soles and face. Mucous membranes are spared. Rarely, subungual splinter haemorrhages have been noted[93,100]. Typically, meningococci cannot be isolated from aspirate or skin biopsy and histology shows allergic vasculitis.

A migratory polyarthralgia, affecting all joints except the spine and temporomandibular joints, commonly waxes and wanes with the febrile episodes. Signs of joint swelling and limitation of movement are relatively frequent but very few cases have joint effusions. When present, effusions are usually purulent but sterile.

In Benoit's review of 148 cases, 37% had had a preceding upper respiratory tract infection[93]. More than 60% suffered headache. Splenomegaly occurred in 20, anaemia in 16 and thrombocytopenia in one. Lymphadenopathy was noted occasionally. Renal involvement, with haematuria or evidence of nephritis, was observed in 16%. Myalgia was recorded in only 2%, but Rosen *et al.*[94] reported a case in which daily fever, headache and severe myalgia over 3 months were the main symptoms. In this case, the serum creatinine phosphokinase and aldolase levels were normal but an EMG showed abnormalities consistent with polymyositis. The patient's condition did not improve with steroid therapy. Treatment with chloramphenicol was started when a meningococcus was isolated from the CSF, and was followed by striking resolution of the chronic symptoms.

In Benoit's series, the two most important focal complications were meningitis and carditis. Other specific features of the infection included epididymitis, conjunctivitis, iritis and retinitis. Angoff et al.[100] reported a patient in whom a pericardial friction rub was heard.

Most patients with chronic meningococcaemia do not have clinical evidence of meningitis. CSF examination is usually normal[101], or shows a sterile low-grade pleocytosis only[98]. However, six of the cases reviewed by Benoit had an episode of acute meningitis preceding the development of chronic meningococcaemia. These included two patients who had survived proven meningococcal meningitis treated with antiserum who then developed chronic meningococcaemia one and four months afterwards[96]. In another 17 cases meningitis occurred late in the course of the illness. This was not a universally terminal event despite the lack of antibiotic treatment[62,63,65,102]. In two more recent cases[94,99], meningitis supervened after prolonged febrile illnesses were treated with corticosteroids. In both cases there had been little clinical evidence of meningeal irritation.

Nineteen of Benoit's cases had evidence of endocarditis. In half, this was manifest by the presence of changing cardiac murmurs in patients who survived their illnesses. In the remainder, endocarditis occurred late in the course of the illness and was the cause of death.

The diagnosis of chronic meningococcaemia can be difficult. Often, of a series of blood cultures, only those taken 2–3 weeks into the illness are positive[93,98]. Usually the ESR and CRP are elevated. The white blood cell count is not dramatically raised, but often a left shift is noted. Autoantibodies are not present.

Benoit found the mean duration of chronic meningococcaemia to be about 7 weeks, with an upper limit of 40 weeks. Well documented recent cases lasted from 14 to 42 days. By convention, the shortest duration is one week, when chronic meningococcaemia merges with the more indolent presentations of acute meningococcaemia. Chronic meningococcaemia responds rapidly to systemic antimicrobial therapy. Fever settles within 12 hours and does not recur and the rash fades over a few days. By contrast, patients treated with corticosteroids prior to establishment of the diagnosis do not improve, and may develop meningitis. Fifteen of 148 cases reviewed by Benoit died. They tended to be older and had a longer duration of illness. Most had localising complications—meningitis and particularly endocarditis. Seven had been treated with serum therapy, one received sulphadiazine and the rest had no therapy. None of the more recently reported cases died, and the single sequela reported was persistent monoarthritis.

REFERENCES

1. Edwards MS, Baker CJ. Complications and sequelae of meningococcal infections in children. J Pediatr 1981; *99*: 540–5.
2. Olcén P, Barr J, Kjellander J. Meningitis and bacteremia due to *Neisseria meningitidis*: clinical and laboratory findings in 69 cases from Orebro county, 1965 to 1977. Scand J Infect Dis 1979; *11*: 111–19.
3. Donald PR, Burger PJ, van Zyl LE. Meningococcal disease at Tygerberg Hospital. S A Med J 1980; *60*: 271–5.
4. Wong VK, Hitchcock W, Mason WH. Meningococcal infections in children: a review of 100 cases. Pediatr Infect Dis J 1989; *8*: 224–7.
5. Voss L, Lennon D, Sinclair J. The clinical features of paediatric meningococcal disease, Auckland, 1985–87. N Z J Med 1989; *102*: 243–5.
6. Werne CS. Gastrointestinal disease associated with meningococcaemia. Ann Emerg Med 1984; *13*: 471–3.
7. Waldum HL, Fuglesang JE. Fulminant meningococcemia starting as an acute gastroenteritis. Scand J Infect Dis 1977; *9*(4): 309–10.
8. Kilpi T, Anttila M, Kallio MJT, Peltola H. Severity of childhood meningitis and duration of illness before diagnosis. Lancet 1991; *338*: 406–9.
9. Wood MJ, Anderson M. *Neurological Infections*. London: Saunders, 1988.
10. Carpenter RR, Petersdorf RG. The clinical spectrum of bacterial meningitis. Am J Med 1962; *33*: 260–75.
11. Wolf RE, Birbara CA. Meningococcal infections at an army training centre. Am J Med 1968; *44*: 243–55.
12. Mahida Y, Noone M. Atypical presentation of meningococcal meningitis. J Infect 1986; *13*: 277–9.
13. Edwards KM, Jones LM, Stephens DS. Clinical features of mild systemic meningococcal disease with characterization of bacterial isolates. Clin Pediatr 1985; *24*: 617–20.
14. Nye FJ. The value of initial laboratory investigations in the management of meningitis. J Infect 1983; *7*: 31–8.
15. Polk DB, Steele RW. Bacterial meningitis presenting with normal cerebrospinal fluid. Pediatr Infect Dis J 1987; *6*: 1040–2.
16. Onorato IM, Wormser GP, Nicholas P. 'Normal' CSF in bacterial meningitis. JAMA 1980; *244*: 1469–71.
17. Marzouk O, Thomson APJ, Sills JA, Hart CA, Harris F. Features and outcome in meningococcal disease presenting with a maculopapular rash. Arch Dis Child 1991; *66*: 485–7.
18. Toews WH, Bass JW. Skin manifestations of meningococcal infection; an immediate indicator of prognosis. Am J Dis Child 1974; *127*: 173–6.
19. Baxter P, Priestley B. Meningococcal rash. Lancet 1988; *i*: 1166–7.
20. Seyfer AE, Kiefer R. The management of dermal necrosis after acute *Neisseria* infection. Milit Med 1989; *154*: 598–600.
21. Robboy SJ, Mihm MC, Colman R, Minna JD. The skin in disseminated intravascular coagulation. Prospective analysis of thirty-six cases. Br J Dermatol 1973; *88*: 221–9.
22. Glauser MP, Zanetti G, Baumgartner J-D, Cohen J. Septic shock: pathogenesis. Lancet 1991; *338*: 732–6.
23. Monsalve F, Rucabado L, Salvador A, Bonastre J, Cunat J, Ruano M. Myocardial depression in septic shock caused by meningococcal infection. Crit Care Med 1984; *12*: 1021–3.

24. Sullivan TD, LaScolea LJ. *Neisseria meningitidis* bacteremia in children: quantitation of bacteremia and spontaneous clinical recovery without antibiotic therapy. Pediatrics 1987; *80*: 63–7.
25. Shapiro ED, Aaron NH, Wald ER, Chiponis D. Risk factors for development of bacterial meningitis among children with occult bacteremia. J Pediatr 1986; *109*: 15–19.
26. Havens PL, Garland JS, Brook MM, Dewitz BA, Stremski ES, Troshynski TJ. Trends in mortality in children hospitalized with acute meningococcal infections, 1957 to 1987. Pediatr Infect Dis J 1989; *8*: 8–11.
27. Tesoro LJ, Selbst SM. Factors affecting outcome in meningococcal infection. Am J Dis Child 1991; *145*: 218–20.
28. Stiehm ER, Damrosch DS. Factors in the prognosis of meningococcal infection. J Pediatr 1966; *68*: 457–67.
29. Leclerc F, Hue V, Martinot A, Delepoulle F. Scoring systems for accurate prognosis of patients with meningococcal infections. Am J Dis Child 1991; *145*: 1090–1.
30. Fallon RJ, Brown WM, Lore W. Meningococcal infections in Scotland 1972–82. J Hyg 1984; *93*: 167–80.
31. Sinclair JF, Skeoch CH, Hallwoth D. Prognosis of meningococcal septicaemia. Lancet 1987; *ii*: 38.
32. Thomson APJ, Sills JA, Hart CA. Validation of the Glasgow Meningococcal Septicaemia Prognostic Score: a 10-year retrospective survey. Crit Care Med 1991; *19*: 26–30.
33. Counts GW, Gregory DF, Spearman GJ, Lee BA, Filice GA, Holmes KK, Griffiss JM, and the Pacific Northwest Study Group. Group A meningococcal disease in the US Pacific Northwest: epidemiology, clinical features, and the effects of a vaccination control program. Rev Infect Dis 1984; *6*: 640–8.
34. Farmer TW. Neurologic complications during meningococcic meningitis treated with sulfonamide drugs. Arch Intern Med 1945; *76*: 201–9.
35. Dodge PR, Hallowell D, Feigin RD, Holmes SJ, Kaplan SL, Jubelirer DP *et al*. Prospective evaluation of hearing impairment as a sequela of acute bacterial meningitis. N Engl J Med 1984; *311*: 869–74.
36. Vienny H, Despland PA, Lutschg J, Deonna T, Dutoit-Marco ML, Gander C. Early diagnosis and evolution of deafness in childhood meningitis: a study using brainstem auditory evoked potentials. Pediatrics 1984; *73*: 579–86.
37. Kaplan SL, Catlin FI, Weaver T, Feigin RD. Onset of hearing loss in children with bacterial meningitis. Pediatrics 1984; *73*: 575–8.
38. Schwartz JF, Ataxia in bacterial meningitis. Neurology 1972; *22*: 1071–4.
39. Yabek SM. Meningococcal meningitis presenting as acute cerebellar ataxia. Pediatrics 1973; *52*: 718–20.
40. Steven NM, Nathwani D. Facial palsy, meningococcal meningitis and HSV re-activation. Clin Infect Dis 1993; *16*: 181.
41. Engber WD, Marti LB, Moore CT. Peripheral neuropathy – an unusual complication of meningococcemia. J Hand Surg [Am] 1977; *2*: 404–5.
42. Gotshall RA. Conus medullaris syndrome after meningococcal meningitis. N Engl J Med 1972; *286*: 882–3.
43. Schaad UB. Arthritis in disease due to *Neisseria meningitidis*. Rev Infect Dis 1980; *2*: 880–7.
44. Whittle HC, Abdillahi MT, Fakunle FA, Greenwood BM, Bryceson AD, Parry EH *et al*. Allergic complications of meningococcal disease. I. Clinical aspects. Br Med J 1973; *ii*: 733–7.

45. Pollet SM, Leek JC. Tenosynovitis in meningococcemia. Arthritis Rheum 1987; *30*: 232–3.
46. Rosen MS, Myers AR, Dickey B. Meningococcemia presenting as septic arthritis, pericarditis and tenosynovitis. Arthritris Rheum 1985; *28*: 576–8.
47. Fam AG, Tenenbaum J, Stein JL. Clinical forms of meningococcal arthritis: a study of five cases. J Rheumatol 1979; *6*: 567–73.
48. Kidd BL, Hart HH, Grigor RR. Clinical features of meningococcal arthritis: a report of four cases. Ann Rheum Dis 1985; *44*: 790–2.
49. Greenwood BM, Whittle HC, Bryceson AD. Allergic complications of meningococcal disease. II. Immunological investigations. Br Med J 1973; *ii*: 737–40.
50. Olivieri I, Pifferi M, Ceccarelli M, Puccetti A, Perri G, Ughi C, Ciompi ML. Erosive immune complex-mediated arthritis associated with meningococcal meningitis. Clin Rheumatol 1986; *5*: 531–4.
51. Hammerschlag MR, Baker CJ. Meningococcal osteomyelitis: a report of two cases associated with septic arthritis. J Pediatr 1976; *88*: 519–20.
52. Schaad UB, Nelson JD, McCracken GH. Primary meningococcal arthritis. Infection 1981; *9*: 170–3.
53. Rompalo AM, Hook EW, Roberts PL, Ramsey PG, Handsfield HH, Holmes KK. The acute arthritis-dermatitis syndrome. The changing importance of *Neisseria gonorrhoeae* and *Neisseria meningitidis*. Arch Intern Med 1987; *147*: 281–3.
54. Ploy-Song-Sang Y, Winkle RA, Phair JP. *Neisseria meningitidis* cellulitis. South Med J 1972; *65*: 1243–4.
55. Williams DN, Geddes AM. Meningococcal meningitis complicated by pericarditis, panophthalmitis, and arthritis. Br Med J 1970; *ii*: 93.
56. Pierce HI, Cooper EB. Meningococcal pericarditis. Arch Intern Med 1972; *129*: 918–22.
57. Morse JR, Oretsky MI, Hudson JA. Pericarditis as a complication of meningococcal meningitis. Ann Intern Med 1971; *74*: 212–17.
58. Blaser MJ, Reingold AL, Alsever RN, Hightower A. Primary meningococcal pericarditis: a disease of adults associated with serogroup C *Neisseria meningitidis*. Rev Infect Dis 1984; *6*: 625–32.
59. Maron BJ, Macoul KL, Benaron P. Unusual complications of meningococcal meningitis. Hopkins Med J 1972; *131*: 64–68.
60. Gersony WM, McCracken GH. Purulent pericarditis in infancy. Pediatrics 1967; *40*: 224–31.
61. Firestone GM. Meningococcus endocarditis. Am J Med Sci 1946; *211*: 556–64.
62. Cecil RL, Soper WB. Meningococcus endocarditis with septicaemia. Arch Intern Med 1911; *8*: 1–16.
63. Hyland CM. Meningococcus endocarditis. JAMA 1929; *92*: 1412.
64. Gwyn NB. Subacute meningococcal endocarditis. Arch Intern Med 1931; *48*: 1110–17.
65. Bray HA. Chronic meningococcus septicaemia associated with pulmonary tuberculosis. Arch Intern Med 1915; *16*: 487–502.
66. Heinle RW. Meningococcic septicaemia. Arch Intern Med 1939; *63*: 575–83.
67. Nye, RB, Semisch CW, Merves L. Chronic meningococcaemia complicated by acute endocarditis. Ann Intern Med 1942; *16*: 1245–52.
68. Master AM. Meningococcaemia with endocarditis. JAMA 1931; *96*: 1640–6.
69. Dennis J, Edwards LD, Fisher TN, Makeever L. Endocarditis on a Bjork-Shiley mitral prosthesis due to *Neisseria meningitidis*. Scand J Thorac Cardiovasc Surg 1977; *11*: 205–9.

70. Levin S, Balagtas R, Susmano A, Edwards L, Dainauskas J. Meningococcus endocarditis at the site of Starr-Edwards mitral prosthesis. Arch Intern Med 1972; 129: 963–6.
71. Gunn J, Gaw A, Trueman AM. A case of meningococcal endocarditis. Eur Heart J 1992; 13: 1004–5.
72. Ødegaard A. Primary meningococcal conjunctivitis followed by meningitis and septicemia. NIPH Ann 1983; 6: 55–7.
73. Brook I, Bateman JB, Petit TH. Meningococcal conjunctivitis. Arch Ophthalmol 1979; 97: 890–1.
74. Zagorzycki MT, Brook I. Primary meningococcal conjunctivitis in an infant. Clin Pediatr 1979; 18: 233–4.
75. Newton DA, Wilson DG. Primary meningococcal conjunctivitis. Pediatrics 1977; 60: 104–6.
76. Kenny JF. Meningococcal conjunctivitis in neonates. Clin Pediatr 1987; 26: 473–6.
77. Werner EB, Herschorn BR. Exogenous endophthalmitis. Am J Ophthalmol 1983; 95: 123–4.
78. Gamel JW, Allansmith MR. Metastatic staphylococcal endophthalmitis presenting as chronic iridocyclitis. Am J Ophthalmol 1974; 77: 454.
79. Jay WM, Schanzlin DJ, Fritz KJ. Medical therapy of metastatic meningococcal ophthalmitis. 1979; 87: 567–8.
80. Jensen AD, Naidoff MA. Bilateral meningococcal ophthalmitis. Arch Ophthalmol 1973; 90: 396–8.
81. Gradon JD, Lutwick LI. Retropharyngeal space infections in a community hospital. Am J Emerg Med 1991; 9: 77–80.
82. Hoppes GM, Ellenbogen C, Gebhart RJ. Group Y meningococcal disease in United States Air Force recruits. Am J Med 1977; 62: 661–6.
83. Kertulla Y, Leinonen M, Koskela M, Makela PH. The aetiology of pneumonia. Application of bacterial serology and basic laboratory methods. J Infect 1987; 14: 21–30.
84. Galpin JE, Chow AW, Yoshikawa TT, Guze LB. Meningococcal pneumonia. Am J Med Sci 1975; 269: 247–50.
85. Davies BI, Spanjaard L, Dankert J. Meningococcal chest infections in a general hospital. Eur J Clin Microbiol Infect Dis 1991; 10: 399–404.
86. Bar-Meir S, Chojkier M, Groszmann RJ, Atterbury CE, Conn HO. Spontaneous meningococcal peritonitis: a report of two cases. Am J Digest Dis 1978; 23: 119–22.
87. Finkelstein R, Hashman N, Klein L, Merzbach D. Primary peritonitis due to *Neisseria meningitidis* serogroup W-135. J Infect Dis 1986; 154: 543.
88. Leggiadro RJ, Lazar LF. Spontaneous bacterial peritonitis due to *Neisseria meningitidis* serogroup Z in an infant with liver failure. Clin Pediatr 1991; 30: 350–2.
89. Hagman M, Forslin L, Moi H, Danielsson D. *Neisseria meningitidis* in specimens from urogenital sites. Is increased awareness necessary? Sex Trans Dis 1991; 18: 228–32.
90. Condé-Glez CJ, Calderon E. Urogenital infection due to meningococcus in men and women. Sex Trans Dis 1991; 18: 72–5.
91. Baker RW, Peppercorn MA. Gastrointestinal ailments of homosexual men. Medicine 1982; 61: 390–405.
92. Fallon RJ, Robinson ET. Meningococcal vulvovaginitis. Scand J Infect Dis 1974; 6: 295–6.
93. Benoit FL. Chronic meningococcaemia; case report and review of the literature.

Am J Med 1963; *35*: 103–12.

94. Rosen MS, Lorber B, Myers AR. Chronic meningococcal meningitis; an association with C5 deficiency. Arch Intern Med 1988; *148*: 1441–2.

95. Jennens ID, O'Reilly M, Yung AP. Chronic meningococcal disease. Med J Aust 1990; *153*: 556–9.

96. Campbell EP. Meningococcaemia. Am J Med Sci 1943; *206*: 566–76.

97. Flaegstad T, Johnsen K, Hvidsten D, Kristiansen BE. Benign meningococcemia with IgG and IgM antimeningococcal antibodies measured by ELISA. Scand J Infect Dis 1987; *19*: 629–33.

98. Neilsen LT. Chronic meningococcaemia. Arch Dermatol 1970; *102*: 97–101.

99. Raman GV. Meningococcal septicaemia presenting as erythema multiforme. Br J Clin Pract 1990; *44*: 508–9.

100. Angoff GH, Czarnetzki B, Wolinsky E. A case of chronic meningococcemia with unusual features. Am J Med Sci 1975; *269*: 243–6.

101. Olcén P, Eeg-Olofsson O, Fryden A, Kernell A, Ansehn S. Benign meningococcemia in childhood. A report of five cases with clinical and diagnostic remarks. Scand J Infect Dis 1978; *10*: 107–11.

102. Appelbaum E. Chronic meningococcus septicaemia. Am J Med Sci 1937; *193*: 96–101.

9
Treatment of Meningococcal Disease in Childhood

SIMON NADEL, MICHAEL LEVIN and PARVIZ HABIBI
Department of Paediatrics, St Mary's Hospital Medical School,
London, UK

INTRODUCTION

Meningococcal infection remains an important cause of childhood morbidity and mortality worldwide. The disease was usually fatal in the pre-antibiotic era[1]. The mortality due to meningococcal infections declined to 10–20% following the introduction of antibiotics. However, it is disappointing that despite the availability of an increasing array of potent antibiotics, together with advances in intensive care management, the overall mortality rate remains at 10%, rising to 50–60% for children who present with meningococcal septicaemia and shock[2].

For many years there has been a fatalistic approach to the treatment of meningococcal infections. Once the condition was recognised and appropriate antibiotics administered, it was felt that the outcome was dependent more on luck or divine intervention than the result of medical care. However, it has become increasingly clear that interventions which aim to correct the disordered physiology present in meningococcal sepsis, if administered promptly and competently, may improve the prognosis significantly. This chapter will review current thoughts on the optimal therapy of meningococcal sepsis in relation to the pathophysiology of the disorder.

Meningococcal Disease. Edited by Keith Cartwright © 1995 John Wiley & Sons Ltd

Meningococcal septicaemia and meningitis

One of the major impediments to the provision of appropriate treatment for meningococcal disease has been lack of recognition that very different pathophysiological processes are operative in the two major clinical forms of the disorder[3]. The meningococcal purpuric rash is often thought, even by experienced clinicians, to be synonymous with the presence of meningococcal meningitis. This may result in failure to deliver effective therapy for patients whose predominant problem is circulatory failure and shock rather than meningitis. The confusion between these conditions has been compounded by the use of the term 'meningococcal meningitis' to describe patients with either septicaemia or meningitis, in public health advice and media reports on the disorder[4].

As discussed in Chapter 8, there are two distinct presentations of meningococcal disease in childhood. The most common form of disease is meningococcal meningitis. Clinical features of this are indistinguishable from those of meningitis caused by other organisms[5]. Older children develop high fever, vomiting and drowsiness, and complain of headache, stiff neck and photophobia. In infants and younger children the features are more subtle or non-specific, and may include fever, vomiting, irritability, drowsiness and confusion. In more severe cases a declining level of consciousness, convulsions and ultimately coma occur. Clinical findings are similar to those found in other forms of meningitis with stiff neck and a positive Kernig's sign, but usually without evidence of circulatory failure unless the child is severely dehydrated due to inadequate fluid intake or vomiting. If a purpuric rash is present this provides a clue to the likelihood of the meningitis being caused by *N. meningitidis*. For patients without a rash, distinction between meningococcal meningitis and other causes of bacterial meningitis depends on the isolation of meningococci from blood, direct visualisation and/or culture of the organism, or detection of meningococcal capsular antigen in the cerebrospinal fluid (CSF).

Although less common than meningococcal meningitis, meningococcal septicaemia with septic shock is the form of meningococcal infection which is associated with greater mortality. The presenting features are those of high fever, vomiting, muscle aches, shivering, frank rigors and confusion. These features may be similar to those seen in many trivial febrile illnesses and the distinction between these and early meningococcal septicaemia may be difficult. In contrast to the predominant neurological features seen in patients with the meningitic form of the disease, children presenting with meningococcal septicaemia usually have a clear sensorium and may be awake and responsive. The lack of central nervous system involvement may prevent recognition of the true severity of the illness. In the early phases of meningococcal septicaemia the clinical findings may just be those of high fever with a flushed or 'toxic' appearance, and tachycardia. However, as the disease progresses clinical features of circulatory failure develop. Peripheral perfusion is impaired, with a prolonged capillary refill time and an increasing gap between central and peripheral temperature. There is a progressive increase in heart rate and the peripheries may become cold and mottled. Oliguria or anuria may develop.

It must be stressed that a low blood pressure is not a feature of shock in children until a pre-terminal stage has been reached. Blood pressure may be maintained by intense vasoconstriction even in the face of a significant reduction in circulating volume and cardiac output[6]. Signs of impending circulatory collapse include rising heart rate and respiratory rate, cyanosis and ultimately a decline in blood pressure. Confusion, somnolence and eventual coma reflect diminished cerebral perfusion.

A petechial or purpuric rash is usually present in patients with meningococcal septicaemia. However, the severity of the rash and the degree of circulatory failure are not closely correlated. Severely shocked patients may have scanty petechiae which may only be seen after a careful search of all areas of the body. In contrast, other patients may have a fulminant purpuric rash with extensive cutaneous involvement and yet may have only moderate circulatory impairment.

A major focus of the discussion in this chapter will be the differences in pathophysiology underlying the meningitic and septicaemic forms of the disease, and therefore the subsequent differences in treatment required. However, in some patients there is an overlap between the two forms of the disease. In such cases, features of meningitis as well as those of septic shock may occur simultaneously. Although there is some overlap in the presentation and management required for the two major forms of meningococcal disease, a distinction between these is essential to understand both the pathophysiology and treatment.

Recognition of severe disease

It has been known since the study of Stiehm and Damrosch that patients presenting without meningitis but with features of septic shock have a very much worse prognosis[7]. The poor prognostic features proposed by Stiehm and Damrosch have been confirmed in subsequent studies and are included in several scoring systems designed to predict severe disease[8-10]. Although occasional patients with a meningitic presentation may develop severely elevated intracranial pressure and die as a result of profound cerebral involvement, most deaths from meningococcal disease occur in patients with profound shock. Clinical and laboratory features which predict poor prognosis at the time of presentation include a rapidly progressive purpuric rash, absence of meningism, the presence of shock (hypotension or evidence of peripheral or organ underperfusion), low peripheral blood white cell count, thrombocytopenia and markedly deranged coagulation indices. Patients with these features have a mortality of 30–60%.

PATHOPHYSIOLOGY OF MENINGOCOCCAL SEPTICAEMIA

Immunopathology

The bacterial and host factors which enable the meningococcus to pass from the nasopharynx into the bloodstream remain poorly understood and are discussed in more detail in Chapter 4. Once within the bloodstream, both bacterial and host factors may be important in allowing bacterial survival and proliferation. The absence of specific antibody and deficiency in properdin or terminal components of the complement pathway facilitate survival of the bacteria and are well known factors predisposing to neisserial infection[11,12]. The studies of Brandtzaeg and his Norwegian group, have been important in defining the immunopathological events which occur in meningococcal sepsis. Meningococci, or products released by the bacteria, including endotoxin and peptidoglycan trigger an intense host inflammatory response (Chapter 4). Endotoxin is probably one of the most important bacterial components contributing to the inflammatory process[13,14]. Levels of endotoxin correlate with the severity of the disease and with elaboration and release of a range of inflammatory mediators[15], including the cytokines tumour necrosis factor and interleukin-1, and the complement components. Activation of macrophages, neutrophils and platelets occurs. Neutrophil activation is demonstrated by the presence of high levels of neutrophil elastase in plasma[16]. Activation of the coagulation system occurs with increased tissue factor expression on monocytes[17] and endothelium[18], platelet activation, depression of the coagulation inhibitors antithrombin III, proteins C and S[19,20], and elevation of plasminogen activator inhibitor[21]. The degree of inflammatory cell activation and levels of these mediators correlate with the severity of the clinical disease. While the link between high levels of endotoxin and an intense inflammatory response is thus established[22,23], the mechanisms by which bacteria and the inflammatory process induce the clinical manifestations of the disease has been much less well studied.

Clinical pathophysiology

There are few medical conditions which present as complex an array of clinical problems as are found in children with meningococcal shock. Although cardiorespiratory failure is the dominant clinical problem, this coexists with multiorgan failure, severe coagulopathy and a complex metabolic derangement with acidosis, electrolyte disturbance and abnormalities in intermediary metabolism[22,23]. Although the precise sequence of events leading to this complex physiological derangement is not well understood, most of the abnormalities are explained by four primary processes:

1. Severe capillary leak resulting in loss of circulating volume.
2. Vasodilatation of some vascular beds coexisting with vasoconstriction of others.
3. Intravascular thrombosis.
4. Severe depression of myocardial function.

Capillary leak

The earliest event in the development of meningococcal shock is probably an increase in vascular permeability. Leakage of albumin and other plasma proteins from the intravascular compartment into the interstitium results in hypovolaemia and therefore diminished venous return to the heart[6] (Figure 9.1). Reduced filling of the left and right ventricles results in diminished cardiac output as predicted by Starling's law (Figure 9.2). The compensatory sympathetic response to hypovolaemia initially maintains cardiac output by increasing heart rate and contractility. Homeostatic responses may maintain blood pressure and vital organ perfusion by intense vasoconstriction of vascular beds in the skin, splanchnic and renal circulation. Children in the early stages of meningococcal septicaemia therefore may have a well-maintained blood pressure. The only signs of impending shock are an increased heart rate and diminished peripheral perfusion. As the capillary leak worsens and severe hypovolaemia develops, these compensatory mechanisms begin to fail, cardiac output falls and hypotension may ensue. If the intense vasoconstriction is sustained, hypoxia occurs in underperfused tissues and organs. Anaerobic metabolism in hypoxic tissues results in increasing acidosis. Myocardial function is further depressed by hypoxia, acidosis and reduced coronary perfusion due to the worsening hypotension. These, together with the severe electrolytic and metabolic derangements which occur in meningococcal sepsis, including hypocalcaemia, hypokalaemia and lack of nutrient substrates, increase the risk of cardiac arrest. Once profound acidosis, hypoxia and hypotension are present, reversal of shock becomes increasingly difficult.

The importance of hypovolaemia in the causation of meningococcal shock has been well documented by Mercier *et al.*[24]. Patients who did not survive were found to have persistently low central venous and pulmonary capillary wedge pressures, increased peripheral and pulmonary vascular resistance, and were resistant to volume replacement. In contrast, patients

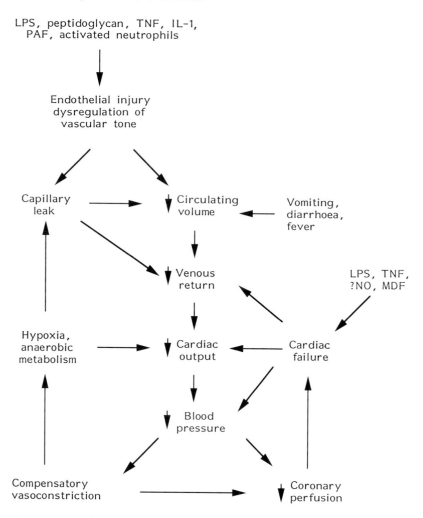

Figure 9.1   Mechanism of shock in meningococcal disease. LPS, lipopolysaccharide; TNF, tumour necrosis factor; IL-1, interleukin-1; PAF, platelet activating factor; NO, nitric oxide, MDF, myocardial depressant factor

who survived meningococcal sepsis had well maintained central venous pressures and at no stage developed as profound volume depletion as occurred in those with a fatal outcome.

It is not uncommon for patients with meningococcal shock to require several times their normal circulating volume of colloid in the first 24–48 hours following admission in order to restore circulating volume. Marked peripheral oedema is the inevitable consequence of the profound capillary leak and develops in virtually all patients (Plate 3).

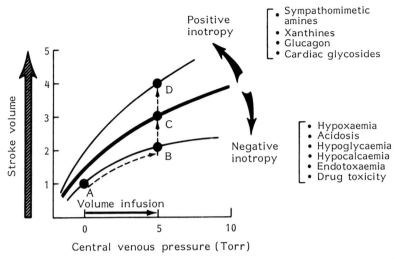

Figure 9.2   *Starling curve. The Starling curve relates cardiac output (or stroke volume) to the filling pressure of the left and right ventricles. Patients presenting with meningococcal septicaemia are usually at point A, with a low central venous pressure (CVP), and low cardiac output. Volume replacement increases cardiac output (point B), but myocardial contractility remains impaired due to the negative inotropic effects of acidosis, electrolyte imbalance and endotoxaemia. Correction of the myocardial depressant factors and the use of exogenous inotropic agents improves the cardiac output achieved at the same filling pressure (points C and D)*

Although the capillary leak and resulting hypovolaemia are probably key events in the initiation of septic shock, their aetiology is not well understood. There is evidence that increased vascular permeability to albumin may be the result of loss of surface glycosaminoglycans and glycoproteins which are normally present on the endothelial surface[25]. Albumin is normally confined within the vasculature not only by its size, but also by its charge[26]. An electrostatic repulsion exists between negatively charged glycosaminoglycans on the endothelial surface and the negative charges present on albumin at physiological pH. Experimental neutralisation or removal of endothelial negatively charged groups results in a profound capillary leak[27]. Endotoxin activated neutrophils have been shown to remove endothelial negative charge experimentally[25]. In view of the intense neutrophil activation and margination of neutrophils seen in meningococcal sepsis, it is likely that a similar process may occur in affected patients.

Vasoconstriction/vasodilatation

Intense vasoconstriction is usually present on admission in patients with meningococcal sepsis[24]. The 'warm' shock sometimes seen in adults with

gram-negative sepsis is extremely uncommon in children with meningococcaemia. Most patients have high peripheral vascular resistance, with cold
peripheries, stagnant capillary refill and diminished peripheral pulses.
However, once circulatory volume has been restored and myocardial
function improved by inotropes, a different picture may emerge which may
more closely resemble so-called 'warm shock' usually seen in adults.
Peripheral vasodilatation, wide pulse pressure, hypotension and progressive
acidosis develop despite evidence of elevated cardiac output.

The mechanisms responsible for the vasoconstriction and inappropriate
vasodilatation of some vascular beds have not been well studied.
Vasoconstrictor substances known to be elevated in patients with shock
include catecholamines, renin, aldosterone, thromboxane A2 and endothelin[22,28,29]. Elevation of these mediators, together with low cardiac
output, may explain the intense vasoconstriction. In vitro studies have
suggested that endothelial cell production of prostacyclin is inhibited by
plasma from patients with meningococcal disease[30]. A reduction in
endothelial production of this vasodilator may also contribute to the platelet
activation and consumption, together with vasoconstriction and small-vessel
thrombosis. The mediators of the vasodilatation seen later in the illness (once
volume replacement has been achieved), and in occasional patients from the
onset of the disease, are less well defined. Excess production of nitric oxide
has been suggested as playing a role in the vasodilatation seen in other forms
of gram-negative sepsis[31,32], but this mediator has not yet been evaluated in
meningococcal disease.

Coagulopathy and intravascular thrombosis

Disturbances in haemostatic parameters are early findings in patients with
meningococcal sepsis[33,34]. Thrombocytopenia, prolonged kaolin partial
thromboplastin time, prothrombin time and thrombin time, together with a
reduction in plasma fibrinogen and elevation of fibrin degradation products,
are usually present on admission. These features have been interpreted as
indicating the presence of disseminated intravascular coagulation. This is
supported by the finding of elevated levels of fibrinopeptide A and depletion
of coagulation pathway factors. Reduction in the coagulation inhibitors
antithrombin III, protein C and protein S as well as extrinsic pathway
inhibitor is commonly seen on admission[19,20]. Severe depression of the
levels of these inhibitors is associated with severe disease. Defective
fibrinolysis has also been documented with low levels of plasminogen and
alpha 2 antiplasmin and high levels of plasminogen activator inhibitor[21].

The mechanisms responsible for the coagulopathy are incompletely
understood. Endotoxin is a potent inducer of tissue factor expression on
endothelial cells and on circulating monocytes[17,18] and the degree of

coagulopathy has been correlated with levels of endotoxin. Congenital deficiencies of protein C and S are associated with purpuric lesions similar to those found in meningococcal disease[35,36], suggesting that depletion of these inhibitors may be involved in the pathogenesis of the purpuric lesions. More recent studies have suggested that loss of the anticoagulant glycosaminoglycans heparan sulphate and dermatan sulphate from the endothelial surface may result in defective thromboresistance due to a failure to bind and activate antithrombin III and heparin cofactor II[37]. As mentioned above, prostacyclin production by the endothelium is also diminished. A defect in endothelial thromboresistance may therefore coexist with up-regulation of endothelial procoagulant activities[34].

The coagulopathy of meningococcal disease is associated with the presence of purpuric lesions which may at times progress to the clinical picture of purpura fulminans. Severely affected patients may progress from having small areas of petechiae to extensive confluent areas of skin necrosis (see Plate 4). Lesions are characteristically sharply demarcated and have a predilection for peripheral sites on the limbs, the ears and the tip of the nose. Although in most patients the purpuric lesions are confined to the skin, in some cases major vessel thrombosis occurs resulting in gangrene of digits or entire limbs (see Plate 5). Peripheral gangrene is most commonly seen in patients who have been profoundly shocked with intense vasoconstriction. Initially, the limbs may appear ice cold, white and bloodless. This appearance may be followed by the development of obvious venous and arterial occlusion with a progressive blackening of the limb. Infarction of organs other than the skin is rare, but in occasional patients microvascular or major vessel thrombosis may be seen at post mortem in the vascular beds of the lungs and kidneys. Areas of thrombosis may coexist with haemorrhage, which for unknown reasons is most common in the adrenals[38].

Myocardial failure

Depressed myocardial function due to hypovolaemia is one of the earliest features of meningococcal sepsis. However, even once circulating volume has been restored, myocardial function may remain severely depressed[29]. Initial echocardiographic studies reveal good myocardial function with a normal ejection fraction and underfilled left and right ventricles. In patients who develop persistent shock, this initial picture may be replaced by one of severe myocardial dysfunction. End diastolic and end systolic volumes are markedly elevated and ejection fraction markedly reduced. A gallop rhythm is usually audible with evidence of elevated central venous and pulmonary wedge pressures and enlargment of the liver.

The depressed myocardial function is probably multifactorial[28]. Coronary artery perfusion may be impaired due to hypotension and myocardial contractility depressed by hypoxia, acidosis, hypocalcaemia, hypokalaemia, hypomagnesaemia and hypophosphataemia. Derangements of glucose and fatty acid metabolism are also recognised in sepsis and may have effects on myocardial function due to inadequate fuel for cardiac myocytes. Direct effects of endotoxin, tumour necrosis factor and nitric oxide have also been proposed as mediators of poor myocardial function. A poorly characterised myocardial depressant factor has been reported to be released in shock[39]. These mediators and metabolic abnormalities alone or in concert result in a poorly functioning myocardium and subsequent myocardial failure.

Other organ dysfunction

Most patients with profound shock will develop evidence of multiorgan dysfunction. Respiratory failure is extremely common in patients with shock. Capillary leak also occurs within the pulmonary vasculature. Pulmonary oedema with leakage of high protein fluid into the alveoli occurs due to both the capillary leak syndrome and to left ventricular failure. Pulmonary vascular occlusion with platelet/thrombin microthrombi and aggregated neutrophils may contribute to the picture of the acute respiratory distress syndrome (ARDS)[40]. Early findings are of tachypnoea, chest wall retraction and hypoxia. Rising respiratory rate suggests the likelihood of impending respiratory failure. Initially, increased respiratory effort may maintain oxygen saturation and a low arterial concentration of carbon dioxide ($PaCO_2$) is commonly seen. Pulmonary oedema may supervene suddenly with the rapid development of cyanosis and with frothy pulmonary oedema fluid filling the airway. Respiratory failure is likely in shocked patients who are not electively ventilated.

Oliguria is one of the earliest events in septic shock. Initially this is prerenal in origin and the findings are those of concentrated urine, with a low urine sodium concentration and elevated urine to plasma urea ratio. If shock persists, intense renal vasoconstriction and reduced renal perfusion result in vasomotor nephropathy[41]. If cardiac output and renal perfusion are restored, renal failure may be reversible but protracted renal failure with acute tubular or cortical necrosis is seen if prolonged shock occurs.

Renal failure was seldom reported in the early literature as most patients with profound shock did not survive the initial days of the illness. However, with improvements in intensive care and better management of circulatory failure, prolonged renal failure is increasingly recognised.

In patients with meningococcal septicaemia but without meningitis, neurological dysfunction is usually the result of impaired cerebral perfusion and metabolism due to hypotension, hypoxia and acidosis. Patients with prolonged hypotension and hypoxia may develop coma, with evidence of hypoxic encephalopathy. The presence of meningitis may compound a neurological deficit induced by hypoperfusion.

MANAGEMENT OF MENINGOCOCCAL SEPTICAEMIA

Recognition and initial therapy

If prognosis is to be improved, a major factor which must be addressed is the speed with which the infection is recognised and treated. Any febrile child with a petechial rash or with suggestive clinical features should be considered to have meningococcal infection and treatment commenced without awaiting further confirmation. If outside the hospital, intravenous benzylpenicillin (75 mg/kg) should be administered and the child transferred to hospital. Penicillin (600 mg) can be given intramuscularly if vascular access is difficult. A number of published studies have suggested that the administration of penicillin by general practitioners outside the hospital improves mortality[42,43]. While not all studies have supported this conclusion[44], the weight of evidence suggests that early administration of antibiotics is of benefit[45]. The first dose of antibiotics should be administered by the first doctor to see the patient. Treatment may be delayed for crucial hours if the first dose of antibiotics is not given until the child has been transferred to the paediatric ward.

If the child is first seen in hospital, blood cultures should be obtained, an intravenous cannula placed immediately and antibiotics administered promptly.

Lumbar puncture

The decision to perform a lumbar puncture should only be made after a full assessment of the severity of the disease. While the organism may be readily seen in, or cultured from, the CSF in meningococcal meningitis, the procedure may be hazardous in patients who are shocked, or in those who have signs of raised intracranial pressure. In no case should antibiotic administration be delayed by performance of a lumber puncture. Patients who show signs of circulatory compromise or deteriorating neurological condition should not undergo a lumbar puncture and antibiotics should be commenced without delay after taking blood cultures.

Microbiological diagnosis

The diagnosis of meningococcal disease will be established by culture of the organism from blood in only 50–60% of cases, even if prior antibiotics have not been administered. Cultures of CSF (if undertaken) or nasopharyngeal cultures may provide additional evidence, and meningococcal antigens may be detected in the CSF or in blood in approximately 60% of culture-negative cases, depending on the serogroup of the causative organism. Antibodies against LOS or outer membrane proteins may help to confirm the diagnosis retrospectively, but will not help in initial management.

Choice of antibiotics

Penicillin remains the treatment of choice for meningococcal sepsis. However, other infections including *Streptococcus pneumoniae*, *Haemophilus influenzae* type b and other gram-negative organisms may occasionally cause a similar clinical picture with shock and a petechial rash. Until cultures are available or the organism is identified by Gram stain or rapid antigen detection tests, the antibiotic regimen should include cover for *Haemophilus influenzae* in children under 5 years[46]. Penicillin resistant strains of *Neisseria meningitidis* have been reported in Spain[47] and South Africa[48], but insensitive strains have not been encountered in the UK.

For many years chloramphenicol and penicillin have been the standard antibiotic combination for initial blind therapy. However, the third generation cephalosporins cefotaxime and ceftriaxone have several advantages over this standard regimen. Although the mortality and long-term morbidity of patients treated with the newer antibiotics are similar to those treated with conventional therapy, the third generation cephalosporins are preferred because of their activity against all three major childhood meningeal pathogens, their excellent penetration into the CSF and their lack of toxicity. They also have the advantage of overcoming the problem of emerging resistance to conventional therapy amongst the three major pathogens. Additional advantages include elimination of the need to monitor serum chloramphenicol levels and the convenience and reliability of using a single agent which can be administered on a 1–3 times daily basis[49]. Our current practice is the use of cefotaxime (200 mg/kg/day) or ceftriaxone (100 mg/kg/day) in divided doses, as initial therapy until microbiological confirmation of the diagnosis has been achieved.

In countries where the cost of third generation cephalosporins precludes their widespread use, the combination of penicillin and chloramphenicol remains a highly satisfactory regimen.

Initial assessment, observation and detection of complications

The course of meningococcaemia is extremely unpredictable. All children with suspected meningococcal septicaemia, whatever their clinical condition on admission, should be considered to have potentially life-threatening illness and should be observed vigilantly during the first 48 hours following admission to hospital. Many children who are alert, well perfused and do not appear acutely ill on admission may deteriorate suddenly in the following hours, with the development of severe shock and vascular compromise. A number of clinical prognostic scoring systems have been developed to identify those at greatest risk of a deteriorating course (see Chapter 7). The original criteria proposed by Stiehm and Damrosch remain useful predictors of severe disease and are based on criteria which are available very soon after admission[7]. Children with evidence of shock or underperfusion, in particular those who have no evidence of meningeal involvement, a low peripheral white cell count and a rapidly progressive purpuric rash are likely to deteriorate in the hours following admission. Ideally, admission to a paediatric intensive care unit should be arranged. If this is not readily available, admission to the hospital's adult intensive care unit or, in less severe cases, close observation on a paediatric ward or high dependency unit is an acceptable alternative.

The most important complication requiring urgent intervention is the development of shock. It must be stressed that hypotension is not necessary to diagnose shock. A fall in blood pressure is a very late sign, and the condition should be recognised on the basis of any sign of impaired skin or organ perfusion. Cold peripheries, poor capillary refill, rising heart rate, rapid breathing and oliguria are all warning signs. The fact that the child is alert or even restless and combative should not be interpreted as indicating that the situation is stable. Restlessness may be a sign of poor cerebral perfusion or hypoxaemia. In addition to non-invasive monitoring of blood pressure, pulse, perfusion and urine output, core and peripheral temperature monitoring is a useful guide to impaired perfusion. Any gradient above $4\,^{\circ}C$ between the rectal temperature and the temperature of the big toe should be interpreted as indicating underperfusion if the ambient temperature is reasonable[6].

Resuscitation

Children who present with meningococcal shock need immediate resuscitation and restoration of circulating volume (Figure 9.3). Firstly the airway must be assessed for patency and security. Supplemental oxygen at high concentration, via face mask or endotracheal tube, should be given even if there is a normal transcutaneous oxygen saturation. Secure and efficient vascular access must be obtained. If necessary, the intraosseous route should be used where venous access is difficult. Even if major signs of shock are not present, almost all children with meningococcaemia will have some clinical evidence of underperfusion. This should be treated promptly by infusing colloid. Typically, 20–40 ml/kg of plasma or 4.5% albumin can be given over 10–30 minutes without risk of pulmonary oedema. If this improves the perfusion a further 20–40 ml/kg can be given over the next hour. The degree of hypovolaemia is usually underestimated and it is not uncommon for children with meningococcal shock to require several times their circulating volume of colloid in the first 24 hours. Such volumes can only be given with monitoring of central venous or pulmonary capillary wedge pressure, along with continuous clinical assessment. This is best undertaken by a paediatric intensive care unit team familiar with the interpretation of haemodynamic

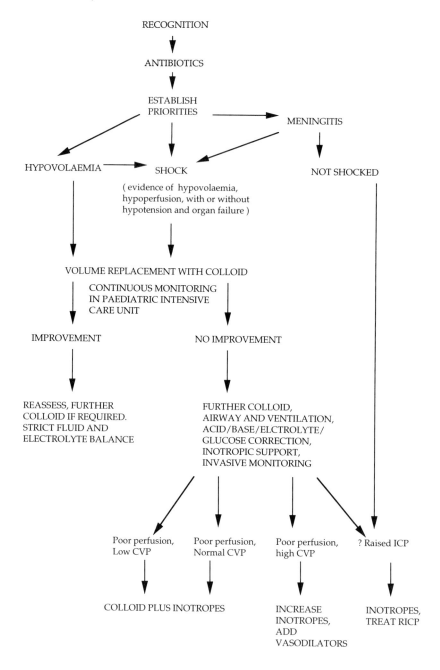

Figure 9.3 *Management of meningococcal sepsis. CVP, central venous pressure. RICP, raised intracranial pressure*

monitoring. If the child fails to respond to two aliquots of 40 ml/kg of colloid, or if continued deterioration occurs, transfer to an intensive care unit and invasive monitoring of central venous pressure and arterial blood pressure are urgently required to guide further volume replacement.

Intensive care management

In children with fulminant meningococcaemia as evidenced by shock unresponsive to 40–80 mls/kg of colloid, there is a severe capillary leak syndrome and myocardinal dysfunction. Thus there is a considerable danger of pulmonary oedema developing (Figure 9.4). Severely shocked children should be electively ventilated, even if they are alert and ventilating adequately, as precipitate deterioration may occur. Elective ventilation allows the patient to be sedated appropriately and, if necessary, paralysed. These measures can reduce greatly the work of breathing and the myocardial workload. However, sedatives may exacerbate hypotension and some muscle relaxants such as pancuronium are myocardial depressants. Depending on the clinical status of the patients, our practice is to use a combination of atropine and either thiopentone or ketamine and suxamethonium or vecuronium for induction of anaesthesia and endotracheal intubation.

Intubation should proceed with caution as these agents, particularly thiopentone, may exacerbate hypovolaemia in children who are already intravascularly depleted. For maintenance of sedation and paralysis we use fentanyl or morphine, together with midazolam and atracurium by infusion.

Strategies to improve circulatory failure include optimising preload, decreasing afterload and improving myocardial contractility. In severely shocked patients, or those who remain underperfused despite volume replacement, inotropic support should be initiated early and concurrently with the continued volume expansion. Low doses of dopamine (5–10 μg/kg/min) or dobutamine (5–10 μg/kg/min) can be administered safely by peripheral infusions before central vascular access has been established. When central venous or pulmonary capillary wedge pressure has been established, further volume expansion can be undertaken to optimise intravascular volume. If shock persists once central venous pressure has been restored, additional inotropic support with higher doses of dobutamine (up to 30 μg/kg/min) or adrenaline (0.01–5 μg/kg/min) may be required to improve myocardial function. It is important to emphasise that there are no definite normal values for optimal central venous and pulmonary capillary wedge pressures in severely shocked children with ongoing capillary leak and myocardial dysfunction. Continuous monitoring of peripheral and core temperature difference, systemic arterial pressure, oxygen saturation, urine

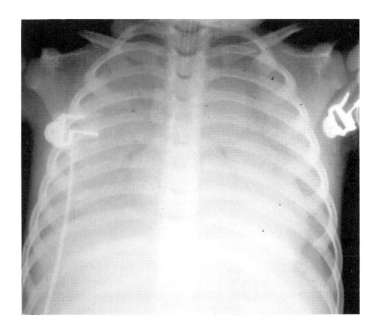

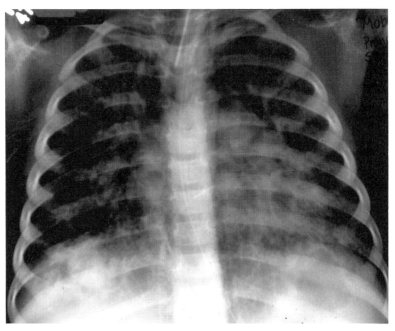

output and repeated clinical assessment are vital in the delivery of optimal resuscitation.

Echocardiographic evaluation is helpful in early detection of myocardial failure in patients who continue to deteriorate despite volume replacement. In patients who have depressed myocardial activity or who remain hypotensive and underperfused despite an adequate filling pressure, myocardial contractility may be improved by using higher doses of dobutamine (15–30 μg/kg/min). In some patients with severe shock, infusions of adrenaline or noradrenaline may be required to maintain blood pressure at a level which produces acceptable coronary perfusion.

In patients with continued peripheral vasoconstriction despite adequate cardiac filling pressures and arterial blood pressure, vasodilators are a logical and effective treatment in improving perfusion and reducing the afterload of the heart. Low-dose prostacyclin (5–20 ng/kg/min) or nitroprusside are the most commonly used vasodilators, and are particularly indicated in patients with severe vasoconstriction and impending peripheral gangrene. Vasodilators, however, should be administered to patients with severe shock with extreme caution. Unless venous filling has already been optimised and careful haemodynamic monitoring is in place, severe hypotension may result. Prostacyclin is not only a vasodilator, but an inhibitor of platelet aggregation. It is a logical form of treatment to reverse vasoconstriction and improve arterial circulation and there have been encouraging reports of its use in patients with severe sepsis[50]. However, there have been no controlled trials of its use in meningococcal sepsis.

The phosophodiesterase inhibitor, enoximone, has also been advocated for its positive inotropic and vasodilator activity in patients with refractory shock. There is limited experience of this agent in children but first reports are promising[51].

Respiratory failure

Pulmonary oedema may occur suddenly in patients with severe meningococcal sepsis. It is our policy to ventilate electively any child with severe shock requiring large volumes of colloid, even if no signs of respiratory failure are present. Control of the airway and administration of positive pressure ventilation allows volume resuscitation to proceed safely with a reduced risk of the sudden development of pulmonary oedema. Some patients present in profound respiratory failure even if they have not received volume resuscitation. Such patients should be ventilated

Figure 9.4 *(opposite)   Respiratory failure in meningococcal sepsis. Top: chest X-ray showing acute pulmonary oedema in a child with profound shock. Bottom: chest X-ray of the same child one week later showing typical changes of the acute respiratory distress syndrome (ARDS)*

immediately to prevent acute respiratory collapse from developing. There are two major patterns of respiratory failure in the initial days of treatment of meningococcal sepsis. Some patients develop pulmonary oedema with frothy, blood-stained fluid welling up in the trachea. The administration of positive pressure ventilation with positive end expiratory pressure and correction of the coagulaopathy are the mainstay of treatment of haemorrhagic pulmonary oedema. Measures to improve left ventricular function will also be of benefit. Pulmonary oedema occurs most commonly in the first 24–48 hours of treatment in children who have severe left ventricular dysfunction and a profound capillary leak.

The second form of respiratory failure is the development of the acute respiratory distress syndrome (ARDS). This pattern of lung injury tends to occur 24–48 hours after onset of the disease and often after the initial resuscitation and correction of hypovolaemia has been undertaken. Development of ARDS is heralded by an increase in oxygen requirement and reduction in pulmonary compliance. In non-ventilated patients there is a progressive increase in respiratory rate and work of breathing. In ventilated patients a progressive increase in the fraction of inspired oxygen required to maintain oxygenation, and in patients who are treated on volume cycle ventilators an increase in respiratory pressures are the earliest signs. The pathophysiology of ARDS in meningococcal disease is not well understood. Aggregation of neutrophils, platelets and fibrin within the pulmonary capillaries may occur in some patients. In others the predominant feature is the accumulation of high protein fluid in the interstitium and alveolar spaces[52]. Pulmonary haemorrhage may be an additional complication in some patients. With the improved management of acute circulatory failure, more patients are developing severe ARDS and this may be a cause of late mortality.

Management of ARDS in meningococcal sepsis depends on measures to improve myocardial function, removal of extravascular fluid accumulation by meticulous fluid management or dialysis and by ventilatory patterns designed to reduce barotrauma to the lung. In general, tolerance of higher than normal levels of arterial CO_2 will allow lowering of the peak inspiratory pressure. Therefore, pressure-limited ventilation with reversed inspiratory to expiratory time ratios and high positive end expiratory pressure has been used to optimise oxygenation and limit barotrauma. A number of experimental treatments are now being assessed, including use of high frequency oscillating ventilation[53], inhaled nitric oxide[54], and extracorporeal membrane oxygenation[55].

Renal function and fluid management

In the face of a continuing capillary leak it may be difficult to maintain effective fluid balance. In general, an attempt should be made to maintain intravascular volume by the administration of colloid or crystalloid according to the central venous pressure and the signs of peripheral and other organ perfusion. Extravascular fluid accumulation can be reduced by restriction of crystalloid to approximately 50% of maintenance requirements. Severely shocked patients usually become oliguric. Initially the renal impairment is prerenal in origin and may respond to measures which improve cardiac output and renal perfusion. However, if hypotension is severe and sustained, vasomotor nephropathy or cortical necrosis may occur.

Dialysis should be instituted early in severely shocked patients. Dialysis is an extremely effective means of preventing or reducing the extravascular fluid accumulation and in normalising electrolytic and acid–base balance. Peritoneal dialysis is probably the preferred modality in severely shocked and haemodynamically unstable patients. However, haemofiltration is preferred in some units. In patients in whom haemodynamic stability has been achieved, haemodialysis and haemofiltration are acceptable alternatives.

Metabolic abnormalities

Patients with severe meningococcal sepsis have a complex derangement in electrolytes, acid–base balance and metabolism. Metabolic acidosis is an inevitable consequence of tissue underperfusion in shock. Plasma sodium is usually normal, but if severe vomiting has occurred in the early phases of the illness hyponatraemia may be present. Surprisingly, hypokalaemia rather than hyperkalaemia is the usual finding in severely shocked patients. The plasma potassium levels may be markedly reduced despite the severe acidosis which would normally be expected to result in a shift of potassium from the intracellular space. Hypocalcaemia, hypophosphataemia and hypomagnesaemia are also often seen[56,57]. Hypoglycaemia is common early in the illness, and conversely hyperglycaemia and glucose intolerance may be problems following initial resuscitation, particularly in patients who require high doses of catecholamines. The precise mechanisms underlying this complex derangement of electrolytes is poorly understood, but collectively the derangement of electrolytes may play a major role in impairing mycocardial function and in predisposing to arrhythmias. The electrolyte abnormalities should be detected early by frequent measurement of plasma electrolytes and acid–base balance. Any departure from normal should be corrected immediately. Many patients will require potassium and calcium supplementation during the initial phase of the illness, and bicarbonate infusions and glucose administration are often required. Correction of the electrolyte and metabolic derangement is often hampered by the presence of oliguria or anuria. Dialysis is often required to facilitate correction of the electrolyte derangement.

Central nervous system involvement

Although correction of shock and haemodynamic stabilisation is the most important initial aspect of treatment, other factors may be important in individual patients. Cerebral oedema and raised intracranial pressure may occur in meningococcal disease as they do in other forms of meningitis. Elective ventilation, control of the $PaCO_2$ and improvements in cardiac output and thus cerebral perfusion are probably the most important aspects of treatment[58]. Administration of mannitol and intracranial pressure monitoring may be hazardous in the presence of severe shock and disseminated intravascular coagulation, and should not be undertaken until shock has been controlled. If neurological findings suggest raised intracranial pressure after resuscitation and correction of shock, infusion of mannitol (0.25–0.5 g/kg), with or without intracranial pressure monitoring, may be considered. Intracranial pressure monitoring, while potentially useful in the management of children with raised intracranial pressure who are not shocked, is of little use until an adequate cardiac output has been achieved.

Management of disseminated intravascular coagulation

Virtually all patients with meningococcaemia show evidence of coagulopathy and thrombocytopaenia. These abnormalities, together with the histological finding of fibrin in blood vessels within the skin and other organs, suggest the presence of disseminated intravascular coagulation (DIC). Heparin was advocated in several early reports as a means of correcting the DIC[59,60], but failed to improve prognosis and was occasionally associated with bleeding complications. Although lowgrade DIC does occur in meningococcaemia, the extent and importance of this process in the pathophysiology of the disease may have been over-stressed, and it is possible that platelet activation has an equally important role. Though there is insufficient evidence to recommend routine heparinisation for all patients with meningococcaemia, in individual patients and in particular those with impending peripheral gangrene and severe coagulation derangements, low dose heparin (10 units/kg/hour), together with fresh frozen plasma, is a logical treatment and is unlikely to be associated with bleeding problems. The administration of large quantities of fresh frozen plasma may also serve to restore depleted levels of the antithrombin III, protein C and protein S. Prostacyclin has been used to treat a number of patients with impending peripheral gangrene, and while it appears a promising treatment its use has not been subjected to controlled trial.

MANAGEMENT OF MENINGOCOCCAL MENINGITIS

Introduction

Meningococcal meningitis carries a lower mortality than the septicaemic form of the illness[2]. Deaths continue to occur in patients presenting with classical meningitis without evidence of septic shock, largely due to the severity of the inflammatory process within the brain. Long-term morbidity including neurological deficits and sensorineural hearing loss occurs in a small proportion of survivors. In recent years there has been a rapid advance in the understanding of the pathophysiological events occurring in the central nervous system in all forms of bacterial meningitis[61]. Much of this knowledge has come from the study of animal models of bacterial meningitis which have been extended into clinical studies. As a result of this new understanding of the pathophysiological events occurring in meningitis, there have been a number of important changes in clinical management, the most important being the introduction of anti-inflammatory treatment.

Pathophysiology and immunopathology

The mechanisms by which bacteria invade through the nasopharyngeal mucosa, survive and multiply in the bloodstream, evading antibacterial immunological mechanisms, and then penetrate through the blood–brain barrier are discussed in some detail in Chapter 4. Once the organism has invaded the CSF, a number of bacterial components, particularly lipopolysaccharide (LPS) or lipo-oligosaccharide (LOS) and peptidoglycan, are the major determinants of meningeal inflammation[61]. The teichoic acid of gram-positive organisms[62] and peptidoglycan components of both gram-positive and gram-negative organisms have been shown to be potent inducers of inflammation in the CSF and to impair blood–brain barrier function on direct intracisternal inoculation in experimental animals[63]. Similarly, direct inoculation of LPS from *H. influenzae*, or the LOS of *N. meningitidis* into the CSF of experimental animals causes an intense inflammatory reaction with influx of leucocytes, increase in protein and lactate and a decline in CSF glucose concentration[64–68]. These studies have provided overwhelming evidence that bacterial endotoxins and other bacterial cell wall constituents are important in the initiation of the inflammatory changes within the CSF, and the disturbance of function of the blood–brain barrier.

Inflammatory changes in the CSF occur several hours after the inoculation of bacteria or cell wall constituents into the meningeal space of experimental animals. This has led to the hypothesis that elaboration and release of host mediators are instrumental in the development of the inflammatory changes. In animal models, tumour necrosis factor alpha (TNF-α) and interleukin-1 beta (IL-1β) are important mediators of the initial meningeal inflammation[69]. Levels of TNF-α and IL-1β together with interleukin-6 (IL-6) increase in the CSF of animals following intracisternal inoculation of meningococcal LOS, and this rise in cytokine levels precedes cellular influx and protein exudation[69-72]. These cytokine mediators have been shown to stimulate the release of other factors in the inflammatory cascade, including platelet activating factor (PAF), interleukin-8 (IL-8) and interferon gamma (IFN-γ). Release of these pro-inflammatory mediators causes up-regulation of various cellular adhesion molecules including integrins, selectins and the IgG superfamily on the surfaces of peripheral blood leucocytes and vascular endothelial cells of the blood–brain barrier, resulting in attraction, attachment and migration of leucocytes into the CSF[61-73]. Once present in the CSF, polymorphonuclear neutrophils (PMNs) are activated and undergo degranulation with release of proteolytic enzymes, cationic proteins and reactive oxygen species[70]. These products further alter the integrity of the blood–brain barrier, thus interrupting its primary functions: active transport and facilitated diffusion of nutrients (including glucose and other metabolites) and secretion of CSF. Increased permeability of the blood–brain barrier results in leakage of albumin and other macromolecules into the CSF, causing vasogenic oedema. The presence of anaphylotoxins (C3a, C5a) in the CSF due to the protein leak also encourages passage of PMNs into the CSF, further accentuating the inflammatory process. Toxic products of neutrophil activation and other inflammatory cells cause cytotoxic oedema and damage to surrounding cells.

The importance of the cytokines, TNF-α and IL-1β, has been confirmed in studies which have shown that the inflammatory response to LPS in the CSF of experimental animals can be almost entirely prevented by the simultaneous inoculation of antibodies to TNF-α, IL-1β, or both[71,72]. However, the use of antibodies against these cytokines does not completely annul the inflammatory response, suggesting that other mediators also have an important role. Furthermore, direct inoculation of TNF-α, IL-1β and IFN-γ induces inflammatory changes which closely resemble those seen with LPS inoculation. In addition to the development of vasogenic and cytotoxic oedema, interstitial oedema may be caused by impaired reabsorption of CSF by the arachnoid villi, a phenomenon which has been demonstrated in experimental models of meningitis[74].

The consequences of increased secretion of CSF, diminished reabsorption, and breakdown of the blood–brain barrier are an increase in brain water content and CSF volume, and the development of severe brain oedema. This leads to an increase in intracranial pressure, which, if severe, will lead to a reduction in cerebral blood flow (CBF). In experimental models of meningitis, CBF at first increases due to local vasodilatation induced by inflammation, and then decreases as a consequence of raised intracranial pressure[75]. These changes are paralleled by an increase in CSF lactate levels indicating tissue hypoxia[76]. Changes in CBF may also be a consequence of a loss of cerebrovascular autoregulation, which has been shown to occur in severe bacterial meningitis[76]. Cerebral blood flow is normally maintained at constant levels irrespective of systemic arterial pressure. Once autoregulation has been lost, CBF is totally dependent on systemic pressure. Inadequate blood flow may occur if there is systemic hypotension. The rise in intracranial pressure, together with the systemic hypotension which is common in meningococcal sepsis, may readily result in cerebral hypoperfusion. Together with the vasculitis and thrombosis of cerebral vessels, ischaemia of areas of the brain may result, leading to neuronal injury and focal or diffuse brain damage.

Understanding the pathophysiological and immunological events leading to cerebral injury, as outlined above, has allowed more rational approaches to therapy, and the introduction of new forms of treatment designed to reduce the intracranial inflammatory process.

Diagnosis and initial therapy

In the absence of a purpuric rash, the distinction between meningitis due to *N. meningitidis* and that caused by other bacteria depends on isolation of the organism from the blood or CSF, or detection of meningococcal antigens in blood or CSF. As is the case for patients with meningococcal septicaemia, blood cultures are positive in less than two-thirds of cases. Blood culture positivity is greatly reduced if antibiotics have been administered prior to referral to hospital[77].

Lumbar puncture remains an essential procedure to establish the presence of meningitis and to define the causative organism. A lumbar puncture should be performed whenever the diagnosis of meningitis is suspected on the basis of clinical signs, or in infants who are irritable, lethargic, off feeds and with an abnormal temperature (either high or low), as the signs of bacterial meningitis in infancy may be non-specific. Lumbar puncture is generally a safe procedure, but there are several recognised contraindications: signs of raised intracranial pressure; infection of the skin at the lumbar puncture site; the presence of bleeding diatheses; and severe cardiovascular compromise in the neonate.

In considering the risks of lumbar puncture in patients with bacterial meningitis and in particular in those with a meningococcal purpuric rash, additional factors should be considered. Elevated intracranial pressure occurs in virtually all patients with bacterial meningitis[78]. It must be stressed that the presence of papilloedema is a late and therefore unreliable sign of severely elevated intracranial pressure. Raised intracranial pressure should be suspected in any patient who has:

- severely depressed or a rapidly declining level of consciousness,
- alterations in blood pressure or heart rate,
- cranial nerve palsies or opisthotonic posturing.

If any of these features are present the risk of cerebral herniation following lumbar puncture is considerable and the procedure should be deferred.

Meningococcal septicaemia without signs of meningitis may itself be a contraindication to lumbar puncture for several reasons. Patients with a meningococcal purpuric rash are often in a state of septic shock. Performing a stressful and perhaps painful procedure may cause an increase in respiratory and cardiovascular workload due to the positioning of the patient and may result in an acute deterioration in the patient's condition. The patient may also have raised intracranial pressure as a consequence of meningitis and reduced cerebral perfusion as a result of hypotension. Lumbar puncture in these circumstances may result in acute brain stem herniation[79].

The diagnosis of meningococcal infection is usually obvious in patients with a characteristic rash. Bacteriological confirmation can be obtained by blood culture or rapid antigen testing in a high proportion of individuals. Meningococcal infection can also be confirmed serologically by the analysis of acute and convalescent sera to detect a rise in antibodies to meningococcal antigens[80,81] and a nasopharyngeal swab will yield a meningococcus in 50% or more of cases (though the isolation of a meningococcus from this site only adds weight to, but does not confirm, invasive meningococcal disease).

The presence or absence of meningitis does not alter the management of patients with meningococcal disease. Although several scoring systems utilise the presence of low CSF white cell counts as a poor prognostic feature, the same poor prognostic implications are derived from a clinical assessment of whether meningism is present and from the child's orientation and level of consciousness. Treatment is rarely changed as a direct consequence of the CSF findings in patients in whom the diagnosis is suspected from the characteristic rash.

If it is felt necessary to obtain laboratory confirmation of meningitis, lumbar puncture should be delayed until circulatory stability has been achieved, and until any features suggesting raised intracranial pressure have been eliminated. The cellular and chemical changes will still be present in the CSF several days after the acute illness, though cultivable organisms may have been cleared, a neutrophil pleocytosis may have given way to a predominance of lymphocytes, and changes in CSF glucose and protein will be less marked.

Based on these considerations, we believe that lumbar puncture should be undertaken with far more caution than has been previously practised. The possible risks of the procedure must be balanced against the benefits of the information which may be derived from the procedure in any patient with evidence of severe meningitis and in all patients with septic shock[80,82].

Antibiotic treatment

Antibiotic recommendations for patients with meningococcal meningitis are similar to those discussed previously for patients presenting with meningococcal septicaemia. Before the results of cultures or antigen tests are available, the antibiotic regimen should cover the other major childhood meningeal pathogens as well as *Neisseria meningitidis*. A combination of penicillin and chloramphenicol remains the most widely used initial therapy worldwide[46]. However, in view of the increasing risk of chloramphenicol resistance in *H. influenzae* strains[83], and the possibility of penicillin resistant meningococci in certain countries[47,48], most authorities in Europe and North America now recommend a third-generation cephalosporin such as cefotaxime or ceftriaxone as first line treatment[49]. Third-generation cephalosporins have the advantage of high activity against all common meningeal pathogens except *Listeria monocytogenes*, current lack of resistance, excellent penetration into the CSF and the ease of use of a single agent which can be given on a three times daily basis (cefotaxime) or once or twice daily (ceftriaxone). Once a meningococcus has been isolated and has been shown to be penicillin sensitive, therapy can be changed to benzylpenicillin.

There is now good evidence that 7 days of parenteral therapy is adequate for both meningococcal meningitis and meningococcal septicaemia, and it is possible that a shorter duration of treatment may also be successful[84]. The duration of therapy may need to be extended if there are complications such as brain abscess or subdural empyaema, prolonged fever, or the development of nosocomial superinfection.

Antibiotic recommendations in developing countries

Third generation cephalosporins are currently far more expensive than penicillin or chloramphenicol. For poorer countries penicillin alone remains the treatment of choice for patients with meningococcal meningitis or septicaemia. Chloramphenicol should be administered to patients without a characteristic purpuric rash until the results of cultures or Gram stain are available. Chloramphenicol alone is also efficacious against all three major meningeal pathogens. Chloramphenicol may be administered intravenously or intramuscularly during the initial phase of treatment and once the patient's condition has improved, the oral route may be used to complete a course of treatment.

Anti-inflammatory treatment

The growing evidence that damage to the brain is mediated by activation of host inflammatory pathways triggered by the release of endotoxin and other bacterial constituents, has led to the hypothesis that injury to the brain may be reduced by the use of anti-inflammatory treatment[61,85-87]. In experimental animals, the inflammatory process can be reduced by using agents which act to neutralise endotoxin such as polymyxin B[64], those which block the binding of endotoxin to macrophages such as bactericidal permeability enhancing factor (BPI)[88] and anti-CD14 antibodies[89], antibodies directed against cytokine mediators such as IL-1β or TNF-α[71,72], antibodies directed against neutrophil adhesion molecules[90,91], or pharmacological agents which inhibit neutrophil and macrophage activation such as steroids, pentoxyphylline, or non-steroidal anti-inflammatory agents[92-94].

While several of these anti-inflammatory mediators have shown benefit in animal experiments, convincing evidence for a beneficial effect from steroids has now emerged from a series of clinical trials[80]. Initial studies conducted in the USA showed a clear benefit from the use of dexamethasone in reducing the severity of neurological sequelae, particularly deafness[87]. Subsequent studies in Costa Rica[78], Egypt[94] and Switzerland[95] have all reported a beneficial effect from the use of dexamethasone in reducing neurological sequelae. Most patients in these published studies have suffered from H. influenzae or S. pneumoniae meningitis. Firm conclusions on the efficacy of dexamethasone in reducing neurological damage in patients with meningococcal meningitis cannot be derived from these studies. However, the pathophysiological events occurring in meningococcal meningitis are unlikely to differ significantly from those seen in other forms of bacterial meningitis. For patients who present with meningococcal meningitis without septic shock, treatment with dexamethasone as for other forms of bacterial meningitis seems appropriate. In both animal studies and in recently published clinical trials, the benefit of dexamethasone appears greatest if it is administered early in the course of the illness, preferably prior to antibiotic administration. Therefore our current recommendation would be to administer dexamethasone in a dose of 0.15 mg/kg, 6 hourly for 4 days starting prior to, or concurrently with, the first dose of antibiotics.

There have been few side effects documented in patients receiving dexamethasone. In particular there have been no reports of delayed CSF sterilisation or treatment failure, although gastrointestinal bleeding has been observed in a small proportion of patients.

Based on studies in animals, a variety of other anti-inflammatory agents are likely to be of benefit in reducing central nervous system injury, but there have been no clinical studies on which to base recommendations for their routine use.

Supportive care

There has been increasing recognition that antibiotic administration is only one component of the overall management of patients with severe meningitis. Neurological derangement often coexists with circulatory insufficiency, impaired respiration, metabolic derangement, and convulsions. Measures to detect and correct any coexisting physiological derangement are important in improving the prognosis.

All patients with invasive meningococcal infection may deteriorate suddenly. They should therefore be managed in a facility which can readily institute intensive care. Patients with severe meningitis or septicaemia who are first admitted to hospitals which lack intensive care facilities should be stabilised and then transferred to more specialised units by staff experienced in resuscitation and transport of critically ill children.

Management of children with raised intracranial pressure

All patients with bacterial meningitis are likely to have raised intracranial pressure as part of their disease process. In a recent study the mean opening pressure at the time of lumbar puncture was 180 ± 70 mm of water, more than twice the upper limit of normal in infants and children[78]. Signs of raised intracranial pressure include an altered level of consciousness, altered pupillary responses, hyper- or hypotension, reduction in resting pulse rate, and altered respiratory pattern. Papilloedema is often a late sign of raised intracranial pressure. Raised intracranial pressure should be suspected in any patient with severely depressed levels of consciousness and measures should be instituted in order to prevent brain stem compression and herniation. Diagnosis of raised intracranial pressure should be based on clinical suspicion rather than the use of computed tomography (CT) or magnetic resonance (MR) scans. Both methods are insensitive in predicting raised intracranial pressure, though they are useful for excluding alternative diagnoses in neurologically impaired patients[96,97]. Central nervous system (CNS) imaging is thus not routinely required in the management of patients with severe meningitis.

The primary therapeutic objective in the management of raised intracranial pressure is to preserve oxygen and nutrient delivery to the brain. Relatively simple interventions to optimise respiration and cardiac output, and prevent metabolic abnormalities, may be as important as measures which reduce intracranial pressure directly. In patients who are comatose and suffering from raised intracranial pressure, obstruction to the airway, cessation of respiration, or convulsions may result in both hypoxia and hypercapnia, with disastrous effects on brain perfusion and enhanced development of cerebral oedema. Maintenance of the airway, elective ventilation to optimise respiration, and control of convulsions are important interventions. Although most decisions on the use of measures to reduce raised intracranial pressure are taken on the basis of clinical criteria, direct measurement of intracranial pressure has been advocated by some authorities, and should logically be of help in defining the therapeutic interventions required. However, there have been no studies which indicate that intracranial pressure monitoring reduces mortality from meningitis[98].

Simple measures to reduce intracranial pressure include nursing the patient in a head-up position of 20–30 degrees from horizontal and nursing in a quiet environment. Other important interventions include the use of osmotic agents, fluid restriction and control of cerebrovascular tone through manipulation of arterial CO_2 concentration.

Extravascular fluid accumulation and thus intracranial pressure can be reduced through the use of osmotically active agents such as mannitol. An infusion of mannitol in a dose of 0.25–1 g/kg results in a rapid shift in fluid from the extravascular to the intravascular space and may be associated with a prompt reduction in intracranial pressure[98]. In view of the rapid action of mannitol, it may be life saving in patients with impending cerebral herniation, and is often of use while other measures such as airway control, artificial ventilation and fluid restriction are being initiated. The use of mannitol is often combined with fluid restriction to 50–70% of maintenance requirements, together with the use of frusemide or other loop diuretics to maintain plasma osmolality between 295 and 305 mOsm/l. In areas of brain with extensive vascular injury, mannitol may accumulate extravascularly, possibly worsening brain oedema. Furthermore, repeated doses may cause a hyperosmolar state. Together with fluid restriction this may impair cardiac output. Therefore mannitol should be used with caution, particularly when administered for prolonged periods.

In children with Cushing's triad (pupillary changes, hypotension and bradycardia, with or without respiratory insufficiency), or a Glasgow Coma Score (modified paediatric coma scale) of less than 8, urgent endotracheal intubation and artificial ventilation should be carried out, both to protect the airway and to prevent an acute rise in intracranial pressure due to further increases in $PaCO_2$. Use of hyperventilation as a treatment for raised intracranial pressure has been the subject of much recent controversy[75,99]. Based on the linear correlation between $PaCO_2$ and cerebral blood flow, hyperventilation to reduce $PaCO_2$ may be effective in decreasing the volume within the vascular compartment of the intracranial cavity, and therefore in reducing intracranial pressure. It is not clear, however, whether such reduction in cerebral blood flow is beneficial, as it may reduce the oxygen supply to critically dependent areas. Moreover there is evidence that cerebral autoregulation and CO_2 reactivity are impaired or absent in injured areas of brain. Hyperventilation as a measure to reduce intracranial pressure should therefore be used with caution and with careful monitoring. Modest reductions in $PaCO_2$ to between 3.5 and 4.5 kPa is usually advocated and should be monitored by repeated blood gases or by end-tidal CO_2 measurement. More severe hyperventilation should only be undertaken in cases where there is evidence of impending brain stem herniation.

In general, fluid intake should be modestly restricted in patients with meningitis who are well hydrated. However, many patients who are admitted with bacterial meningitis have been vomiting or have experienced reduced fluid intake in the days preceding admission. Further restriction of fluid intake may severely impair circulating volume and reduce cardiac output.

Most children with meningococcal meningitis are hypovolaemic at presentation due to increased capillary permeability, reduced fluid intake prior to presentation, and increased fluid losses due to vomiting and fever. In the past, emphasis on the possibility of inappropriate antidiuretic hormone secretion has led to the practice of fluid restriction in all patients with meningitis, even in the face of severe hypovolaemia. Recent studies indicate that the increased levels of antidiuretic hormone seen in individuals with meningitis represent an appropriate response to dehydration[100]. With adequate rehydration these levels return to normal. Correction of hypovolaemia, preferably with colloid infusions, will improve cardiac output and may have a beneficial effect on cerebral blood flow. In patients with incipient shock, the use of inotropic agents as well as colloid infusions may be important in optimising cerebral perfusion.

Sedation and control of convulsions

A child who has a significantly reduced level of consciousness due to bacterial meningitis should not be sedated, even if extremely irritable or combative. Irritability or combativeness may indicate hypoxia due to reduced respiratory drive. The addition of hypnotic or tranquillising agents may precipitate acute respiratory failure or respiratory arrest, or cause a further rise in intracranial pressure. Simple analgesics or antipyretic agents alone should be used in those children who are not critically ill. Patients who require endotracheal intubation and artificial ventilation should receive a combination of drugs to provide analgesia, amnesia and sedation, together with a muscle relaxant. This combination will decrease intracranial pressure. A commonly used combination is morphine in a dose of 0.02 mg/kg/h, midazolam (2–6 μg/kg/min), and atracurium at 10–30 μg/kg/min.

Barbiturates have been used to treat severely raised intracranial pressure that is refractory to other forms of therapy[98]. However, large doses of agents such as thiopentone may severely impair cardiac output and should only be used in patients with adequate cardiovascular stability and with extremely careful monitoring. Thiopentone is particularly useful for induction of anaesthesia prior to endotracheal intubation in patients with acutely raised intracranial pressure.

Seizures occur within 48 hours of presentation in 20–30% of patients with bacterial meningitis. Seizures are especially dangerous in patients with raised intracranial pressure, as they will result in extreme metabolic demands and an increase in cerebral blood flow and may precipitate a further rise in intracranial pressure. Convulsions may be difficult to detect in patients who are pharmacologically paralysed to permit artificial ventilation. In such patients electrical monitoring should be used to detect seizure activity. The use of anticonvulsant treatment in non-ventilated patients may precipitate respiratory arrest and careful observation of respiration and ventilation should be undertaken during the treatment of seizures. Short-acting agents such as diazepam or paraldehyde can be used to control acute seizures, and barbiturates or phenytoin are generally used for longer-term control.

EXPERIMENTAL FORMS OF THERAPY FOR MENINGITIS AND SEPTICAEMIA

There are a number of experimental forms of therapy which have shown promise in animal models of either meningitis or septicaemia. These are designed to reduce the inflammatory process, or reverse the disordered physiology and are currently being evaluated in animal models or clinical trials. A full discussion is beyond the scope of this chapter, but some of these therapeutic possibilities are listed in the Table 9.1.

It is essential that the introduction of any new form of therapy is based on the results of well-conducted randomised, placebo-controlled trials. Several such trials are currently in progress and results are eagerly awaited.

PREVENTION OF SECONDARY CASES

The risk of secondary cases occurring in family members or close contacts of patients with meningococcal meningitis or septicaemia is well known. Fear and anxiety within the family, school or the community frequently follows the occurrence of a case of meningococcal disease. Careful handling of the family, as well as of the contacts, is required. Close collaboration between the physicians caring for the affected patient and those responsible for community and public health advice is always essential. Rifampicin should be administered to all household contacts as soon as possible after the index case has been diagnosed, and to the index case prior to discharge from hospital. Ciprofloxacin or ceftriaxone are alternative, though less widely used, prophylactic agents[101,102].

Both bivalent (A and C) and tetravalent (A, C, Y and W-135) polysaccharide vaccines have proved effective in the containment of both small and large outbreaks of meningococcal disease in defined communities[103]. These vaccines do not control disease due to meningococci of serogroup B. They

Table 9.1 *New and experimental therapeutic modalities in meningococcal septicaemia*

Anti-endotoxin agents
 Monoclonal antibodies against endotoxin/lipid A
 Lipopolysaccharide binding protein
 Bactericidal permeability increasing factor
 CD14 receptor antagonists
 Novel antimicrobials

Anti-cytokine response agents
 Monoclonal antibodies against tumour necrosis factor.
 Monoclonal antibodies against interleukin-1
 Tumour necrosis factor receptor antagonist
 Interleukin-1 receptor antagonist
 Soluble TNF receptor

Leucocyte activation antagonists
 Monoclonal antibodies against leucocyte adhesion molecules (e.g. CD11/CD18)
 Non-steroidal anti-inflammatory agents (e.g. ibuprofen)
 Phosphodiesterase inhibitors (e.g. pentoxyfylline)
 Corticosteroids
 Phospholipase A2 antagonists

Cardiovascular supportive agents
 New inotropes (e.g. dopexamine)
 Both inotropic and vasodilating agents (e.g. enoximone)
 Nitric oxide antagonists (e.g. L-NMMA)
 Vasodilators (e.g. prostacyclin, sodium nitroprusside)
 Thromboxane synthetase inhibitors (e.g. imidazole)

Agents for the treatment of disseminated intravascular coagulation
 Heparin
 Antithrombin III
 Plasminogen activators
 Monoclonal antibodies against tissue factor
 Proteins C and S

Agents for the treatment of the acute respiratory distress syndrome
 Inhaled nitric oxide
 High frequency oscillating ventilation
 Extracorporeal membrane oxygenation
 Extracorporeal membrane CO_2 removal
 Intravenous membrane oxygenation
 Surfactant therapy
 Liquid ventilation

Miscellaneous agents
 Superoxide dismutase
 Platelet activating factor antagonists
 N-acetylcysteine
 Monoclonal antibodies to activated complement components
 Kinin receptor antagonists
 Monoclonal antibodies to tissue factor
 Oxygen free radical scavengers
 Protease inhibitors
 Calcium channel blockers

appear to have limited effect on nasopharyngeal carriage of the meningococci and therefore may not prevent spread of infection to unimmunised individuals[104]. The use of vaccines in the prevention of meningococcal disease is examined in greater detail in Chapter 11.

The risk of secondary cases occurring in nursery schools or children's day-care centres is sufficiently high to warrant administration of rifampicin prophylaxis to children in the same class. Rifampicin is not offered routinely to class contacts of older children or adults unless contact with the affected patient has been intimate. Contacts should be advised to seek medical care promptly should they develop fever or any other suspicious symptoms. Prompt notification of all cases and involvement of the public health authorities in the tracing and management of contacts is essential for control of disease in the community. A detailed account of control of meningococcal disease in the community will be found in Chapter 11.

REFERENCES

1. Noah ND. Epidemiology of bacterial meningitis: UK and USA. In: Williams JD, Burnie J, eds. *Bacterial Meningitis*. London: Academic Press, 1987; 93–115.
2. Havens PL, Garland JS, Brook MM, Dewitz BA, Stremski ES, Troshynski TJ. Trends in mortality in children hospitalised with meningococcal infections, 1957 and 1987. Pediatr Infect Dis J 1989; *8*: 8–11.
3. Heyderman RS, Klein NJ, Levin M. Pathophysiology and management of meningococcal septicaemia. Recent Adv Paediatr 1992; *11*: 1–18.
4. Thompson APJ, Hayhurst GK. Press publicity in meningococcal disease. Arch Dis Child 1993; *69*: 166–9.
5. Levin M, Heyderman RS. Bacterial meningitis. Rec Adv Paediatr 1990; *9*: 1–19.
6. Levin M. Shock. In: Black D, ed. *Paediatric Emergencies*. 2nd edition. London: Butterworths, 1987; 87–116.
7. Stiehm RS, Damrosch DS. Factors in the prognosis of meningococcal infection. J Pediatr 1966; *68*: 457–67.
8. Gedde-Dahl TW, Bjark P, Høiby EA, Høst JH, Brunn JN. Severity of meningococcal disease: assessment by factors and scores and implications for patient management. Rev Infect Dis 1990; *12*: 973–91.
9. Sinclair JF, Skeoch CH, Hallworth D. Prognosis of meningococcal septicaemia. Lancet 1987; *ii*: 38.
10. Leclerc F, Beuscart R, Guillois B, Diependaele JF, Krim G, Devictor D *et al.* Prognostic factors of severe infectious purpura in children. Intensive Care Med 1985; *11*: 140–3.
11. Fijen CAP, Kuijper EJ, Hannema AJ, Sjöholm AG, van Putten JPM. Complement deficiencies in patients over ten years old with meningococcal disease due to uncommon serogroups. Lancet 1989; *ii*: 585–8.
12. Nurnberger W, Pietsch H, Seger R, Bufon T, Wahn V. Familial deficiency of the seventh component of complement associated with recurrent meningococcal infections. Eur J Pediatr 1989; *148*: 758–60.

13. Brandtzaeg P, Kierulf P, Gaustad P, Skulberg A, Bruun JN, Halvorsen S *et al.* Plasma endotoxin as a predictor of multiple organ failure and death in systemic meningococcal disease. J Infect Dis 1989; *159*: 195–204.
14. Brandtzaeg P, Mollnes TE, Kierulf P. Complement activation and endotoxin levels in systemic meningococcal disease. J Infect Dis 1989; *160*: 58–65.
15. Waage A, Brandtzaeg P, Halstensen A, Kierulf P, Espevik T. The complex pattern of cytokines in serum from patients with meningococcal septic shock. J Exp Med 1989; *169*: 333–8.
16. Speer CP, Rethwilm M, Gahr M. Elastase-alpha-l-proteinase inhibitor: an early indicator of septicaemia and bacterial meningitis in children. J Pediatr 1987; *111*: 667–71.
17. Gregory SA, Morrissey JH, Edginton TS. Regulation of tissue factor gene expression in the monocyte procoagulant response to endotoxin. Mol Cell Biol 1989; *9*: 2752–5.
18. Colucci M, Balconi G, Lorenzet R, Pietra A, Locati D. Cultured human endothelial cells generate tissue factor in response to endotoxin. J Clin Invest 1983; *71*: 1893–6.
19. Brandtzaeg P, Sandset PM, Joø GB, Øvstebø R, Abildgaard U, Kierulf P. The quantitative association of plasma endotoxin, antithrombin, protein C, extrinsic pathway inhibitor and fibrinopeptide A in systemic meningococcal disease. Thromb Res 1989; *55*: 459–70.
20. Powars DR, Rogers ZR, Patch MJ, McGehee WG, Francis RB. Purpura fulminans in meningococcemia: association with acquired deficiencies of proteins C and S. N Engl J Med 1987; *317*: 571–2.
21. Brandtzaeg P, Joø G, Brusletto B, Kierulf P. Plasminogen activator inhibitor 1 and 2, alpha-2-antiplasmin, plasminogen and endotoxin levels in systemic meningococcal disease. Thromb Res 1990; *57*: 271–8.
22. Bone RC. The pathogenesis of sepsis, Ann Inter Med 1991; *115*: 457–69.
23. Jafari HS, McCracken GH. Sepsis and septic shock: a review for clinicians. Pediatr Infect Dis J 1992; *11*: 739–49.
24. Mercier J-C, Beaufils F, Hartman J-F, Azéma D. Hemodynamic patterns of meningococcal shock in children. Crit Care Med 1988; *16*: 27–33.
25. Klein N, Shennan G, Heyderman R, Levin M. Alteration in glycosaminoglycan metabolism and surface charge on human umbilical vein endothelial cells induced by cytokines, endotoxin and neutrophils. J Cell Science 1992; *102*: 821–32.
26. Brenner BM, Hostetter MD, Humes HD. Molecular basis of proteinuria of glomerular origin. N Engl J Med 1978; *298*: 826–33.
27. Kanwar YS. Biophysiology of glomerular filtration and proteinuria. Lab Invest 1984; *51*: 7–21.
28. Parrillo JE. Pathogenetic mechanisms of septic shock. N Engl J Med 1993; *328*: 1471–7.
29. Voerman HJ, Stehouwer CDA, van Kamp GJ, van Schijndel RJMS, Groeneveld ABJ, Thijs LG. Plasma endothelin levels are increased during septic shock. Crit Care Med 1992; *20*: 1097–101.
30. Heyderman RS, Klein NJ, Shennan GI, Levin M. Deficiency of prostacyclin production in meningococcal shock. Arch Dis Child 1991; *66*: 1296–9.
31. Lorente JA, Landin L, de Pablo R, Renes E, Liste D. L-arginine pathway in the sepsis syndrome. Crit Care Med 1993; *21*: 1287–95.
32. Cobb JP, Cunnion RE, Danner RL. Nitric oxide as a target for therapy in septic shock. Crit Care Med 1993; *21*: 1261–3.

33. McGehee WG, Rapaport SI, Hjort PF. Intravascular coagulation in fulminant meningococcemia. Ann Intern Med 1967; 67: 250–60.
34. Heyderman RS. Severe sepsis and intravascular thrombosis. Arch Dis Child 1993; 68: 621–5.
35. Esmon CT, Taylor FB, Snow RT. Inflammation and coagulation: linked processes potentially regulated through a common pathway mediated by protein C. Thromb Haemost 1991; 66: 160–5.
36. Comp PC, Nixon RR, Cooper MR, Esmon CT. Familial protein S deficiency is associated with recurrent thrombosis. J Clin Invest 1984; 74: 2082–8.
37. Heyderman RS, Klein NJ, Shennan GI, Levin M. Modulation of the anticoagulant properties of glycosaminoglycans on the surface of the vascular endothelium by endotoxin and neutrophils: evaluation by an amidolytic assay. Thromb Res 1992; 67: 677–85.
38. Ferguson JH, Chapman OD. Fulminating meningococcic infections and the so-called Waterhouse–Friedrichsen Syndrome. Am J Pathol 1947; 24: 763–95.
39. Parrillo JE, Burch C, Shelhamer JH et al. A circulating myocardial depressant substance in humans with septic shock. Septic shock patients with a reduced ejection fraction have a circulating factor that depresses in vitro myocardial cell performance. J Clin Invest 1985; 76: 1539—53.
40. Repine JE. Scientific perspectives on adult respiratory distress syndrome. Lancet 1992; 399: 466–9.
41. Linton AL, Cumming AD. Acute renal failure in sepsis. In: Solez K, Racusen LC, eds. Acute Renal Failure. Diagnosis; Treatment and Prevention. New York: Marcel Dekker, 1991, 87–91.
42. Cartwright K, Reilly S, White D, Stuart J. Early treatment with parenteral penicillin in meningococcal disease. Br Med J 1992; 305: 143–7.
43. Strang JR, Pugh EJ. Meningococcal infections: reducing the case fatality rate by giving penicillin before admission to hospital. Br Med J 1992; 305: 141–3.
44. Sørenson HT, Moller-Petersen J, Krarup HB, Pedersen H, Hansen H, Hamburger H. Early treatment of meningococcal disease. Br Med J 1992; 305: 774.
45. Gedde-Dahl TW, Høiby EA, Brandtzaeg P, Eskerud JR, Bøvre K. Some arguments on early hospital admission and treatment of suspected meningococcal disease cases. NIPH Ann 1990; 13: 45–60.
46. Klein NJ, Heyderman RS, Levin M. Antibiotic choices for meningitis beyond the neonatal period. Arch Dis Child 1992; 67: 157–61.
47. van Esso D, Fontanals D, Uriz S, Morera MA, Juncosa T, Latorre et al. Neisseria meningitidis strains with decreased susceptibility to penicillin. Pediatr Infect Dis J 1987; 6: 438–9.
48. Botha P. Penicillin-resistant Neisseria meningitidis in Southern Africa. Lancet 1988; i: 54.
49. Peltola H, Anttila M, Renkonen O-V. Randomised comparison of chloramphenicol, ampicillin, cefotaxime and ceftriaxone for childhood bacterial meningitis. Lancet 1989; i: 1281–7.
50. Bihari DJ, Tinker J. The therapeutic value of vasodilator prostaglandins in multiple organ failure associated with sepsis. Intensive Care Med 1988; 15: 3–7.
51. Dage RC, Okerholm RA. Pharmacology and pharmacokinetics of enoximone. Cardiology 1990; 77 (suppl 3): 2–13.
52. Martin MA, Silverman HJ. Gram-negative sepsis and the adult respiratory distress syndrome. Clin Infect Dis 1992; 4: 1213–28.
53. Anon. High frequency ventilation. Lancet 1991; 337: 706–7.
54. Roissaint R, Falke KJ, Lopez F, Slama K, Pison U, Zapol WM. Inhaled nitric

oxide for the adult respiratoy distress syndrome. N Engl J Med 1993; *328:* 399–405.

55. Villar J, Winston B, Slutsky AS. Non-conventional techniques of ventilatory support. Crit Care Clin 1990; *6:* 579–603.

56. Mallet E, Lanse X, Devaux AM, Ensel P, Basuyau JP,. Brunelle P. Hypercalcitonemia in fulminating meningococcemia in children. Lancet 1983; *i:* 294.

57. Sanchez GJ, Venkataraman PS, Pryor RW, Parker MK, Fry HD, Blick KE. Hypercalcitonemia and hypercalcemia in acutely ill children: studies in serum calcium, blood ionised calcium, and calcium regulating hormones. J Pediatr 1989; *114:* 952–6.

58. Ashwal S, Stringer W, Tomasi L, Schneider S, Thompson J, Perkin R. Cerebral blood flow and carbon dioxide reactivity in children with bacterial meningitis. J Pediat 1990; *117:* 523–30.

59. Gérard P, Moriau M, Bachy A, Malvaux P, De Meyer R. Meningoccocal purpura: report of 19 patients treated with heparin. J Pediatr 1973; *82:* 780–6.

60. Corrigan JJ, Jordan CM. Heparin therapy in septicemia with disseminated intravascular coagulation. Effect on mortality and on correction of hemostatic defects. N Engl J Med 1970; *283:* 778–82.

61. Quagliarello V, Scheld WM. Bacterial meningitis: pathogenesis, pathophysiology and progress. N Engl J Med 1992; *327:* 864–72.

62. Tuomanen E, Liu H, Hengstler B, Zak O, Tomaz A. The initiation of meningeal inflammation by components of the pneumococcal cell wall. J Infect Dis 1985; *151:* 859–68.

63. Roord JJ, Apicella MA, Scheld WM. The role of *Haemophilus influenzae* type b peptidoglycan in the initiation of subarachnoid space inflammation and blood-brain barrier permeability during experimental meningitis. In: *Program and abstracts of the 31st Interscience Conference on Antimicrobial Agents and Chemotherapy, Chicago, September 29 – October 2 1991.* Chicago: American Society of Microbiology, 1991; 251.

64. Wispelwey B, Lesse AJ, Hansen EJ, Scheld WM. *Haemophilus influenzae* lipopolysaccharide-induced blood–brain barrier permeability during experimental meningitis in the rat. J Clin Invest 1988; *82:* 1339–46.

65. Wispelwey B, Hansen EJ, Scheld WM. *Haemophilus influenzae* outer-membrane vesicle-induced blood-brain barrier permeability during experimental meningitis. Infect Immun 1989; *57:* 2559–62.

66. Mustafa MM, Ramilo O, Syrogiannopoulos GA, Olsen KD, McCracken GH, Hansen EJ. Induction of meningeal inflammation by outer membrane vesicles of *Haemophilus influenzae* type b. J Infect Dis 1989; *159:* 917–22.

67. Burroughs M, Prasad S, Cabellos C, Mendelman PM, Tuomanen E. The biologic activities of peptidoglycan in experimental *Haemophilus influenzae* meningitis. J Infect Dis 1993; *167:* 464–8.

68. Burroughs M, Cabellos C, Prasad S, Tuomanen E. Bacterial components and the pathophysiology of injury to the blood–brain barrier: does cell wall add to the effects of endotoxin in gram-negative meningitis? J Infect Dis 1992; *165:* S82–85.

69. Waage A, Halstensen A, Shalaby R, Brandtzaeg P, Kierulf P, Espevik T. Local production of tumor necrosis factor alpha, interleukin 1 and interleukin 6 in meningococcal meningitis: relation to the inflammatory response. J Exp Med 1989; *170:* 1859–67.

70. Saukkonen K, Sande S, Cioffe C, Wolpe S, Sherry B, Cerami A *et al.* The role of cytokines in the generation of inflammation and tissue damage in experimental

gram-positive meningitis. J Exp Med 1990; *171*: 439–48.

71. Ramilo O, Sáez-Llorens X, Mertsola J, Jafari H, Olsen KD, Hansen EJ *et al.*
    Tumor necrosis factor alpha/cachectin and interleukin 1-beta initiate meningeal
    inflammation. J Exp Med 1990; *172*: 497–507.

72. Sáez-Llorens X, Romilo O, Mustafa MM, Mertsola J, McCracken GH.
    Molecular pathophysiology of bacterial meningitis: current concepts and
    therapeutic implications. J Pediatr 1990; *116*: 671–84.

73. Arditi M, Manogue KR, Caplan M, Yogev R. Cerebospinal fluid cachectin/tumor
    necrosis factor alpha and platelet activating factor concentrations and severity
    of bacterial meningitis in children. J Infect Dis 1990; *162*: 139–47.

74. Niemoller VM, Täuber MG. Brain edema and increased intracranial pressure in
    the pathophysiology of bacterial meningitis. Eur J Clin Microbiol Infect Dis
    1989; *8*: 107–17.

75. Tureen JH, Dworkin RJ, Kennedy SL, Sachdeva M, Sande MA. Loss of
    cerebrovascular autoregulation in experimental meningitis in rabbits. J Clin
    Invest 1990; *85*: 577–81.

76. Tureen JH, Täuber MG, Sande MA. Effect of hydration status on cerebral
    blood flow and cerebrospinal fluid lactic acidosis in rabbits with experimental
    meningitis. J Clin Invest 1992; *89*: 947–53.

77. Cartwright K, Jones DM. Investigation of meningococcal disease. J Clin Pathol
    1989; *42*: 634–9.

78. Odio CM, Faingezicht I, Paris M, Nassar M, Baltodano A, Rogers J *et al.* The
    beneficial effects of early dexamethasone administration in infants and children
    with bacterial meningitis. N Engl J Med 1991; *324*: 1525–31.

79. Duffy GP. Lumbar puncture in the presence of increased intracranial pressure.
    Br Med J 1969; *i*: 407–9.

80. Feigin RD, McCracken GH, Klein JO. Diagnosis and management of
    meningitis. Pediatr Infect Dis J 1992; *11*: 785–814.

81. Talan DA, Hoffman JR, Yoshikawa TT, Overturf GD. Role of empiric
    antibiotics prior to lumbar puncture in suspected bacterial meningitis: state of
    the art. Rev Infect Dis 1988; *10*: 365–76.

82. Dezateux C, Dinwiddie RJ. Dangers of lumbar puncture. Br Med J 1986; *i*: 827–8.

83. Campos J, Garcia-Tornel S, Gairi JM, Fabregues I. *Haemophilus influenzae* type
    b causing meningitis: comparative clinical and laboratory study. J Pediat 1986;
    108: 897–902.

84. Radetsky M. Duration of treatment in bacterial meningitis: a historical inquiry.
    Pediatr Infect Dis J 1990; *9*: 2–9.

85. Täuber MG, Sande MA. Pathogenesis of bacterial meningitis: contributions by
    experimental models in rabbits. Infection 1984; *12*: 3–10.

86. Kadurugamuwa J, Hengstler B, Zak O. Cerebrospinal fluid protein profile in
    experimental pneumococcal meningitis and its alteration by ampicillin and
    anti-inflammatory agents. J Infect Dis 1989; *159*: 26–34.

87. Lebel MH, Freij BJ, Syrogiannopoulos GA, Chrane DF, Hoyt J, Stewart SM *et
    al.* Dexamethasone therapy for bacterial meningitis: results of two double-blind,
    placebo-controlled trials. N Engl J Med 1988; *319*: 964–71.

88. Weiss J, Elsbach P, Shu C, Castillo J, Grinna L, Horwitz A *et al.* Human
    bactericidal/permeability-increasing protein and a recombinant NH2-terminal
    fragment cause killing of serum resistant gram-negative bacteria in whole
    blood and inhibit tumor necrosis factor release induced by the bacteria. J Clin
    Invest 1992; *90*: 1122–30.

89. von Asmuth EJU, Dentener MA, Bazil V, Bouma MG, Leeuwenberg JFM,

Buurman WA. Anti-CD14 antibodies reduce responses of cultured endothelial cells to endotoxin. Immunology 1993; *80*: 78–83.

90. Tuomanem EI, Saukkonen K, Sande S, Cioffe C, Wright SO. Reduction of inflammation, tissue damage, and mortality in bacterial meningitis in rabbits treated with monoclonal antibodies against adhesion-promoting receptors of leukocytes. J Exp Med 1989; *170*: 959–69.

91. Sáez-Llorens X, Jafari HS, Severien S, Parras F, Olsen KD, Hansen EJ *et al.* Enhanced attenuation of meningeal inflammation and brain edema by concomitant administration of anti-CD18 monoclonal antibodies and dexamethasone in experimental haemophilus meningitis. J Clin Invest 1991; *88*: 2003–11.

92. Sáez-Llorens X, Ramilo O, Mustafa MM, Mertsola J, De Alba C, Hanse E *et al.* Pentoxifylline modulates meningeal inflammation in experimental bacterial meningitis. Antimicrob Agents Chemother 1990; *34*: 837–43.

93. Tureen JH, Täuber MG, Sande MA. Effect of indomethacin on the pathophysiology of experimental meningitis in rabbits. J Infect Dis 1991; *163*: 647–9.

94. Girgis NI, Farid Z, Mikhail IA, Farrag I, Sultan Y, Kilpatick ME. Dexamethasone treatment for bacterial meningitis in children and adults. Pediatr Infect Dis J 1989; *8*: 848–51.

95. Mertsola J, Kennedy WA, Waagner DC, Sáez-Llorens X, Olsen K, Hansen EJ *et al.* Endotoxin concentrations in cerebrospinal fluid correlate with clinical severity and neurologic outcome of *Haemophilus influenzae* type by meningitis. Am J Dis Child 1991; *145*: 1099–103.

96. Pike MG, Wong PKH, Bencivenga R, Flodmark O, Cabral DA, Speert DP *et al.* Electrophysiologic studies, computed tomography and neurological outcome in acute bacterial meningitis. J Pediatr 1990; *116*: 702–6.

97. Chang KH, Han MH, Roh JK, Kim IO, Han MC, Kim CW. Gd-DTPA-enhanced MR imaging of the brain in patients with meningitis: comparison with CT. Am J Neuroradiol 1990; *11*: 69–76.

98. Dean JM, Rogers MC, Traystman RJ. Pathophysiology and clinical management of the intracranial vault. In: Rogers MC ed. *Textbook of Pediatric Intensive Care.* Baltimore: Williams and Wilkins, 1992; 639–66.

99. Bouma GJ, Muizelaar JP. Relationship between cardiac output and cerebral blood flow in patients with intact and impaired autoregulation. J Neurosurg 1990; *73*: 368–74.

100. Powell KR, Sugarman LI, Eskenazi AE, Woodin KA, Kays MA, McCormick KL *et al.* Normalisation of plasma arginine vasopressin concentrations when children with meningitis are given maintenance plus replacement fluid therapy. J Pediatr 1990; *117*: 515–22.

101. Visakorpi R. Ciprofloxacin in meningococcal carriers. Scand J Infect Dis 1989; *60*: S108–11.

102. Schwartz B, Al-Tobaiqi A, Al-Ruwais A, Fontaine RE, A'ashi J, Hightower AW *et al.* Comparative efficacy of ceftriaxone and rifampicin in eradicating pharyngeal carriage of group A *Neisseria meningitidis.* Lancet 1988; *i*: 1239–42.

103. Frasch CE. Vaccines for prevention of meningococcal disease. Clin Microbiol Rev 1989; *2*: S134–8.

104. Hassan-King MKA, Wall RA, Greenwood BM. Meningococcal carriage, meningococcal disease and vaccination. J Infect 1988; *16*: 55–9.

10
Meningococcal Vaccines: Past, Present and Future

CARL E. FRASCH
Bacterial Polysaccharides Laboratory, Center for Biologics
Evaluation and Research, Bethesda, Maryland, USA

INTRODUCTION

Epidemic meningococcal meningitis is often extremely disruptive to the
healthcare system, and in some countries overwhelms the infectious disease
hospitals. Meningococcal disease has in the past caused substantial public
health problems in the military as it did in the great epidemics during World
Wars I and II in Europe and in the United States. Prevention of the disease
through immunoprophylaxis has been practiced for nearly 100 years.

Meningococcal vaccines produced and clinically evaluated over the last
85 years were not developed *de novo*, but were based on discoveries and
developments occurring in other areas of medicine and medical microbiology.
Earlier reviews on meningococcal vaccines include few details concerning
the impact that research on vaccines and chemotherapy for other bacterial
diseases had on the development and use of meningococcal vaccines[1,2]. This
review traces the development of meningococcal vaccines from early
attempts at the beginning of this century up to the present.

HISTORY

Before the days of serum therapy and later chemotherapy mortality from
meningococcal meningitis was between 60 and 80%[3,4]. The introduction of

---

Meningococcal Disease. Edited by Keith Cartwright © 1995 John Wiley & Sons Ltd serum therapy in Europe in 1906–7 by Wassermann and in the United States by Flexner[3,5] led to a reduction in mortality to between 13 and 30% in treated patients, depending upon how promptly serum therapy was initiated[3]. Attempts at immunoprophylaxis began a few years later. Since then, there have been many attempts to produce effective vaccines, first using whole cell preparations, then with soluble toxins, leading up to the purified polysaccharide (PS) and outer membrane protein (OMP) vaccines being used today.

Whole cell vaccines

Successes in the prevention of typhoid fever using killed whole cell vaccines, first by Wright around 1900 in Great Britain and then by Russell in 1912 in the US Army, showed the potential for the prevention of meningococcal disease through immunoprophylaxis[6,7]. Sophian and Black[8] vaccinated 11 medical students with a heat-killed whole cell meningococcal vaccine, using three increasing doses of bacteria given at weekly intervals. The volunteers developed adverse reactions similar to those seen with typhoid vaccine. All individuals developed agglutinating and complement fixing antibodies. The investigators went on to vaccinate 280 family case contacts and 100 nurses. Two nurses, who received two of the three doses, developed meningitis but survived. No other cases were seen in other vaccinated individuals. A number of other clinical trials with varying success followed[4].

The Great War 1914–18

Greenwood described an uncontrolled vaccination campaign carried out during an outbreak of cerebospinal fever in Salisbury, Great Britain during the winter of 1914–15[9]. A polyvalent vaccine, containing six freshly isolated strains from the Salisbury outbreak, was used in a two dose series. The vaccine was given to over 4000 individuals, of whom 983 were aged between 5 and 15 years. After approximately one year of observation there were 7 cases amongst 5040 unvaccinated children in Salisbury compared with no cases in the vaccinated children.

Following outbreaks of type I (serogroup A) meningococcal meningitis in US Army camps a mass vaccination trial was undertaken in 1917 by Gates[10]. His vaccine was prepared from type I and type II (serogroup B) strains grown for 16 hours on solid agar, washed off with saline and heated to 65 °C for 30 minutes. A graded three dose immunisation series was given at 8 day intervals. Again, significant adverse reactions occurred, comparable to those seen following typhoid vaccination. Some reactions even simulated meningitis, leading to spinal taps being performed on some vaccinees; all cultures were negative. Gates immunised 4700 officers and men (3700 received all three doses) out of a total of 25 000 men at Fort Riley, Kansas.

Over a 5 month interval between January and June, 1917, following the immunisation campaign, 43 cases occurred among those not vaccinated, compared to 1 case in a fully vaccinated soldier and 2 in partially vaccinated individuals. Thus efficacy was 87% in fully vaccinated troops.

Lack of evidence of protection by whole cell vaccines

In 1940 Underwood reviewed a number of efficacy trials conducted primarily in Africa and the Near East in the 1920s and 1930s; he concluded that most were not adequately controlled, and that none provided conclusive evidence to support the use of the vaccines tested[4]. On re-analysing the seven trials that he considered adequately controlled he found two that showed evidence of protection ($p < 0.04$) and four that did not. Later, Lapeyssonie reported on the results of 11 efficacy trials (one of which was included in Underwood's analysis) conducted in the so-called "meningitis belt" of Africa between 1915 and 1950[11]. In only two was there good evidence of protection.

The uncertain efficacy of whole cell meningococcal vaccines combined with generally unacceptable levels of adverse reactions led to their falling into disuse. However, some whole cell vaccines prepared from freshly isolated strains provided good evidence of protective efficacy, probably due in large part to the presence of capsular polysaccharide. Maintaining strains to be used in vaccines or for production of hyperimmune therapeutic serum posed major problems. The only known means of strain preservation was repeated passage (about weekly) on special media, such as Dorset egg yolk medium, and it was soon realised that repeated subculture resulted in loss of serogroup specific antigens. The freeze-dry process (lyophilisation) did not become available until 1935, when it was developed for preservation of serum[12].

"Exotoxin" vaccines

Meningococcal disease is often associated with high toxicity. Though meningococci had long been known to possess cell-associated endotoxin, exotoxins had not been demonstrated. However, a report in 1931 of the successful use of diphtheria toxin-antitoxin for immunisation[13], and the publication of similar studies with tetanus toxoid, led to a search for possible meningococcal exotoxins. Subsequently, investigations into possible use of soluble toxins for immunoprophylaxis in prevention of meningococcal meningitis took place.

Studies undertaken by Ferry and Steele[14,15] and by Kuhns[16,17] in the 1930s were of particular interest. In 1931 Ferry *et al.* described the presence of an extracellular toxin in 4 days old glucose broth culture filtrates[14]. Only cultures that grew as heavy pellicles over a clear culture broth seemed to produce the toxin and Gram stains of these 4 day cultures showed only intact bacteria. When dilutions of the culture filtrates were injected intradermally in sensitive individuals, an erythema with induration was induced within 24 hours. The skin reactions were similar to those seen following intradermal injections of scarlet fever streptococcal toxin. In 1924 Dick and Dick described the test that would subsequently bear their name[18]. In the Dick test, culture filtrates of a group A streptococcal strain producing erythrogenic exotoxin were injected intradermally, inducing an erythematous reaction in the skin which appeared within 6 to 12 hours, reaching a maximum by 24 hours. Heating to 96 °C for 45 minutes inactivated the streptococcal toxin. Ferry *et al.* reported that the meningococcal toxin was not inactivated by exposure to 80 °C for 30 minutes, but was rendered inert by boiling for 30 minutes[14]. However, Kuhns reported later that autoclaving was required to inactivate the meningococcal toxin[16].

The test for sensitivity to diphtheria toxin was also well known when Ferry *et al.* were conducting their studies with the meningococcus. The Schick test had been used to assess susceptibility to diphtheria since 1913[19]. The Schick test is often positive by 24 hours, but is best read 4 to 7 days after injection. Thus, the meningococcal 'toxin' behaved more like streptococcal toxin.

Clinical trials of 'exotoxin' vaccines

Ferry and Steel used their meningococcal toxin for active immunisation of children aged 12 to 18[15]. Over 600 children were skin tested of whom 47% had positive reactions. Children who were skin test positive received three or four graded injections of toxin with doses at weekly intervals. Eight weeks later, when the immunised children were retested, up to 70% had become skin test negative. Ferry and Steel did not examine the relationship, if any, between skin test reactivity and protection. However, a positive Schick test indicates susceptibility to the disease, and diphtheria vaccination converts the Schick test to negative.

Kuhns working in 1935–7 with the Civilian Conservation Corps in Kansas extended the initial observations of Ferry and Steel[14,15]. They produced meningococcal culture filtrate toxin from 4 day stationary cultures as described by Ferry, and compared the skin test reactivity of this material to killed whole cultures, whole cell lysates, and extracted endotoxin. Both endotoxin and autoclaved toxin gave uniformly negative skin tests, whereas all other preparations were skin test positive in sensitive individuals. In the local Schwartzman reaction, first described in 1928, intradermal injection of endotoxin causes no visible erythema. Thus, the erythrogenic toxin does not appear to be an endotoxin, but may be related to the recently described iron-regulated meningococcal RTX toxin-like exoprotein[20] (see also Chapter 2). Like the RTX cytotoxins, Kuhns' meningococcal filtrate toxin caused *in vitro* haemolysis of red blood cells[17].

Kuhns *et al.* evaluated the predictive value of skin testing in protection against meningococcal disease and the effect of prophylactic immunisation with toxin filtrates[17]. They skin tested 7339 young men in Civilian Conservation Corps camps and found that 53.3% were positive (erythema ≥ 1 cm in diameter). These individuals were selectively immunised with four graded doses of the toxin; two months later 79% were skin test negative. Three cases of meningitis occurred among unimmunised skin test negative individuals, indicating that skin testing had not identified all susceptibles. Kuhns and his colleagues went on to immunise all individuals in 20 camps after 1–12 cases (average 3) had occurred in a given camp. An average of 84% of those initially skin test positive became negative. Significantly, while 60 cases occurred prior to the vaccination campaign, only one case occurred afterwards and this was in an unimmunised skin test negative individual.

We now know that the soluble toxin prepared by Kuhns *et al.* would also have contained capsular polysaccharide, OMPs and lipopolysaccharide (LPS), but that the LPS would not have caused the skin reactions. It is interesting to speculate whether the protection observed was due to antibodies to capsular polysaccharide or to other antigens.

Chemoprophylaxis; early polysaccharide vaccines

Two discoveries in the late 1930s impacted significantly on the future of meningococcal vaccines; these were the development of sulphadiazine and the identification of the serogroup-specific antigens of serogroups A and C as polysaccharides. By 1940 sulpha drugs were being used routinely to treat meningococcal meningitis, and a few years later penicillin would become widely available. These developments led to the rapid discontinuation of serum therapy, and to a waning of interest in the development and use of meningococcal vaccines.

The advent of World War II meant large increases in throughput of military recruits at training camps in the United States and England. These were accompanied by large epidemics of serogroup A meningococcal meningitis within the military, heightening interest once more in the prevention of meningococcal disease. The use of sulphonamide prophylaxis became widespread, and the search for a safe and effective serogroup A vaccine led to clinical studies of the recently identified serogroup A polysaccharide[21,22].

Development of polysaccharide vaccines

In 1935 Scherp and Rake had purified the type I (serogroup A) specific substance from 10 to 18 day old broth cultures and identified the substance as a polysaccharide. Later, Scherp and Rake observed that the mouse protective power of anti-serogroup A meningococcal horse serum was directly related to its content of anti-polysaccharide antibodies[23]. Studies by Kabat to develop an effective meningococcal vaccine were strongly influenced by the then recent success of a multivalent pneumococcal polysaccharide vaccine. MacLeod *et al.* had been working on such vaccines since 1937 and in 1945 published studies on a pneumococcal outbreak at an Army air base in South Dakota that was effectively halted by use of a 6-valent pneumococcal polysaccharide vaccine[24]. The serogroup A meningococcal polysaccharide vaccine produced by Kabat for clinical evaluation was based on purification methods developed by Scherp and Rake[21,22]. However, the Kabat vaccine failed to induce antibodies in most recipients.

Later studies on a serogroup C meningococcal polysaccharide vaccine prepared by Watson and Scherp using a similar method gave similarly disappointing results[25]. Twenty years later it would be shown that meningococcal polysaccharides purified using the methods employed by these investigators were degraded, having a low molecular size[26]. In 1958 Kabat clearly demonstrated the relationship between the molecular size of a polysaccharide and its ability to induce an immune response in man[27]. His studies using different sizes of dextrans showed that low molecular weight dextrans were poorly immunogenic, while those of high molecular weight were good immunogens. This provided an explanation for the disappointing results obtained with the first serogroup A and serogroup C polysaccharide vaccines.

Outbreaks due to sulphonamide-resistant meningococci

Use of sulphadiazine had greatly reduced the danger of meningococcal outbreaks in defined populations such as the military and this, combined with the use of penicillin for treatment of meningococcal meningitis, effectively delayed further concerted efforts to develop an effective vaccine. All this changed in 1963, when outbreaks of sulphonamide-resistant serogroup B meningococcal meningitis occurred in the US Army, then training large numbers of recruits for the Vietnam war[28]. These outbreaks led Artenstein at the Walter Reed Army Medical Center to assemble a group of investigators to work on the meningococcal disease problem. A careful analysis by Gotschlich[26] of meningococcal polysaccharide purification methods used by earlier investigators led to development of a new purification method, critical to the success of most future polysaccharide vaccines.

Effective polysaccharide preparations

Gotschlich hypothesised that the A and C polysaccharides purified by Kabat and later by Watson and Scherp[22,25] were enzymatically depolymerised due either to the long culture period or to the long broth concentration steps used in the purification. He solved these problems by using the cationic detergent cetavlon to precipitate rapidly the polyanionic polysaccharide from 12 to 15 hour broth cultures[29]. The resulting polysaccharides were of high molecular size and were contaminated with less than 1% of nucleic acid or protein.

Safe and effective immunisation against meningococcal disease became a reality with the accomplishments of Gotschlich *et al.*[26,30]. The purified capsular polysaccharide vaccines against serogroup A and serogroup C were among the first chemically pure bacterial vaccines. The serogroup A polysaccharide is a polymer of N-acetyl mannosamine phosphate, while the serogroup C polysaccharide is a homopolymer of α 2→9 linked N-acetyl neuraminic acid (sialic acid). After these polysaccharides were shown to be immunogenic in adults and older children they were subjected to efficacy trials in North and South America, Europe and Africa.

POLYSACCHARIDE VACCINES

First clinical trials

Meningococcal polysaccharide vaccines were first demonstrated to be immunogenic in humans by Gotschlich *et al.*[30], after failure to induce antibodies detectable by indirect haemagglutination in several animal species including monkeys. Gotschlich and his coworkers went on to immunise US Army recruits with the A and C polysaccharides, inducing both haemagglutinating and bactericidal antibodies. These studies were done in the midst of serogroup C outbreaks on several bases, with outbreak strain carrier rates of up to 80%. The researchers were able to document a significantly reduced acquisition rate of serogroup C carriage among vaccinated recruits compared with unvaccinated individuals[31]. A similar reduction in serogroup A meningococcal carriage was seen among Finnish army recruits following administration of the serogroup A vaccine. Thus both polysaccharides, when purified as high molecular size antigens, were safe and immunogenic.

Vaccine dosage, delivery and stability

Artenstein *et al.* evaluated different dosages of the serogroup C vaccines and immunisation routes in preparation for large-scale efficacy studies at a number of US Army recruit training centres[32]. They tested 10, 50 and 100 μg doses given intradermally, subcutaneously, and by jet injector. The 50 μg dose was more immunogenic than the 10 μg dose and similar to the 100 μg dose. There were no differences in immunogenicity between the three routes of immunisation, and a second vaccination 3–4 weeks later did not boost antibody levels. Using the 50 μg dose given subcutaneously or by jet injector they conducted two large field trials in recruit camps between 1969 and 1970[33,34]. In the first trial over 13 500 recruits were vaccinated representing 20% of the recruit population; efficacy was 87%. The second trial in a larger number of recruits showed an efficacy of 90% over the 8 weeks of recruit training.

Interestingly, vaccine recipients who were injected intradermally had marked erythema. The reaction began within 4–6 hours, reached a maximum by 24 hours and was gone by 48 hours. There was a direct correlation between dose and size of the skin reaction. Those who were reinjected by the intradermal route had erythema not unlike that seen after the primary injection. Artenstein et al. concluded that the skin reaction was not due to the polysaccharide content, nor to antibody levels to polysaccharide[32].

An early study in Nigeria, using a low molecular weight (< 25 000) serogroup A vaccine, showed no protection[35]. The vaccine lot (V-1) used in this trial was inadvertently exposed to high ambient temperatures prior to its administration. Unfortunately, the tendency of the serogroup A polysaccharide to depolymerise at ambient temperatures in the absence of a stabiliser such as lactose had yet to be appreciated.

Vaccine efficacy

Efficacy of serogroup A vaccines was shown in a number of trials in Africa and in a Finnish trial in 1974. In 1973 Wahdan et al.[36] conducted field trials in Egyptian school children aged 6 to 15 years using two lots of serogroup A vaccine. The molecular sizes of the serogroup A polysaccharides in the two lots were significantly different (about 75 000 and 170 000). Both vaccines gave 90% or greater protection during the first year after immunisation, but the lower molecular weight vaccine provided no protection in the second year. In contrast, the high molecular weight vaccine provided protection for at least 3 years.

A serogroup A meningococcal epidemic began in Finland in 1973 and a randomised controlled mass immunisation trial with serogroup A polysaccharide vaccine was conducted during the winter of 1974–5[37]. The vaccine was highly effective in children aged over 3 months. Although the number of serogroup A cases overall declined greatly, statistical calculations suggested 90% to 100% protection for 3 years[38]. During and after the trial the incidence of meningococcal disease due to serogroups B and C did not differ between the vaccinated and control populations.

In late 1977, an epidemic of serogroup A meningococcal disease began in Rwanda. In response, a limited vaccination campaign was undertaken using a bivalent A/C polysaccharide vaccine in an area experiencing up to 80 cases per 100 000 population per month[39]. Within 2 weeks of vaccine administration there was a complete cessation of meningococcal disease in the population, yet the serogroup A carrier rate remained unchanged.

Duration of protection

The duration of protection following immunisation with serogroup A polysaccharide is highly dependent on age. In studies in Burkina Faso, Reingold et al. estimated the efficacy of the vaccine 1, 2 and 3 years after vaccination[40]. Approximately 90% efficacy was seen after one year in all age groups, but by the second year little protection remained in children who had been vaccinated at age 3 years or less. In children aged 4 to 16 significant protection (67%) persisted for 3 years.

The only efficacy studies of serogroup C polysaccharide in young children were those conducted in Brazil[41,42] during a serogroup C meningococcal epidemic which began in 1971. Because of the epidemic Brazil obtained one of the first lots of serogroup C polysaccharide vaccine produced by Merck Sharp & Dohme. This vaccine was administered to 67 300 children aged 6 to 36 months in Greater São Paulo, and a similar number of controls received tetanus and diphtheria toxoids. The children were followed for approximately 17 months (January 1973 to June 1974). The study was terminated in 1974 because a massive serogroup A meningococcal epidemic began in that year. The serogroup C vaccine was not effective in children under 24 months of age, and only 52% effective in those aged 24–36 months.

Immunogenicity studies with the Merck vaccine lot used in São Paulo indicated that the vaccine was less immunogenic than other batches of similar vaccine that had been used in US children[41,43]; also, molecular sizing of the vaccine showed that it was smaller than the serogroup C polysaccharide in the present vaccine. It is therefore quite probable that the current serogroup C polysaccharide vaccine is more effective.

THE CURENT POLYSACCHARIDE VACCINE

The current tetravalent vaccine containing the A, C, Y and W-135 polysaccharides was licensed in the United States in 1981, and is also manufactured in Belgium and France. Each 0.5 ml dose of the vaccine contains 50 μg of each of the four polysaccharides; the vaccine is administered subcutaneously. The serogroup Y and W-135 polysaccharides were added to the vaccine because up to 20% of meningococcal disease was due to these serogroups. The low incidence of disease due to serogroup Y and W-135 strains made efficacy studies impractical, but several lines of evidence clearly demonstrated that protection against meningococcal disease is due to serum bactericidal antibodies[44,45], allowing use of immunological surrogates. The importance of bactericidal antibodies is evident from the following observations:

1. The peak incidence of meningococcal disease is in children aged under one who have little or no bactericidal antibody.
2. Gotschlich *et al.* showed that serogroup C disease among military recruits occurred only in individuals lacking bactericidal antibodies to the virulent strain[44].
3. Individuals with an inherited deficiency of one of the terminal complement components have a high susceptibility to repeated attacks of meningococcal disease.

A condition of vaccine licensure was that the Y and W-135 polysaccharides should stimulate a four-fold or greater increase in bactericidal antibodies in at least 90% of adults 3 to 4 weeks after vaccination. The safety of the tetravalent vaccine was comparable with that seen with the earlier bivalent vaccine[46].

Effect of age on response to vaccine

The antibody response to meningococcal polysaccharide is age-dependent. Like other polysaccharides, they are T-cell independent immunogens and the ability to respond to such immunogens shows age-specific maturation. Unlike a number of other polysaccharides, serogroup A meningococcal polysaccharide is immunogenic in children aged 6 months or more[43]. Gold found that the peak antibody response following immunisation with serogroup A polysaccharide inceased in a linear manner with the logarithm of age between 7 months and 21 years. It was also found that children aged between 3 and 17 months who received a second injection of serogroup A polysaccharide had a booster response[47,48]. Booster responses are not normally seen with T-cell independent antigens. However, the booster response was seen only if the primary injection was given before 12 months of age. Goldschneider observed that when infants aged 3 months were given a serogroup A vaccine, a negligible antibody response occurred. When these infants were reinjected at age 7 months, a significantly higher antibody response was seen in primed infants compared with previously unvaccinated 7 month old infants. Gold *et al.*[1,43] suggested that since the peak antibody levels were the same following either primary or booster immunisation in children aged over 2, the serogroup A (and C) polysaccharides did not induce immunological memory, but stimulated pre-existing memory B lymphocytes generated by prior contact with cross-reactive antigens.

Persistence of antibodies

Persistence of vaccine-induced antibodies is age-dependent. An estimation of the minimum antibody level required for protection against meningococcal disease was needed before a meaningful assessment of the persistence of anti-polysaccharide antibodies could be made. Although such estimations are difficult, between 1 and 2 µg/ml of antibody is apparently required[37]. This estimate is based on the mean antibody levels found in adults (2 µg/ml) and in young children in whom the serogroup A polysaccharide vaccine was shown to be nearly 100% effective. Antibody persistence has been followed for over 5 years[38,43]. By two years post vaccination, antibody levels in children immunised when aged under one had declined to those of unimmunised controls. In Finnish studies, elevated antibody levels persisted for only one year in children aged 17 to 24 months when immunised, and for 2 years in children aged 2 to 3 years. Older children had elevated antibody levels for at least 5 years. These immunological data correlate well with the observed age-related fall in protection.

Persistence of vaccine-induced meningococcal polysaccharide antibodies is markedly affected by the presence of malaria in the population. Studies in Nigeria and Burkina Faso, where malaria incidence is high, indicated a more rapid decline in serogroup A and C polysaccharide antibodies following immunisation, than observed elsewhere. Greenwood found that malaria-infected individuals in Nigeria had a depressed immune response, and that treatment with chloroquine one week before immunisation enhanced peak antibody levels[49,50].

Differences in immune responses to serogroup A and C polysaccharides

Serogroup C meningococcal polysaccharide induces significant increases in antibodies in infants aged 3 months, but antibody levels fall rapidly. In contrast to serogroup A polysaccharide, no evidence of a booster effect is seen; in fact there is a decreased immune response in infants who are re-immunised at age 7 or 12 months following primary vaccination at age 3 months. By age 18 months the immune response returns to normal. Antibody levels decline rapidly following immunisation of young children with the serogroup C vaccine[51]. One year after immunisation of children aged 6 to 8 years antibody levels declined by over 60% and only 55% had antibody levels presumed to be protective (> 2 µg/ml).

There are large differences in the age-related acquisition of natural antibodies to serogroup A and serogroup C polysaccharides[43]. By age five to six, over 50% of children have more than 2 µg/ml of anti-serogroup A antibodies, whereas similar levels of anti-serogroup C antibodies do not develop until adolescence. Bacterial antigens cross-reactive with the serogroup A polysaccharide are much commoner than those cross-reacting with the serogroup C polysaccharide; they are thought to account for most of the natural antibody.

Serogroups Y and W-135

Immunogenicity of the serogroup Y and serogroup W-135 polysaccharides has been evaluated in both adults and children[52-54] and found to be comparable with that of the A and C polysaccharides. Over 90% of adults responded to immunisation with fourfold or greater increases in bactericidal antibody levels. The bactericidal titres to Y and W-135 polysaccharides increased from less than four to approximately 512. As expected, children responded less well, but seroconversion rates were not different from the response to the serogroup A polysaccharide[53,54].

RECOMMENDATIONS FOR CURRENT USAGE

The Immunization Practices Advisory Committee (ACIP) of the US Public Health Service has made recommendations for the use of the meningococcal polysaccharide vaccines[55]. Routine vaccination of civilian populations in industrialised countries is not currently recommended for the following reasons:

- The risk of infection is low.
- An approved vaccine against serogroup B is not available.
- Most endemic disease occurs in young children.

Vaccination is advised to control outbreaks due to meningococcal serogroups covered by the vaccine. Routine vaccination is recommended for travellers to countries recognised as having hyperendemic or epidemic meningococcal disease such as Nepal, Saudi Arabia, Kenya and the "meningitis belt" of sub-Saharan Africa, which extends from Mauritania in the west to Ethiopia in the east.

High risk groups

The American Academy of Pediatrics does not recommend routine childhood vaccination but advocates vaccinating children aged 2 or more who are in high risk groups, including those with asplenia and those with terminal complement deficiencies[56]. Galazka observed that the currently available meningococcal polysaccharide vaccines should not be included within the routine World Health Organization recommended immunisation progammes because of the relatively short duration of protection, the irregularity of epidemics, the changing importance of serogroups causing disease, and, not least, the high cost of immunisation for developing countries[57]. Vaccination of individuals with a deficiency in one of the terminal complement components or with properdin deficiency may be effective in preventing disease. Patients with deficiencies in C5, C6, C7, or C8 have a prolonged increased susceptibility to meningococcal disease[58]. The low mortality rate (4%) in such infections suggests that presence of antibodies that can promote opsonophagocytosis is important. It follows that vaccination could provide some protection.

Normal properdin function appears to be necessary for resistance to meningococcal disease. Properdin promotes bactericidal killing through activation of the alternative complement pathway by stabilising the C3 convertase, C3b,Bb[59]. Many individuals with meningococcal disease associated with properdin deficiency are young children, who would not be expected to have developed protective antibodies[59]. Vaccination of properdin-deficient individuals with meningococcal polysaccharide vaccines has been shown to induce antibodies that permit bacterial killing via the classical complement pathway[60].

Control of epidemics

Although major epidemics of meningococcal disease occur regularly in the meningitis belt of Africa, especially during the dry season, it was not certain how meningococcal vaccines should be used under these circumstances. Studies by Greenwood and Wali in 1979 in northern Nigeria indicated that selective vaccination could be both effective and economically feasible in outbreak control[61]. They vaccinated all individuals aged over one year in nine villages where a second case of disease had occurred and compared these with seven control villages. The spread of meningococcal disease in the affected villages quickly came to a halt. They suggested that since vaccine may be in limited supply and that most disease occurred in individuals aged 5 to 15, selective vaccination of this age group in affected areas could reduce considerably the incidence of meningococcal disease. They emphasised, however, that for selective vaccination to be effective, good disease surveillance is required.

Control of localised outbreaks

In recent years there has been an increased use of the currently available meningococcal vaccines to control localised outbreaks in Europe and North America. The ACIP has recently provided guidance for the control of localised outbreaks[62]. The ACIP recommended that the trigger for action limit should be a rate of confirmed meningococcal disease 10 times the normal endemic rate. To determine whether an outbreak is occurring, the increased disease should be within a population defined both by age and location. To be considered an outbreak the increased disease rate should be shown to be due to a single meningococcal strain. This can be confirmed by serological analysis or by multi-locus enzyme electophoresis (MLEE).

Use of polysaccharide vaccine in Canada, 1992

Beginning in 1991, Canada experienced a series of serogroup C meningococcal outbreaks. A serogroup C serotype 2a outbreak occurred during the early winter of 1991–2 in Ottawa-Carleton[63,64]. During this time there were seven cases of meningococcal disease among teenagers, four of them fatal. As a result, a mass immunisation campaign was carried out. The decision to immunise was based on a number of factors:

• Disease due to a single serogroup.
• A higher than expected number of cases in a defined population over a short period of time.
• A high case fatality rate.
• Cases occurring early in the meningococcal season.
• The behavioural patterns of the teenage population.

Use of vaccine in New Zealand, 1987

A selective mass vaccination campaign was carried out in Auckland, New Zealand in 1987[65]. During the winters of 1985 and 1986 a large serogroup A meningococcal epidemic occurred in Auckland with rates of 41/100 000 in children younger than 5 years. The public health authorities elected to immunise, and defined the vaccine-eligible population as those individuals between 3 months and 13 years of age (67% of cases had been within this age range in 1986). Children aged 2 to 13 years received a single dose of monovalent serogroup A polysaccharide vaccine. Children aged 3 to 23 months received two doses separated by at least one month. Over 90% of the children received the first dose, but only 26% of the younger children received the second dose. After 2.5 years of surveillance, there was 100% efficacy in those fully vaccinated for their age. In the under twos, who received only a single dose, the estimated efficacies at 3 months and 1 year were 52% and 16% respectively. Although other studies have shown efficacy in young children[37,40] this was the first study to provide data for protective efficacy of serogroup A polysaccharide vaccine in children under 2.

Use of vaccine for outbreak control in developed countries

Based on these experiences, some general recommendations for control of outbreaks in developed countries can be made. Three or more epidemiologically linked cases occurring within a geographically defined population may constitute an outbreak in which vaccine intervention could be considered. The at-risk population can be defined broadly by the age range of cases, such as school children or college students, but would include all case contacts. It can be delineated further by school, institution or community. In the military it has been repeatedly observed that most meningococcal cases occur during recruit training, where a large number of susceptibles are brought together. The same has been observed among incoming college students[66]. At-risk children aged over one should receive the vaccine. When the goal is to control the outbreak, and not to provide long-term protection, duration of protection is of lesser importance. Booster immunisation would need to be considered only if an outbreak persisted.

POLYSACCHARIDE CONJUGATE VACCINES

Problems with non-conjugated polysaccharides

The currently licensed polysaccharide vaccines are T-cell independent immunogens as are other polysaccharides. They are poorly immunogenic in young children, the age group at greatest risk. Serogroup A polysaccharide is protective in children as young as 3 months provided two doses are given; serogroup C polysaccharide may not be protective in children aged less than 18 months, although data addressing this issue are accumulating in Canada. A further consequence of T-cell independence is that the antibody response is not boosted by natural exposure. Therefore duration of protection in children aged under 4 may be 2 years or less[40,65]. Thus, while the current polysaccharide vaccines are very effective in controlling outbreaks and epidemics, they do not induce long-term protection. These problems can all be overcome by conversion of the serogroup A and C polysaccharides into T-cell dependent immunogens through covalent linkage to proteins. It remains to be seen whether a similar approach will be effective for protection against serogroup B disease.

The *Haemophilus influenzae* type b polysaccharide vaccine was not effective in children under 18–24 months of age, whereas *H. influenzae* type b polysaccharide–protein conjugate vaccines have been shown to be highly effective in children as young as 2 months[67,68]. The marked success of these conjugates has led to the development of similar meningococcal serogroup A and C conjugate vaccines[69].

Development of meningococcal polysaccharide conjugates

In early studies, meningococcal A, B and C polysaccharides and oligosaccharides were covalently attached to tetanus toxoid[70–72]. Jennings *et al.*[72] produced conjugates of the serogroup A, B and C polysaccharides by periodate oxidation and direct attachment through the lysine residues in tetanus toxoid. In addition, they prepared oligosaccharides from serogroup C polysaccharide and linked them through a spacer molecule to bovine serum albumin. These conjugates were used to hyperimmunise mice. The serogroup A and C conjugates were highly immunogenic but the serogroup B conjugate was not. Beuvery et al. also produced serogroup A and serogroup C polysaccharide conjugates by attachment to tetanus toxoid[70,71]. These were compared with native polysaccharides for their immunogenicity in mice. The native polysaccharides were essentially non-immogenic when administered in two doses ten weeks apart. In contrast, a single injection of the conjugates elicited high antibody levels. A second injection at week 10 elicited a booster response, typical of a T-cell dependent response. Adsorption of the conjugates to aluminium phosphate significantly increased the primary immune response, but did not affect the booster response[70,71]. Thus, conjugation of serogroup A and C polysaccharides to a protein carrier converted the polysaccharides from T-cell independent to T-cell dependent antigens.

Clinical trials of meningococcal protein–polysaccharide conjugates

Serogroup A and serogroup C polysaccharide–protein conjugate vaccines have now been evaluated in phase I clinical trials[69]. Oligosaccharides (short-chain sugars) derived from the two polysaccharides were covalently coupled to a non-toxic mutant of diphtheria toxin (CRM 197) using a six carbon adipic acid spacer. The vaccine was administered to eight adults at doses of 11 μg of each oligosaccharide and 88 μg of CRM 197 protein per dose. A second injection was given 6 weeks later. There were no significant adverse reactions. All individuals had a significant increase in antibodies following the first dose, but antibody levels were not significantly boosted by the second dose. Due to higher pre-immunisation antibody levels, adults often do not show a booster response to conjugate vaccines. Clinical studies in children are expected to parallel earlier results with the haemophilus conjugate vaccines.

SEROGROUP B VACCINES—POLYSACCHARIDES

Problems of poor immunogenicity

Serogroup B strains have been responsible for most meningococcal disease in developed countries since the late 1940s, yet forty years later only partly effective vaccines are available. Although the serogroup B polysaccharide, a homopolymer of α 2–8 linked sialic acid, appears to be the logical choice for production of a serogroup B meningococcal vaccine, clinical studies to date have failed to confirm this. Serogroup B polysaccharide was first purified in the mid 1960s by Gotschlich *et al.*[29], but it was Wyle *et al.*, also of the Walter Reed Army Medical Center, who first evaluated a serogroup B polysaccharide vaccine in humans[73]. They purified high molecular weight serogroup B polysaccharide from young cultures and evaluated the polysaccharide over a broad dose range from 10 to 250 μg. The vaccine failed to induce measurable increases in antibodies. Most adults have relatively high levels of IgM antibody to the B polysaccharide[74]. Although children have lower antibody levels, the purified polysaccharide was not immunogenic in young children[1]. A number of possible explanations have been given for the observed poor immunogenicity including sensitivity to neuraminidases, and the polysaccharide's similarity to sialic acid moieties on human tissues inducing immunotolerance.

Zollinger has shown that antibodies to the serogroup B polysaccharide induced during natural infection are mostly IgM and of low avidity[75]. These antibodies are highly bactericidal in the presence of rabbit complement, but show no bactericidal activity with human complement, indicating that induction of functionally active antibodies in an animal model with the serogroup B polysaccharide–protein conjugates may not be indicative of the response of humans.

Attempts to enhance immunogenicity

Serogroup B polysaccharide, when non-covalently complexed with meningococcal outer membranes, does induce transient increases in IgM anti-polysaccharide antibodies[76]. Moreno *et al.* have attempted to improve the immunogenicity of the serogroup B polysaccharide by non-covalently complexing it to OMPs and by adsorption of the complexed vaccine to aluminium hydroxide[77,78]. These two vaccines were used to immunise mice and were compared with the pure polysaccharide. While the pure polysaccharide was non-immunogenic, both of the other formulations induced transient increases in IgM antibodies peaking on day 7. A similar serotype 2b protein serogroup B polysaccharide vaccine adsorbed to aluminium hydroxide stimulated increases in serogroup B polysaccharide antibodies measured on week 4 in a few individuals[79]. However, these IgM antibodies are unlikely to be protective since they do not appear to be bactericidal with human complement[80]. There is, however, evidence that serogroup B polysaccharide antibodies may be opsonic[81].

Chemical modification and conjugation to proteins

Alternative approaches in the preparation of immunogenic serogroup B polysaccharide vaccines are to link the polysaccharide covalently to a protein carrier, or to modify the polysaccharide by chemical means. Protein–polysaccharide conjugates prepared using the native serogroup B polysaccharide were found to be essentially non-immunogenic. Jennings *et al.* then made a number of chemical modifications to the polysaccharide[82]; the only modification that did not abrogate the ability of serogroup B specific antibodies to recognise the polysaccharide was substitution of N-propionyl groups for the N-acetyl groups.

The N-propionylated polysaccharide and its tetanus toxoid conjugate were used to immunise mice using Freund's complete adjuvant in a series of three injections[83]. When given alone, the modified polysaccharide failed to induce serogroup B reactive antibodies. In contrast, two injections of the conjugate induced antibody levels substantially above background, and the third injection gave a good booster response. The antibody response was mostly IgG. These antibodies were bactericidal against serogroup B strains of different serotypes[84], but did not kill meningococci of other serogroups. Quantitative precipitin experiments indicated that about half of the antibodies induced to the N-propionylated polysaccharide were specific for the altered polysaccharide[83]. Unexpectedly, only adsorption of the sera with the N-propionylated polysaccharide removed the serogroup B bactericidal antibodies, even though the native polysaccharide adsorbed all radioimmunoassay reactive antibodies. Thus, the N-propionylated serogroup B polysaccharide mimics a bactericidal epitope on the serogroup B organism. They found that the bactericidal antibodies were adsorbed by intact serogroup B meningococci or *E. coli* K1 (which possesses a chemically identical capsular polysaccharide), but not by cells of other meningococcal serogroups[84]. It remains to be seen whether functionally active serogroup B polysaccharide antibodies are induced in primates without strong adjuvants.

Structural differences between native and chemically modified serogroup B polysaccharides

Studies were conducted in Jennings' laboratory to elucidate the structural basis for the selective induction of bactericidal antibodies in mice by N-propionylated serogroup B polysaccharide–tetanus toxoid conjugates[84,85]. When the purified serogroup B polysaccharide was covalently bound to an affinity column using a long spacer molecule, the column-bound IgG_{2a} and IgG_{2b} antibodies were both shown to be bactericidal. In contrast, serogroup B polysaccharide bound to the column via a short spacer bound only non-bactericidal IgG_1 antibodies. In further studies they showed that at least 10 sialic acid residues were required to form a conformational epitope capable of binding bactericidal antibodies[86]. Two structural studies have demonstrated that serogroup B polysaccharide forms helical structures, although at any point in time most of the molecule exists as a random coil[84,87]. Only the helical structures appear to be responsible for antibody binding. Brisson *et al.* found that the helices have nine residues per turn, and that the N-propionylated polysaccharide adopts the same extended helical structure[85].

Cross-reactivity between serogroup B polysaccharide and human neural cells

Polysialosyl chains are present on a neural cell adhesion molecule (N-CAM) found primarily in human and animal fetal brain tissue. Only sialylated N-CAM specifically binds serogroup B polysaccharide antibodies. This observation has led to considerable concern over possible induction of IgG antibodies to the serogroup B polysaccharide through the use of conjugates[88]; though no evidence has been found to date to substantiate these concerns, the possibility of an autoimmune response due to reactivity with polysialosyl glycopeptides in human tissues must be clearly established before such serogroup B conjugates can be considered for clinical evaluation in women and children.

Homology between meningococcal and *E. coli* polysaccharides

Another sialic acid homopolymer is produced by *E. coli* K92. This polysaccharide resembles both the serogroup B and serogroup C meningococcal polysaccharides in that it consists of an alternating α 2–8 and α 2–9 linked sialic acid polymer. The polysaccharide alone induces antibodies cross-reactive only with the α 2–9 linked serogroup C polysaccharide. However, Devi *et al.* found that a tetanus toxoid conjugate of the K92 polysaccharide induced antibodies in mice without adjuvants which reacted with both serogroup C and serogroup B meningococcal polysaccharides[89]. The K92 conjugate induced both IgM and IgG antibodies, but studies of functional activity were not presented.

SEROGROUP B VACCINES—PROTEINS

Outer membrane proteins (OMPs) as vaccine candidates

A promising approach to development of an effective serogroup B meningococcal vaccine is the use of LPS-depleted OMP vaccines. There is considerable antigenic diversity among serogroup B meningococcal strains, with approximately 20 different serotypes, based on variations in the class 2 and class 3 OMPs. However, only a limited number of serotypes are associated with most serogroup B and serogroup C meningococcal disease. Additional antigenic diversity is seen amongst class 1 proteins, which contain the subtype-specific antigens. Class 1 proteins appear to be more immunogenic than class 2 or class 3 proteins and may be more important for induction of protective antibodies. Other OMPs also show antigenic diversity. In spite of the multiplicity of antigens, cross-reactivity apparently exists between many different strains, and preliminary results from efficacy trials (see below) and bactericidal assays suggest that cross-protection may occur if carefully selected vaccine strains are employed.

The idea of using OMPs in a meningococcal vaccine arose from observations that protection against meningococcal disease is correlated with the presence of bactericidal antibodies[30], and that in the case of serogroup B infections, bactericidal antibodies are directed against non-capsular surface antigens[90,91].

The first such vaccines, prepared in the late 1970s, consisted of meningococcal outer membranes depleted of LPS by solubilisation with detergent. The vaccine protein was then separated from the detergent by ethanol precipitation and resuspended in 0.9% sodium chloride. These vaccines were visibly particulate and contained aggregated outer membranes as confirmed by electron microscopy. The early particulate vaccines (as well as later vaccines) contained considerable amounts of LPS (about 5 to 10 μg/100 μg protein), yet were much less pyrogenic in rabbits than would be expected[92]. The LPS that remained was strongly membrane-associated, probably accounting for its lower toxicity.

The particulate outer membrane vaccines were evaluated in adults then in children using a two or three dose immunisation schedule previously evaluated in animal studies[1]. Zollinger et al.[93] found that such a vaccine failed to induce bactericidal antibodies in five adults after three doses. A similar particulate vaccine prepared by Frasch et al. induced low levels of antibody in both adults and children as measured by enzyme-linked immunosorbent assay (ELISA), but also failed to stimulate bactericidal antibodies. Thus, although particulate vaccines were found to be safe in both adults and children, they were poorly immunogenic, an outcome not predicted by animal studies.

Soluble outer membrane vesicle (OMV) vaccines

Zollinger et al. in 1978 were the first to prepare soluble outer membrane vaccines[76]. They found that outer membrane vaccines could be made soluble by combination with a meningococcal polysaccharide. Electron microscopy of similar vaccines prepared in our laboratory showed some aggregation of outer membrane vesicles without the polysaccharide and individual vesicles in vaccines containing polysaccharide[94]. Meningococci release large amounts of essentially pure outer membranes into the culture broth as blebs or vesicles during normal growth[94,95]. These membranes may be purified from the broth and used as the starting material for preparation of a vaccine. Since the natural orientation of the proteins in the outer membrane may be important, we have developed methods to remove LPS selectively, leaving the membranes intact and soluble as confirmed by electron microscopy[94]. Soluble vaccines were prepared with and without the serogroup B polysaccharide non-covalently complexed with the vesicles and were tested in animals[96,97].

Soluble OMV vaccines containing meningococcal polysaccharide have been clinically evaluated[1,76]. They induced bactericidal antibodies after primary immunisation but with only modest increases in antibody titres after a second dose. The immunogenicities of soluble OMV vaccines with and without serogroup B polysaccharide have been compared[1,98,99]. Addition of the polysaccharide results in a significant increase in bactericidal antibodies to a serogroup C serotype 2a strain. Giving a second dose 6 to 8 weeks later results in an increase in the proportion of individuals responding to the vaccine.

The attack rate for serogroup B disease is highest in young children. When the immune responses of children were compared with those of older children and adults, by either OMV ELISA or bactericidal assay, children under 6 years old responded less well[99]. Adsorption of the vaccine into aluminium hydroxide or aluminium phosphate significantly increased the bactericidal response of mice to the OMPs[97]. These vaccines were therefore evaluated in human adults[79]. The aluminium hydroxide adsorbed vaccine was found safe and more immunogenic than the same vaccine without the adjuvant. Vaccine with adjuvant induced significantly higher bactericidal titres. More recently, studies in Norway suggest that adjuvant can be added directly to LPS-depleted membranes[100].

Efficacy trials of serogroup B OMP vaccines

A number of efficacy trials with serogroup B OMP vaccines have been conducted (Table 10.1). The first was conducted in Cape Town, South Africa in the early 1980s using a serotype 2a OMP vaccine containing serogroup B meningococcal polysaccharide, but no adjuvant[101]. The vaccine was immunogenic in all age serogroups including infants. Although the incidence of serogroup B disease in the study population was 175/100 000 and 4400 children were enrolled and vaccinated with either a meningococcal A + C polysaccharide vaccine or the serotype 2a vaccine, an insufficient number of cases occurred to obtain a clear-cut estimate of efficacy. Successful trials were subsequently conducted in Cuba, Chile, Norway and Brazil.

Cuban OMV vaccine

The Cuban B + C meningococcal vaccine contained LPS-depleted outer membranes from a serotype 4, subtype P1.15 strain, serogroup C

Table 10.1 *Field trials of group B meningococcal outer membrane vaccines*

Years	Vaccine formulation	Location	Estimated efficacy	Reference
1981	2a:P1.2 + B polysaccharide	Cape Town, South Africa	Too few cases	101
1987–9	4:P1.15 + C polysaccharide + Al(OH)$_3$	Cuba	83%	102
1989–90	Cuban BC vaccine	São Paulo	47/74%*	103
1990–91	Cuban BC vaccine	Rio de Janeiro	58/71%†	104
1988–90	4:P1.3 + C polysaccharide + Al(OH)$_3$	Iquique, Chile	51%	106
1989–91	15:P1.16 + Al(OH)$_3$	Norway	57%	105

*The efficacy was 47% in children between 24 and 47 months of age, and 74% in children over 47 months of age.
†The overall efficacy was 58% and 71% for children over 47 months of age.

meningococcal polysaccharide and a 'high molecular weight protein complex', all combined with aluminium hydroxide[102]. Each 0.5 ml dose of the vaccine contained 50 μg protein and 50 μg of serogroup C polysaccharide adsorbed to 2 mg aluminium hydroxide. It was administered in two doses separated by 6 to 8 weeks. In a randomised double-blind study in school children, an efficacy of 83% was observed. The most important finding of the Cuban vaccine trial was the demonstration that antibodies induced to non-capsular surface antigens can protect against meningococcal disease.

The Cuban vaccine was used between 1989 and 1991 in two case–control studies in Brazil[103,104]. In greater São Paulo 2.4 million children aged between 3 months and 7 years were vaccinated[103]. This study, in which four controls were matched with each case, demonstrated efficacy that varied with age. For children older than 48 months, efficacy was 74% (95% confidence intervals (CI) 16% to 92%), whereas in younger children, no protective efficacy was shown. In the second Brazilian trial[104], approximately 1.7 million children aged between 6 months and 9 years received two doses of the same Cuban vaccine. The children were followed up for 12 months after the second dose. One control matched for age and location was obtained for each case. The overall efficacy against all meningococcal disease, both laboratory and clinically diagnosed, was 57.7% (95% CI 31% to 74%), compared with 54.1% (95% CI 20% to 73%) for serogroup B cases only. The efficacy estimate was higher (74.4%; 95% CI 42% to 88%) if the city of Rio de Janeiro was analysed separately. Efficacy was also better in older children, 71% (95% CI 38% to 87%) for those aged 48 months or more, compared with 28% (95% CI −45% to 65%) in children aged under 48 months. There was a trend towards better protection in the first 6 months of observation than in the second 6 months; the investigators also observed that the highest protection was seen among children who lived in areas of highest risk.

Norwegian OMV vaccine

A Norwegian serogroup B protein vaccine was studied in a double-blind, placebo-controlled trial in 171 800 secondary school students[105]. Randomisation, as in the Cuban trial, was by school. The vaccine contained LPS-depleted outer membranes from a serotype 15 subtype P1.16 strain, 3% to 6% of high molecular weight proteins, but no meningococcal polysaccharide. The protein was stabilised in 3% sucrose and adsorbed to aluminium hydroxide. The vaccine was formulated to contain 25 μg protein per dose and was administered as two injections 6 weeks apart. After 30 months of observation, an efficacy of 57% was observed (lower confidence limit 28%). No cases were observed in the first 7 months after the second dose in vaccinated individuals, suggesting that a booster dose may improve the protection rate significantly.

Purified OMP vaccine in Chile

A controlled, double-blind randomised efficacy trial of a serogroup B vaccine was conducted in Iquique, Chile, from 1987 until 1989[106]. The vaccine was prepared from a serogroup B serotype 15 subtype P1.3 strain and contained purified OMPs, essentially free of LPS, non-covalently complexed to an equal amount of meningococcal polysaccharide. The vaccine was adsorbed to aluminium hydroxide and was administered in two doses of 100 μg protein with an interval between doses of 6 weeks. The study population of 40 000 included subjects aged one to 21 years and surveillance was continued for 20 months. Overall efficacy was 50%, but protection was age-dependent. Efficacy was 70% in individuals aged 5 to 21 years, but there was no protection in younger children.

OMP and OMV vaccines in prevention of serogroup B disease

These efficacy studies demonstrate that antibodies to non-capsular surface antigens can provide significant protection against serogroup B meningococcal disease. The studies all showed age-dependent protection in the range of 50% to 80%. Protection was shortlived and was greatest for the first 6 to 8 months. Interestingly, protection did not appear to be serotype-specific. The immunisation schedule in all studies consisted of two doses separated by about 6 weeks. Many other vaccines, including diphtheria and tetanus toxoids, pertussis vaccine and the new *Haemophilus influenzae* type b conjugate vaccines, require three or more injections. The data from Brazil and Norway suggest that a third dose given 6 to 8 months after the primary immunisation series can extend the short-term protection. Protection of children aged under 4, in whom most disease occurs, remains a major problem and a three dose primary immunisation schedule should be considered.

Another approach to development of an improved OMV-based vaccine is to include a number of surface proteins strongly upregulated during *in vivo* growth. These include the high molecular weight iron regulated OMPs (IRPs) of molecular weights between 70 000 and 110 000. Studies are in progress in my laboatory and in Brazil to develop and clinically evaluate such a vaccine. The vaccine would include OMVs containing IRPs, serogroup C meningococcal polysaccharide, and alkaline detoxified LPS[107,108]. Detoxified LPS is about 1000-fold less toxic than native LPS and appears to help stabilise bactericidal epitopes on membrane vesicles (Frasch *et al.*, unpublished studies).

ALTERNATIVE APPROACHES TO VACCINE DEVELOPMENT

Optimising OMP vaccines

Improved OMP vaccines can be produced. First, such vaccines should induce broadly protective antibodies, but these antibodies should not be type specific. However, selection of the best proteins for inclusion in a vaccine is complicated since it now appears that most OMPs have antigenic variants. Second, current OMP vaccines do not contain a number of important cell surface proteins that are expressed during infection. These *in vivo* induced proteins include the iron regulated OMPs[109,110], and probably heat-shock proteins[111]. Third, OMV vaccines do not apear to induce a clear booster response as would be expected of a protein antigen when the second immunisation is given 6 weeks after the first. However, data have been presented showing that a two dose primary immunisation series primes for a booster response if the child is reimmunised 6 months to 1 year later[112]. Lastly, it may be necessary to use genetic engineering to remove the class 4 protein from vaccine strains. These proteins are equivalent to gonococcal protein III, which has been shown to induce blocking antibodies[113]. The class 4 protein can be removed from meningococci without affecting the growth properties[114].

Immunogenicity and efficacy studies conducted with different outer membrane vaccines highlight a number of physical characteristics that are important for optimal immunogenicity including the use of soluble vaccines, and the maintenance of the OMPs in their native configuration. A number of studies have shown that isolated OMPs induce few antibodies reactive against surface exposed epitopes. These proteins have loop structures crossing the cell membrane several times[115] (see Chapter 2), which are not conserved upon removal from a membrane environment. In addition, antibodies to any single protein are unlikely to provide broad protection against serogroup B meningococcal disease, and we do not yet know to which proteins the critical protective antibodies are directed.

Improving the immunogenicity of vaccine proteins

The native configuration of OMPs is critical to the induction of functionally active antibodies. It is possible to isolate and purify either from meningococci or as recombinant proteins most of the OMPs that have been considered for inclusion in alternative vaccines. The critical problem is how to package these antigens as vaccine candidates. The work of Wetzler *et al.* with gonococcal proteins suggests that liposomes can be used to present OMPs in a native configuration[116]. Gonococcal porin vaccines were formulated as proteosomes or liposomes. Proteosomes are hydrophobic protein aggregates, and induce high levels of antibodies in rabbits, but these antibodies are primarily against non-surface-exposed hydrophobic epitopes. In contrast, porin proteins incorporated into liposomes induce high levels of antibody to surface-exposed epitopes. The studies of Petrov *et al.* suggest that incorporation of LPS into the liposomes may further increase the antibody response to OMPs contained in liposomes[108].

Alternative vaccine candidates

A number of meningococcal cell surface antigens have been considered for use in a vaccine including pili, the H.8 protein, class 5 proteins, and purified class 2 and class 3 proteins. Antigens under strong consideration include the class 1 protein[117,118], detoxified LPS[118], the 5C protein[119], IRPs[109,120,121] and the class 2/3 proteins incorporated into liposomes[116] (Table 10.2). Non-capsular antigens shown to stimulate bactericidal antibodies should be the prime vaccine candidates.

H.8 antigen

The H.8 antigen is a surface exposed lipoprotein of 20 to 30 KDa[122,123]. Initially it appeared to be an attractive vaccine candidate because almost all meningococcal strains express the protein, whereas most non-pathogenic neisserial species do not[122,123]. However, antibody to H.8 is not bactericidal and is thus unlikely to be protective. Pilus (or fimbrial) protein is another surface antigen of little value as a vaccine candidate, because, although pili are expressed on the surface of almost all freshly isolated meningococcal strains, and antibodies to pili are bactericidal, the surface exposed antigenically dominant epitopes are highly variable.

Class 1 OMPs

Class 1 proteins are the best candidates for an OMP-specific meningococcal protein vaccine. They show much less antigenic heterogeneity than class 2 or class 3 proteins. Seven class 1 serosubtypes represent over 80% of the serogroup B disease isolates[124]. Class 1 protein is present in all the OMV vaccines, and consistently induces functionally important antibodies[107,118,125]. Saukkonen *et al.* showed that four of four monoclonal antibodies directed against class 1 OMP were bactericidal and protective in an infant rat model[125]. These observations have been extended to include data on the human immune response. Zollinger, using class 1 negative mutants of a P1.3 strain, showed that convalescent sera killed the parent strain at substantially higher titres than the P1.3 isogenic mutant. In contrast, the proteosome-like vaccine Zollinger and coworkers used in Iquique, Chile induced class 1

Table 10.2 *Alternative non-capsular antigens as candidates for inclusion in meningococcal vaccines*

Candidate vaccine immunogen	Antigenic variability, number of types	Induces opsonic or bactericidal antibody	Importance in a vaccine	Key references
H.8	1	No	Low	122,123
Pili	Many	Yes	Low	107
Class 1	10–15	Yes	High	116,117
Class 5	Many	Yes	Low	107
5C	1	Yes	High	118
LPS (LOS)	12	Yes*	High?	134
IRPs†	Unknown	Yes	High?	137–140

* LOS vaccines induced opsonic antibody, but failed to induce bactericidal antibody.
† IRPs are iron regulated proteins, some of which are more immunogenic, and all show antigenic variability.

specific antibodies that were not bactericidal[107,108]. Studies with synthetic peptides of the class 1 protein also failed to induce bactericidal antibodies[126]. These results indicate that the native configuration of the class 1 protein is critical to induction of bactericidal antibodies.

The class 1 protein has two immunodominant epitopes (VR1, VR2) associated with serotype specificity and probably induction of bactericidal antibodies[115]. Experimental vaccines containing OMVs with multiple class 1 proteins have been produced[117]. This was done to avoid use of several OMV preparations and the associated increased amounts of toxic LPS. Variants of the serogroup B serotype 15 strain 44/76 were constructed by transformation to contain no class 3 protein and two different class 1 proteins. OMV purified from these constructs induced class 1 serosubtype specific bactericidal antibodies in mice, which were directed against the VR1 and VR2 epitopes of both serosubtypes.

5C protein

Studies on the 5C protein suggest that future OMV vaccines should be prepared from strains expressing the 5C protein, but that the 5C protein alone will not provide broad protection[119,127]. This protein is probably not a true class 5 protein, although Achtman et al. considered it a class 5 variant[128]. Whereas class 5 proteins are heat modifiable, antigenically diverse, and their expression is controlled by multiple repeats of the nucleotide sequence CTCTT, the 5C protein is not heat modifiable, is antigenically conserved, and is not controlled by the CTCTT sequence. The level of 5C expression is variable, a fact which led Achtman et al. to designate strains as 5c and 5C according to the quantity of protein expressed[128]. The 5C protein is expressed on about 20% of serogroup B disease isolates[119].

The 5C protein is a possible vaccine candidate because it induces bactericidal antibodies. These antibodies may also block tissue invasion[129]. The protein appears to be involved in adherence to, and invasion of, endothelial and epithelial cells[129]. In an in vitro model, Virji et al. showed that strains lacking the 5C protein were largely unable to invade cells, and that antibodies to 5C could interfere with attachment and penetration.

The OMV vaccine used in the Norwegian efficacy trial[106] contained 5C protein[119]. Rosenqvist et al. therefore compared the IgG antibody response of vaccine recipients and meningococcal disease patients to this protein. Purified 5C protein was incorporated into liposomes for the antibody assays. Ninety per cent of vaccine recipients responded with a threefold or greater increase in anti-5C antibodies. Using serogroup A meningococcal strains differing primarily in levels of 5C expression and sera from the serogroup B vaccine recipients, Rosenqvist et al. found that antibodies to 5C were strongly bactericidal only for strains expressing large amounts of 5C.

Identical results were obtained with two human monoclonal antibodies to the 5C protein[130]. Elevated 5C antibodies were also seen in convalescent sera, but not in acute sera from meningococcal disease patients. Thus, the 5C protein is antigenically conserved and immunogenic in humans, inducing potentially protective antibodies.

Lipo-oligosaccharide

Meningococcal LPS or lipo-oligosaccharide (LOS) is an important vaccine candidate. Zollinger found that 65% to 90% of serogroup B meningococcal disease isolates express the L3 or L3,7 LOS immunotype[118]. L3,7 LOS exhibits the lacto-N-neotetraose structure, equivalent to paragloboside, and therefore tends to be less immunogenic than other immunotypes. However, sera from infants and children convalescent from meningococcal disease contain antibodies to two different common epitopes on a smaller 3.6 kDa LOS molecule[131].

There are two approaches to the use of LOS in a meningococcal vaccine, namely use of alkaline detoxified LOS, and LOS oligosaccharide conjugate vaccines. In addition, all OMV-based vaccines must contain about 50 to 100 μg of native membrane-bound LOS per mg protein to preserve the membrane structure. Alkaline treatment removes all ester linked fatty acids from the LOS resulting in a 1000- to 10 000-fold reduction in toxicity[107]. Zollinger has suggested several possible advantages of using detoxified LOS in a vaccine in combination with detergent treated OMVs including effective solubilisation of the detergent-treated OMVs, inclusion of additional antigens capable of inducing bactericidal antibodies, and increased vaccine specificity.

The alternative approach is to prepare LOS-derived oligosaccharide–protein conjugates[132,133]. In early studies, Jennings *et al.* produced conjugates by first removing the phosphoethanolamine groups from lipid A-free oligosaccharides. The treated oligosaccharide was then conjugated to tetanus toxoid. However, removal of the phosphoethanolamine adversely affected the L3,7 oligosaccharide. This problem was solved by Verheul *et al.* who introduced free thiol groups into the oligosaccharide, which were then conjugated to a bromacetylated protein carrier[134]. The resulting L3,7,9–tetanus toxoid conjugate was highly immunogenic in rabbits and mice, with and without adjuvant, inducing antibodies of several specificities[133]. Although none of the antibodies induced were bactericidal, they were opsonic for the homologous L3,7,9 immunotype. In follow-up studies L3,7,9 LOS was conjugated to the P1.7,16 class 1 protein[135]. This conjugate induced bactericidal antibodies in mice to the class 1 protein when given with adjuvant, but not to the LOS. Thus, use of LOS vaccines to induce bactericidal antibodies may be difficult.

Iron-regulated proteins

The extremely low concentrations of inorganic iron in the *in vivo* host environment necessitates production of receptor proteins by the meningococcus. The level of expression of these proteins is controlled by the level of inorganic iron. These proteins are therefore referred to as iron-regulated proteins or IRPs. Meningococci express four or five high molecular weight IRPs with sizes between about 70 and 110 kDa. These proteins include receptors specific for human transferrin and lactoferrin[136]. Dyer *et al.*, using isogenic mutants, showed that transferrin binding protein 2 (TBP2) was required for *in vivo* survival[137]. Antibodies to IRPs may function by blocking iron uptake and thus bacterial growth without actually inducing complement-mediated killing. IRPs should therefore be explored as possible vaccine immunogens, though there are problems with this approach.

TBPs are expressed by all meningococcal strains[138]. The molecular sizes of these proteins vary between about 70 and 90 kDa, and they show considerable antigenic heterogeneity, even amongst TBPs of the same molecular size[120]. This presents problems in attempting to develop TBPs for use in a vaccine, although surface exposed conserved antigenic domains may be found, such as the transferrin binding site. Ferron *et al.* examined antigenic heterogeneity among TBPs[139]. They produced antibodies in mice to OMVs containing TBP2s from five selected strains. TBP2s in 35 different strains reacted with at least one of these antibodies, indicating limited heterogeneity. They also observed that in mice TPB2 appeared to be the most consistently immunogenic high molecular weight IRP.

Pettersson *et al.* showed that several monoclonals and a polyclonal serum prepared against the 70 kDa IRP of strain H.44/76 (B15:P1.7,16) were bactericidal, but strain specific[121]. Thus, antigenic heterogeneity has been shown for most IRPs. However, IRP-containing vaccines do hold promise, because meningococcal OMP vaccines containing IRPs induce anti-IRP antibodies in mice, and such antibodies are bactericidal[109]. In addition, rabbit antibodies against IRPs protect young turkeys from *E. coli* septicemia, probably by interfering with iron uptake[140], and vaccines containing IRPs enhance protection of lambs against *Pasteurella haemolytica* septicaemia[141].

REFERENCES

1. Zollinger WD, Moran E. Meningococcal vaccines – present and future. Trans Roy Soc Trop Med Hyg 1991; 85 (Suppl): 37–43.
2. Zollinger WD. Meningococcal meningitis. In: Cruz SJJ, ed. *Vaccines and Immunotherapy*. New York: Pergamon Press, 1991; 113.
3. Zinsser H. *A Textbook of Bacteriology*. New York: Appleton and Co, 1924.

4. Underwood EA. Recent knowledge of the incidence and control of cerebospinal fever. Br Med J 1940; *i*; 757–63.

5. Flexner S. The results of the serum treatment in thirteen hundred cases of epidemic meningitis. J Exp Med 1913; *17*: 553–76.

6. Wright AE, Semple D. Remarks on vaccination against typhoid fever. B Med J 1897; *1*: 256–9.

7. Russell FF. Antityphoid vaccination. Am J Med Sci 1913; *146*: 803–33.

8. Sophian A, Black J. Prophylactic vaccination against epidemic meningitis. JAMA 1912; *59*: 527–32.

9. Greenwood M. The outbreak of cerebrospinal fever at Salisbury in 1914–15. Proc Roy Soc Med 1916; *10* (part 2): 44–60.

10. Gates FL. A report on antimeningitis vaccination and observations on agglutinins in the blood of chronic meningococcus carriers. J Exp Med 1918; *28*: 449–74.

11. Lapeysonnie L. La méningite cérébro-spinale en Afrique. Bull WHO 1963; *28* (Suppl): 3–114.

12. Flosdorf EW, Mudd S. Procedure and apparatus for preservation on "lyophile" form of serum and other biological substances. J Immunol 1935; *29*: 389–425.

13. Glenny AT, Buttle GAH, Stevens MF. Rate of disappearance of diphtheria toxoid injected into rabbits and guinea-pigs: toxoid precipitated with alum. J Pathol Bacteriol 1931; *34*: 267–76.

14. Ferry NS, Norton J, Steele AH. Studies of the properties of buillon filtrates of the meningococcus: production of a soluble toxin. J Immunol 1931; *21*: 293–312.

15. Ferry NS, Steele AH. Active immunization with meningococcus toxin. JAMA 1935; *104*: 983–4.

16. Kuhns DM. The control of meningococcic meningitis epidemics by active immunization with meningococcus soluble toxin: a preliminary report. JAMA 1936; *107*: 5–11.

17. Kuhns DW, Kisner P, Williams MP, Moorman PL. The control of meningococcic meningitis epidemics by active immunization with meningococcus soluble toxin: further studies. JAMA 1938; *110*: 484–7.

18. Dick GF, Dick GH. A skin test for susceptibility to scarlet fever. JAMA 1924; *82*: 265–6.

19. Shick B. Die Diphtherietoxin-hautreaktion des Menschen als Vorprobe der prophylakischen Diphtherieheilseruminjektion. Münch Med Wschr 1913; *60*: 2608–10.

20. Thompson SA, Wang LL, West A, Sparling PF. *Neisseria meningitidis* produces iron-regulated proteins related to the RTX family of exoproteins. J Bacteriol 1993; *175*: 811–18.

21. Scherp H, Rake G. Studies on meningococcus infection. VIII. The type I specific substance. J Exp Med 1935; *61*: 753–69.

22. Kabat EA, Kaiser H, Sikorski H. Preparation of the type-specific polysaccharide of the type I meningococcus and a study of its effectiveness as an antigen in human beings. J Exp Med 1945; *80*: 299–307.

23. Scherp HW, Rake G. Studies on meningococcal infection. XIII. Correlation between antipolysaccharide and the antibody which protects mice against infection with type I meningococci. J Exp Med 1945; *81*: 85–92.

24. MacLeod CM, Hodges RG, Heidleberger M, Bernhard WG. Prevention of pneumococcal pneumonia by immunization with specific capsular polysaccharides. J Exp Med 1945; *82*: 445–65.

25. Watson RG, Scherp HW. The specific hapten of serogroup C (serogroup II

alpha) meningococcus. I. Preparation and immunological behavior. J Immunol 1958; 81: 331–6.
26. Gotschlich EC. Meningococcal serogroup specific polysaccharides. In: Corum CJ, ed. Developments in Industrial Microbiology. Washington DC: American Institute of Biological Sciences, 1970; 92–8.
27. Kabat EA, Bezer AE. The effect of variation on molecular weight on the antigenicity of dextran in man. Arch Biochem 1958; 78: 306–13.
28. Millar JW, Siess EE, Feldman HA, Silverman C, Frank P. In vivo and in vitro resistance to sulfadiazine in strains of Neisseria meningitidis. JAMA 1963; 186: 139–41.
29. Gotschlich EC, Liu TY, Artenstein MS. Human immunity to the meningococcus III. Preparation and immunochemical properties of the serogroup A, serogroup B, and serogroup C meningococcal polysaccharides. J Exp Med 1969; 129: 1349–65.
30. Gotschlich EC, Goldschneider I, Artenstein MS. Human immunity to the meningococcus IV. Immunogenicity of serogroup A and serogroup C polysaccharides in human volunteers. J Exp Med 1969; 129: 1367–84.
31. Gotschlich EC, Goldschneider I, Artenstein MS. Human immunity to the meningococcus. V. The effect of immunization with meningococcal serogroup C polysaccharide on the carrier state. J Exp Med 1969; 129: 1385–95.
32. Artenstein MS, Gold R, Zimmerly JG, Wyle FA, Branche WCJ, Harkins C. Cutaneous reactions and antibody response to meningococcal serogroup C polysaccharide vaccines in man. J Infect Dis 1970; 121: 372–7.
33. Artenstein MS, Gold R, Zimmerly JG, Wyle FA, Schneider H, Harkins C. Prevention of meningococcal disease by serogroup C polysaccharide vaccine. N Engl J Med 1970; 282: 417–20.
34. Gold R, Artenstein MS. Meningococcal infections. 2. Field trial of serogroup C meningococcal polysaccharide vaccine in 1969–70. Bull WHO 1971; 45: 279–82.
35. Sanborn WR, Bencic Z, Cvjetanovic B, Gotschlich EC, Pollock TM, Sippel JE. Trial of a serogroup A meningococcus polysaccharide vaccine in Nigeria. Prog Immunol Stand 1972; 5: 497–505.
36. Wahdan MH, Sallam SA, Hassan MN, Gawad AA, Rakha AS, Sippel JE. A second controlled field trial of a serogroup A meningococcal polysaccharide vaccine in Alexandria. Bull WHO 1977; 55: 645–51.
37. Peltola H, Mäkelä PH, Käyhty H, Jousimies H, Herva E, Hallstrom K et al. Clinical efficacy of meningococcus serogroup A capsular polysaccharide vaccine in children three months to five years of age. N Engl J Med 1977; 297: 686–91.
38. Käyhty H, Karanko V, Peltola H, Sarna S, Mäkelä PH. Serum antibodies to capsular polysaccharide vaccine of serogroup A Neisseria meningitidis followed for three years in infants and children. J Infect Dis 1980; 142: 861–8.
39. Bosmans E, Vimont-Vicary P, Andre FE, Crooy PJ, Roelants P, Vandepitte J. Protective efficacy of a bivalent (A+C) meningococcal vaccine during a cerebrospinal meningitis epidemic in Rwanda. Ann Soc Belg Med Top 1980; 60: 297–306.
40. Reingold AL, Broome CV, Hightower AW, Ajello GW, Bolan GA, Adamsbaum C et al. Age-specific differences in duration of clinical protection after vaccination with meningococcal polysaccharide A vaccine. Lancet 1985, ii: 114–18.
41. Amato NV, Finger H, Gotschlich EC, Feldman RA, de Avila CA, Konichi SR et al. Serologic response to serogroup C meningococcal vaccine in Brazilian

preschool children. Rev Inst Med Trop Sao Paulo 1974; *16*: 149–53.
42. Taunay AE, Feldman RA, Bastos CO, Galvao PAA, Morais JS, Castro IO. Avaliacao do efeito protetor de vacina polissacaridica antimeningococica do serogroupo C, em criancas de 6 a 36 meses. Rev Inst Adolfo Lutz 1978; *38*: 77–82.
43. Gold R. Immunogenicity of meningococcal polysaccharide in man. In: Rudbach J, Baker P, eds. *Immunology of Bacterial Polysaccharides*. New York: Elsevier, 1979; 121–51.
44. Goldschneider I, Gotschlich EC, Artenstein MS. Human immunity to the meningococcus I. The role of humoral antibodies. J Exp Med 1969; *129*: 1307–26.
45. Goldschneider I, Gotschlich EC, Artenstein MS. Human immunity to the meningococcus II. Development of natural immunity. J Exp Med 1969; *129*: 1327–48.
46. Lepow ML, Beeler J, Randolph M, Samuelson JS, Hankins WA. Reactogenicity and immunogenicity of a quadravalent combined meningococcal polysaccharide vaccine in children. J Infect Dis 1986; *154*: 1033–6.
47. Goldschneider I, Lepow ML, Gotschlich EC, Mauck FT, Bachl F, Randolph M. Immunogenicity of serogroup A and serogroup C meningococcal polysaccharides in human infants. J Infect Dis 1973; *128*: 769–76.
48. Mäkelä PH, Peltola H, Käyhty H, Jousimies H, Pettay O, Rouslahti E *et al.* Polysaccharide vaccines of serogroup A *Neisseria meningitidis* and *Haemophilus influenzae* type b: a field trial in Finland. J Infect Dis 1977; *136* (Suppl): S43–50.
49. Williamson AW, Greenwood BM. Impairment of the immune response to vaccination after acute malaria. Lancet 1978; *i*: 1328–9.
50. Greenwood AM, Greenwood BM, Bradley AK, Ball PA, Gilles HM. Enhancement of the immune response to meningococcal polysaccharide vaccine in a malaria endemic area by administration of chloroquine. Ann Trop Med Parasitol 1981; *75*: 261–3.
51. Lepow ML, Goldschneider I, Gold R, Randolph M, Gotschlich EC. Persistence of antibody following immunization of children with serogroups A and C meningococcal polysaccharide vaccines. Pediatrics 1977; *60*: 673–80.
52. Hankins WA, Gwaltney JM, Hendley JO, Farquhar JD, Samuelson JS. Clinical and serological evaluation of a meningococcal polysaccharide vaccine serogroups A, C, Y, and W135. Proc Soc Exp Biol Med 1982; *169*: 54–7.
53. Cadoz M, Armand J, Arminjon F, Gire R, Lafaix CH. Tetravalent (A,C,Y,W135) meningococcal vaccine in children: immunogenicity and safety. Vaccine 1985; 3: 340–2.
54. Peltola HA, Safary A, Käyhty H, Karanko V, Andre FE. Evaluation of 2 tetravalent (ACYW135) meningococcal vaccines in infants and small children – a clinical study comparing immunogenicity of O-acetyl-negative and O-acetyl-positive serogroup C polysaccharides. Pediatrics 1985; *6*: 91–6.
55. Anon. Recommendations of the Immunization Practices Advisory Committee (ACIP)—Meningococcal vaccines. MMWR 1985; *34*: 255–9.
56. Peter G, Hall CB, Lepow ML, Phillips CF eds. *1992 Red Book. Report of Committee on Infectious Diseases*. Elk Grove Village: American Academy of Pediatrics, 1991; 323–6.
57. Galazka A. Meningococcal disease and its control with meningococcal polysaccharide vaccines. Bull WHO 1982; *60*: 1–8.
58. Ross SC, Densen P. Complement deficiency states and infection: Epidemiology, pathogenesis and consequences of Neisserial and other infections in an immune deficiency. Medicine 1984; *63*: 243–73.
59. Sjöholm AG, Kuijper EJ, Tijssen CC, Jansz A, Bol P, Spanjaard L *et al.*

Dysfunctional properdin in a Dutch family with meningococcal disease. N Engl J Med 1988; 319: 33–7.

60. Densen P, Weiler JM, Griffiss JM, Hoffmann LG. Familial properdin deficiency and fatal meningococcemia: correction of the bactericidal defect by vaccination. N Engl J Med 1987; 316: 922–6.

61. Greenwood BM, Wali SS. Control of meningococcal infection in the African meningitis belt by selective vaccination. Lancet 1980; i: 729–32.

62. Anon. Recommendations of the Advisory Committee on Immunization Practices (ACIP). Prevention and control of meningococcal diseases; evaluation and management of outbreaks. MMWR (in press).

63. Gemmill I. An outbreak of meningococcal disease in Ottawa-Carleton December 1991 – February 1992. Can J Pub Hlth 1992; 83: 134–7.

64. Lavigne P, Boulianne N, Fortin C, Naccache H, Douville-Fradet M. Meningococcal infections in Quebec – 1991–92. Can Comm Dis Rep 1992; 18: 113–16.

65. Lennon D, Gellin B, Hood D, Voss L, Heffernan H, Thakur S. Successful intervention in a serogroup A meningococcal outbreak in Auckland, New Zealand. Pediatr Infect Dis J 1992; 11: 617–23.

66. McLaughlin GL, Howe DK, Biggs DR, Smith AR, Ludwinski P, Fox BC et al. Amplification of rDNA loci to detect and type Neisseria meningitidis and other eubacteria. Mol Cell Probes 1993; 7: 7–17.

67. Black SB, Shinefield HR, Kaiser Permanente Ped Vaccine Stdy Grp. Immunization with oligosaccharide conjugate Haemophilus influenzae type b (HbOC) vaccine on a large health maintenance organization population: Extended follow-up and impact on Haemophilus influenzae disease epidemiology. Pediatr Infect Dis J 1992; 11: 610–13.

68. Adams WG, Deaver KA, Cochi SL, Plikaytis BD, Zell ER, Broome CV et al. Decline of childhood Haemophilus influenzae type b (Hib) disease in the Hib vaccine era. JAMA 1993; 269: 221–6.

69. Costantino P, Viti S, Podda A, Velmonte MA, Nencioni L, Rappuoli R. Development and phase 1 clinical testing of a conjugate vaccine against meningococcus A and C. Vaccine 1992; 10: 691–8.

70. Beuvery EC, Miedema F, van Delft R, Haverkamp K. Preparation and immunochemical characterization of meningococcal serogroup C polysaccharide–tetanus toxoid conjugates as a new generation of vaccines. Infect Immun 1983; 40: 39–45.

71. Beuvery EC, Kaaden A, Kanhai V, Leussink AB. Physiochemical and immunological characterization of meningococcal serogroup A polysaccharide–tetanus toxoid conjugates prepared by two methods. Vaccine 1983; 1: 31–6.

72. Jennings HJ, Lugowski C. Immunochemistry of serogroups A, B, and C meningococcal polysaccharide-tetanus toxoid conjugates. J Immunol 1981; 127: 1011–18.

73. Wyle FA, Artenstein MS, Brandt BL, Tramont EC, Kasper DL, Altieri PL et al. Immunologic response of man to serogroup B meningococcal polysaccharide vaccines. J Infect Dis 1972; 126: 514–22.

74. Leinonen M, Frasch CE. Class-specific antibody response to serogroup B Neisseria meningitidis capsular polysaccharide: Use of polylysine precoating in an enzyme-linked immunosorbent assay. Infect Immun 1982; 38: 1203–7.

75. Mandrell RE, Zollinger WD. Measurement of antibodies to meningococcal serogroup B polysaccharide: Low avidity binding and equilibrium binding constants. J Immunol 1982; 129: 2172–7.

76. Zollinger WD, Mandrell RE, Griffiss JM, Altieri P, Berman S. Complex of

meningococcal serogroup B polysaccharide and type 2 outer membrane protein immunogenic in man. J Clin Invest 1979; *63*: 836–48.

77. Moreno C, Lifely MR, Esdaile J. Immunity and protection of mice against *Neisseria meningitidis* serogroup B by vaccination using a polysaccharide complexed with outer membrane proteins: a comparison with purified B polysaccharide. Infect Immun 1985; *47*: 527–33.

78. Moreno C, Lifely MR, Esdaile J. Effect of aluminium ions on chemical and immunological properties of meningococcal serogroup B polysaccharide. Infect Immun 1985; *49*: 587–92.

79. Frasch CE, Zahradnik JM, Wang LY, Mocca LF, Tsai C-M. Antibody response of adults to an aluminium hydroxide adsorbed *Neisseria meningitidis* serotype 2b protein serogroup B-polysaccharide vaccine. J Infect Dis 1988; *158*: 700–8.

80. Zollinger WD, Mandrell RE. Importance of complement source in bactericidal activity of human antibody and murine monoclonal antibody to meningococcal serogroup B polysaccharide. Infect Immun 1983; *40*: 257–64.

81. Lehmann AK, Halstensen A, Naess A, Vollset SE, Sjursen H, Bjune G. Immunization against serogroup B meningococci – Opsonin response in vaccinees as measured by chemiluminescense. APMIS 1991; *99*: 769.

82. Jennings HJ, Roy R, Gamian A. Induction of meningococcal serogroup B polysaccharide-specific IgG antibodies in mice using an N-propionylated B polysaccharide-tetanus toxoid conjugate vaccine. J Immunol 1986; *137*: 1708–13.

83. Jennings HJ, Gamian A, Ashton FE. N-propionylated serogroup b meningococcal polysaccharide mimics a unique epitope on serogroup B *Neisseria meningitidis*. J Exp Med 1987; *165*: 1207–11.

84. Jennings HJ, Gamian A, Michon F, Ashton FE. Unique intermolecular bactericidal epitope involving the homosialopolysaccharide capsule on the cell surface of serogroup B *Neisseria meningitidis* and *Escherichia coli* K1. J Immunol 1989; *142*: 3585–91.

85. Brisson JR, Baumann H, Imberty A, Perez S, Jennings HJ. Helical epitope of the serogroup B meningococcal α(2–8)-linked sialic acid polysaccharide. Biochemistry 1992; *31*: 4996–5004.

86. Jennings HJ, Roy R, Michon F. Determinant specificities of the serogroups B and C polysaccharides of *Neisseria meningitidis*. J Immunol 1985; *134*: 2651–7.

87. Yamasaki R, Bacon B. Three-dimensional structural analysis of the serogroup B polysaccharide of *Neisseria meningitidis* 6275 by two-dimensional NMR: the polysaccharide is suggested to exist in helical conformations in solution. Biochemistry 1991; *30*: 851–7.

88. Finne JM, Leinonen M, Mäkelä PH. Antigenic similarities between brain components and bacteria causing meningitis. Implications for vaccine development. Lancet 1983; *ii*: 355–7.

89. Devi SJN, Robbins JB, Schneerson R. Antibodies to poly[(2→8)-α-N-acetylneuraminic acid] and poly[(2→9)-α-N-acetylneuraminic acid] are elicited by immunization of mice with *Escherichia coli* K92 conjugates: Potential vaccines for serogroups B and C meningococci and *E. coli* K1. Proc Natl Acad Sci USA 1991; *88*: 7175–9.

90. Frasch CE, Chapman SS. Classification of *Neisseria meningitidis* serogroup b into distinct serotypes. III. Application of a new bactericidal inhibition technique to distribution of serotypes among cases and carriers. J Infect Dis 1973; *127*: 149–54.

91. Jones DM, Eldridge J. Development of antibodies to meningococcal protein and lipopolysaccharide antigens in healthy carriers. J Med Microbiol 1979; *12*: 107–11.

92. Tsai CM, Frasch CE, Rivera E, Hochstein HD. Measurements of lipopolysaccharide (endotoxin) in meningococcal protein and polysaccharide preparations for vaccine usage. J Biol Stand 1989; *17*: 249–58.

93. Zollinger WD, Mandrell RE, Altieri P, Berman S, Lowenthal J, Artenstein MS. Safety and immunogenicity of a meningococcal type 2 protein vaccine in animals and human volunteers. J Infect Dis 1978; *137*: 728–39.

94. Frasch CE, Peppler MS. Protection against serogroup B *Neisseria meningitidis* disease: Preparation of soluble protein and protein-polysaccharide immunogens. Infect Immun 1982; *37*: 271–80.

95. Devoe IW, Gilchrist JE. Release of endotoxin in the form of cell wall blebs during in vitro growth of *Neisseria meningitidis*. J Exp Med 1973; *138*: 1156–67.

96. Peppler MS, Frasch CE. Protection against serogroup B *Neisseria meningitidis* disease: effect of serogroup B polysaccharide and polymyxin B on immunogenicity of serotype protein preparations. Infect Immun 1982; *37*: 264–70.

97. Wang L-Y, Frasch CE. Development of a *Neisseria meningitidis* serogroup B serotype 2b protein vaccine and evaluation in a mouse model. Infect Immun 1984; *46*: 408–14.

98. Rosenqvist E, Tjade T, Frøholm LO, Frasch CE. An ELISA study of the antibody response after vaccination with a combined meningococcal serogroup B polysaccharide and serotype 2 outer membrane protein vaccine. NIPH Ann 1983; *6*: 139–49.

99. Frasch CE, Coetzee GJ, Wu L, Wang L-Y, Rosenqvist E. Immune response of adults and children to serogroup B *Neisseria meningitidis* outer membrane protein vaccines. In: Robbins JB ed. *Bacterial Vaccines*. New York: Praeger, 1987; 262–72.

100. Rosenqvist E, Høiby EA, Bjune G, Closs O, Feiring B, Klem A et al. Human antibody responses after vaccination with the Norwegian serogroup B meningococcal outer membrane vessicle vaccine: results from ELISA studies. NIPH Ann 1991; *14*: 169–81.

101. Frasch CE, Coetzee G, Zahradnik JM, Feldman HA, Koornhof HJ. Development and evaluation of serogroup b serotype 2 protein vaccines: report of a serogroup B field trial. Med Trop 1983; *43*: 177–83.

102. Sierra VG, Campa C, Garcia L et al. Efficacy evaluation of the Cuban vaccine VA-MENGOC-BC against disease caused by serogroup B *Neisseria meningitidis*. In: Achtman M, ed. *Neisseria 1990*. Berlin: Walter de Gruyter, 1991; 129–34.

103. De Moraes JC, Perkins BA, Camargo MCC, Hidalgo NTR, Barbosa HA, Sacchi CT et al. Protective efficacy of a serogroup B meningococcal vaccine in Sao Paulo, Brazil. Lancet 1992; *340*: 1074–8.

104. Noronha CP. Avaliacao da eficacia da vacina anti-meningococicia BC no Rio de Janeiro: un estudo caso-controle (thesis), Rio de Janeiro, 1993: 1–232.

105. Bjune G, Høiby EA, Gronnesby JK, Arnesen O, Fredriksen JH, Halstensen A et al. Effect of outer membrane vesicle vaccine against serogroup B meningococcal disease in Norway. Lancet 1991; *338*: 1093–6.

106. Zollinger WD, Boslego J, Moran E, Garcia J, Cruz C, Ruiz S et al. Meningococcal serogroup B vaccine protection trial and follow-up studies. NIPH Ann 1991; *14*: 211–13.

107. Zollinger WD. New and improved vaccines against meningococcal disease. In: Woodrow GC, Levine MM, eds. *New Generations Vaccine*. New York: Marcel Dekker, 1990: 325–48.

108. Petrov AB, Semenov BF, Vartanyan YP, Zakirov MM, Torchilin VP, Trubetskoy VS et al. Toxicity and immunogenicity of *Neisseria meningitidis*

lipopolysaccharide incorporated into liposomes. Infect Immun 1992; *60*: 3897–903.

109. Bhatnagar NB, Frasch CE. Expression of *Neisseria meningitidis* iron-regulated outer membrane proteins, including a 70-Kilodalton transferrin receptor, and their potential for use as vaccines. Infect Immun 1990; *58*: 2875–81.

110. Black JR, Dyer DW, Thompson MK, Sparling PF. Human immune response to iron-repressible outer membrane proteins of *Neisseria meningitidis*. Infect Immun 1986; *54*: 710–13.

111. Woods ML, Bonfiglioli R, McGee ZA, Georgopoulos C. Synthesis of select serogroup of proteins by *Neisseria gonorrhoeae* in response to thermal stress. Infect Immun 1990; *58*: 719–25.

112. Sierra GVG, Campa HC, Varcacel NM, Izquierdo PL, Sotolongo PF, Casanueva GV *et al*. Vaccine against serogroup B *Neisseria meningitidis*: Protection trial and mass vaccination results in Cuba. NIPH Ann 1991; *14*: 195–210.

113. Rice PA, Vayo HE, Tam MR, Blake MS. Immunoglobulin G antibodies directed against protein III block killing of serum-resistant *Neisseria gonorrhoeae* by immune serum. J Exp Med 1986; *164*: 1735–48.

114. Klugman KP, Gotschlich EC, Blake MS. Sequence of the structural gene (rmpM) for the class 4 outer membrane protein of *Neisseria meningitidis*, homology of the protein to gonococcal protein III and *Escherichia coli* OmpA, and construction of meningococcal strains that lack class 4 protein. Infect Immun 1989; *57*: 2066–71.

115. McGuinness B, Barlow AK, Clarke IN, Farley JE, Anilonis A, Poolman JT, Heckels JE. Deduced amino acid sequence of class 1 protein (PorA) from three strains of *Neisseria meningitidis*. Synthetic peptides define the epitopes responsible for serosubtypes specificity. J Exp Med 1990; *171*: 1871–82.

116. Wetzler LM, Blake MS, Barry K, Gotschlich EC. Gonococcal porin vaccine evaluation: Comparison of Por proteosomes, liposomes, and blebs isolated from rmp deletion mutants. J Infect Dis 1992; *166*: 551–5.

117. van der Ley P, Poolman JT. Construction of a multivalent meningococcal vaccine strain based on the class 1 outer membrane protein. Infect Immun 1992; *60*: 3156–61.

118. Zollinge WD, Moran E. Meningococcal vaccines—present and future. Trans R Soc Trop Med Hyg 1991; *85* (Suppl): 37–43.

119. Rosenqvist E, Høiby EA, Wedege E, Kusecek B, Achtman M. The 5C protein of *Neisseria meningitidis* is highly immunogenic in humans and induces bactericidal antibodies. J Infect Dis 1992; *167*: 1065–73.

120. Griffiths E, Stevenson P, Ray A. Antigenic and molecular heterogeneity of the transferrin-binding protein of *Neisseria meningitidis*. FEMS Microbiol Lett 1990; *69*: 31–6.

121. Pettersson A, Kuipers B, Pelzer M, Verhagen E, Tiesjema RH, Tommassen J *et al*. Monoclonal antibodies against the 70-kilodalton iron-regulated protein of *Neisseria meningitidis* are bactericidal and strain specific. Infect Immun 1990; *58*: 3036–41.

122. Cannon JG, Black WJ, Nachamkin I, Stewart PW. Monoclonal antibody that recognizes an outer membrane antigen common to the pathogenic *Neisseria* species. Infect Immun 1984; *43*: 994–9.

123. Bhattacharjee AK, Moran EE, Zollinger WD. Antibodies to meningococcal H.8 (Lip) antigen fail to show bactericidal activity. Can J Microbiol 1990; *36*: 117–22.

124. Abdillahi H, Poolman JT. *Neisseria meningitidis* serogroup B serotyping using

282   C.E. Frasch

monoclonal antibodies in whole-cell ELISA. Microb Path 1988; 4: 27–32.
125. Saukkonen K, Leinonen M, Abdillahi H, Poolman JT. Comparative evaluation of potential components fo serogroup B meningococcal vaccine by passive protection in the infant rat and in vitro bactericidal assay. Vaccine 1989; 7: 325–8.
126. Polman JT, van der Ley PA, Wiertz EJHJ, Hoogerhout P. Second generation meningococcal OMP-LPS vaccines. NIPH Ann 1991; 14: 233–41.
127. Achtman M, Kusecek B, Morelli G, Eickmann K, Jianfu W, Crowe B et al. A comparison of the variable antigens expressed by clone IV-1 and subserogroup III of Neisseria meningitidis serogroup A. J Infect Dis 1992; 165: 53–68.
128. Achtman M, Neibert M, Crowe BA, Strittmatter W, Kusecek B, Weyse E et al. Purification and characterization of eight class 5 outer membrane protein variants from a clone of Neisseria meningitidis serogroup A. J Exp Med 1988; 168: 507–26.
129. Virji M, Makepeace K, Ferguson DJP, Achtman M, Sarkari J, Moxon ER. Expression of the Opc protein correlates with invasion of epithelial and endothelial cells by Neisseria meningitidis. Mol Microbiol 1992; 6: 2785–95.
130. Fernandez de Cossio ME, Ohlin M, Llano M, Selander B, Cruz S, Del Valle J et al. Human monoclonal antibodies against an epitope on the class 5c outer membrane protein common to many pathogenic strains of Neisseria meningitidis. J Infect Dis 1992; 166: 1322–8.
131. Estabrook MM, Baker CJ, Griffiss JM. The immune response of children to meningococcal lipopolysaccharides during disseminated disease is directed primarily against two monoclonal antibody-defined epitopes. J Infect Dis 1993; 167: 966–70.
132. Jennings HJ, Lugowski CH, Ashton FE. Conjugation of meningococcal R-type oligosaccharides to tetanus toxoid as route to a potential vaccine against serogroup B Neisseria meningitidis. Infect Immun 1984; 43: 407–12.
133. Verheul AFM, Snippe H, Poolman JT. Meningococcal lipopolysaccharides: virulence factor and potential vaccine component. Microbiol Rev 1993; 57: 34–49.
134. Verheul AFM, Braat AK, Leenhouts JM, Hoogerhout P, Poolman JT, Snippe H et al. Preparation, characterization, and immunogenicity of meningococcal immunotype L2 and L3,7,9 phosphoethanolamine serogroup-containing oligosaccharide–protein conjugates. Infect Immun 1991; 59: 843–51.
135. Verheul AFM, van Gaans JAM, Wiertz EJH, Snippe H, Verhoef J, Poolman JT. Meningococcal lipopolysaccharide (LPS)-derived oligosaccharide-protein conjugates evoke outer membrane protein but not LPS-specific bactericidal antibodies in mice: Influence of adjuvants. Infect Immun 1993; 61: 187–96.
136. Schryvers AB, Lee BC. Comparative analysis of the transferrin and lactoferrin binding proteins in the family Neisseriaceae. Can J Microbiol 1989; 35: 404–15.
137. Dyer DW, West EP, McKenna W, Thompson SA, Sparling PF: A pleiotropic iron-uptake mutant of Neisseria meningitidis lacks a 70-kDa iron-regulated protein. Infect Immun 1988; 56: 977–83.
138. Ferreiros CM, Criado MT, Pintor M, Ferron L. Analysis of the molecular mass heterogeneity of the transferrin receptor in Neisseria meningitidis and commensal Neisseria. FEMS Microbiol Lett 1991; 83: 247–54.
139. Ferron L, Ferreiros CM, Criado MT, Pintor M. Immunogenicity and antigenic heterogeneity of a human transferrin-bindin 2 protein in Neisseria meningitidis. Infect Immun 1992; 60: 2887–92.
140. Bolin CA, Jensen AE. Passive immunization with antibodies against iron-regulated outer membrane proteins protects turkeys from Escherichia coli septicemia. Infect Immun 1987; 55: 1239–42.

141. Gilmour NJL, Donachie W, Sutherland AD, Gilmour JS, Jones GE, Quirie M. Vaccine containing iron-regulated proteins of *Pasteurella haemolytica* A2 enhances protection against experimental pasteurellosis in lambs. Vaccine 1991; 9: 137–40.

11
Outbreak Management

NORMAN BEGG

PHLS Communicable Disease Surveillance Centre, London, UK

INTRODUCTION

Effective control of meningococcal disease outbreaks is important because of the high morbidity and mortality associated with the disease. The incubation period is short (2–10 days) and epidemics may develop rapidly, demanding timely intervention. Outbreaks often generate considerable alarm, and the management of public relations is almost as important as the management of cases and their contacts. In this chapter the rationale for, and the principles of, control of outbreaks of meningococcal disease will be considered. The main emphasis will be placed on the control of serogroup B and C meningococcal disease in technologically advanced countries rather than on the control of epidemic serogroup A disease in Africa.

RECOGNITION AND INVESTIGATION OF AN OUTBREAK

Prompt recognition of outbreaks is necessary if control measures are to be effective. In the United Kingdom (UK), meningococcal septicaemia and meningitis are both notifiable conditions. During an outbreak cases may present with either (or both) clinical manifestations, and it is important that general practitioners (GPs), casualty (or emergency room) officers, microbiologists and others who may see cases understand the importance of notification to the appropriate public health authority. Notification should be immediate (by telephone). While every effort should be made to obtain laboratory confirmation in suspected cases, notification should never be delayed while results of laboratory tests are awaited.

During an outbreak, active surveillance should be established to ensure that no cases are missed. In practice this means that the public health physician who has responsibility for outbreak control should make daily contact with the local microbiologist, physicians and paediatricians. A register of all suspected cases should be kept and epidemiological and laboratory information recorded for each case. The dataset should include age, sex, onset date, travel history, attendance at school, nursery, playgroup or crèche, attendance at social gatherings, and a list of all the close contacts, together with a note of their respective relationships with the case. The control measures applied to the case and the contacts should also be recorded on the register together with all laboratory results.

Case definitions for meningococcal disease have been developed in a number of countries, notably the United States and Canada[1,2]. They are most useful in large, geographically widespread outbreaks that involve several public health departments where standardisation of data collection is important. Case definitions have not been widely used in the UK.

In those parts of the world where serogroup A meningococcal disease is rare (including Europe, North America and Australia) there are three main types of outbreak: family, community and institutional. Family and community outbreaks are the most common, and are usually caused by serogroup B meningococci. Institutional outbreaks involve schools, military establishments and occasionally hospitals. They are comparatively uncommon, and serogroup C strains predominate. Between 1985 and 1992, 18 institutional outbreaks were reported in England and Wales (Table 11.1).

What is an outbreak?

An outbreak has been defined as "two or more cases associated in time and place"[3]. Approximately 1300 cases of meningococcal disease are notified each year in England and Wales; thus each health district might expect to receive an average of 10 notifications a year, with the greatest concentration during the winter months. Though most of these cases will be sporadic, a sensitive surveillance system will inevitably identify apparent clusters. It is important to determine whether two or more cases associated in time and place constitute an outbreak, or are merely sporadic. In some cases, a history of recent close contact between two cases may be sufficient to confirm an outbreak. Thus a laboratory confirmed case in a household, followed one week later by a second case in the same household, would almost certainly constitute a family outbreak. In contrast, two cases a month apart in different classes of a large secondary school may well be unrelated.

Detailed characterisation of the infecting organism is necessary to determine whether two or more epidemiologically linked cases constitute a genuine outbreak. In addition, the public health physician needs to know

Table 11.1 Institutional outbreaks of meningococcal disease, England and Wales, 1985–92

Group	Number of outbreaks reported (number of cases)			
	School	Military	Other	Total
B	5 (11)	0	0	5 (11)
C	8 (24)	4 (11)	1* (3)	13 (38)
Total	13 (35)	4 (11)	1 (3)	18 (49)

* Homeless families unit.

whether the disease-producing strain is potentially vaccine-preventable (i.e. of serogroup A or serogroup C). All meningococcal isolates should therefore be sent to a reference laboratory for serogrouping, serotyping and determination of sulphonamide sensitivity. In many cases, no isolate is available from the patient. The trend towards giving penicillin as early as possible in the management of suspected meningococcal disease, compounded by a growing reluctance to undertake lumbar puncture in young children with symptoms of meningitis (see Chapter 9), is producing an increasing proportion of cases in which a meningococcus is not isolated from a deep site, such as cerebrospinal fluid (CSF) or blood[4].

Nasopharyngeal swabs from cases and contacts

A well-taken nasopharyngeal swab from the patient will provide a relevant isolate in about 50% of cases, regardless of whether parenteral penicillin has already been administered[5] and antigen detection methods and antibody estimation in convalescent serum may also give diagnostic information. Non-culture diagnostic methods such as detection of meningococcal DNA following amplification by the polymerase chain reaction (PCR)[6] are likely to come into wider use in the near future. Approximately one-third of family contacts living at the same address as a younger index case will be carriers of meningococci[7], and of these strains over 90% will be the same as the index case strain[8]. Swabbing of these contacts before commencing chemoprophylaxis may thus also provide further diagnostic clues in cases with no isolate.

A problem arises when meningococcal disease caused by the same serogroup and serotype of meningococcus is identified in two cases living in close proximity but separated by a long time interval. Does this constitute an outbreak? There are no hard and fast rules. In a school, it is very likely that two or more cases of the same strain within the same term constitute an outbreak, whereas if they occur in different terms they are less likely to indicate transmission in the school environment. In such cases, knowledge of the incidence of meningococcal disease in the community at large, and of the prevalent serogroups and serotypes, may be helpful in determining the significance of possible clusters of cases.

The situation presenting the greatest difficulty is where two or more cases of the same serogroup and serotype occur in a neighbourhood, e.g. the same street or village, but with no other direct links between them. Meningococci of the same serogroup and serotype tend to cluster geographically, causing disease in a local community which may persist for several years (see Chapter 6). Slow transmission which persists for long periods is a feature particularly associated with serogroup B meningococci. During the 1980s, community-wide outbreaks of meningococcal disease due to B15:P1.16 sulphonamide-resistant organisms occurred in Gloucestershire[9], Plymouth[10] and north-west England[11]. The point at which a local increase in a community may be considered an outbreak has not been defined. There are, however, certain features which should alert the public health physician to the possibility of an emerging community outbreak.

These are:

1. The appearance of a strain not recently seen in that community.
2. An increase in the age distribution of cases[12].
3. A change in the clinical presentation of cases when compared with non-epidemic periods.
4. An increase in the case fatality ratio.

THE SCIENTIFIC BASIS FOR OUTBREAK MANAGEMENT

Increased risk in close contacts

Studies in Europe[13] and the USA[7,14] have demonstrated that secondary attack rates among household contacts of meningococcal disease are approximately 1000 fold greater than in the general population. The risk is highest in the first week after the index case presents but an increased risk persists for several months, especially when chemoprophylaxis has been given[15]. Though the relative risk of meningococcal disease amongst contacts of index cases is high, the absolute risk is still very small and secondary cases are comparatively rare in comparison with sporadic cases. Only 44 of 5593 cases (0.8%) of meningococcal infection in England and Wales from 1978–87 were reported to be secondary cases[16]. In 19 of these, the onset was within 2 days of the presentation of the index case, seven were within 3–7 days, seven within 8–28 and eight between 1 and 15 months later[16]. The attack rate in household members for the period 1984–7 was 2.3 per 1000, a relative risk of 144 compared with the general population[17].

The size of the risk for other contacts is less well established. A study in Belgium found a relative risk of 76 for children aged under 3 years whose contact was in day-care centres and 23 for 3–5 year old contacts in nursery schools[13]. The risk of secondary disease among pre-school children attending playgroups, nurseries or crèches is not known precisely, but there is evidence from several studies in the USA that children in these settings play an important role in the transmission of pathogenic meningococci[7,18–20].

There is no consensus concerning the importance of school attendance in transmission of meningococci. A study during an epidemic of serogroup C disease in Brazil found no increased risk among classroom contacts[21]. Increased carriage rates among classroom contacts have, however, been documented in outbreaks in both the UK[22] and the USA[23]. Increased carriage in a school may reflect an increased carriage rate in the local community and does not necessarily implicate the school as the main setting for transmission, which may be through social contacts outside the school. Proximity of contact within the classroom was found to be a risk factor in a school outbreak in Texas[24], although the possibility of other confounding variables could not be ruled out in this study. In another outbreak, school activities that involved prolonged close contact (a ski trip and a poster-making session) were both associated with an increased risk of infection[25].

Although there are anecdotal accounts of meningococcal disease developing in health care staff who have been in contact, such contact is normally very brief and is not normally intimate. Hospital contacts are not generally thought to be at increased risk of infection, although nosocomial transmission of serogroup C disease has been described[26]. There may be an increased risk to staff who perform mouth to mouth resuscitation on patients with meningococcal disease.

CHEMOPROPHYLAXIS

The aim of chemoprophylaxis

Ultimately, the aim of chemoprophylaxis is to reduce the incidence of secondary cases of disease and to arrest outbreaks. No prospective controlled trials of the value of chemoprophylaxis for the prevention of secondary meningococcal disease have ever been undertaken. Three possible mechanisms have been suggested by which chemoprophylaxis of contacts might reduce the rate of secondary disease[16]:

1. By elimination of meningococcal carriage in household members, thereby reducing transmission to susceptibles who are not carriers[27,28]. This requires the simultaneous dosing of the whole contact network. Therefore an arbitrary definition of that network has to be made for

logistical reasons. This approach can only be successful either if there is no re-acquisition of pathogenic meningococci from the wider contact network, or if immunity is induced (e.g. by vaccination) before re-exposure to the same pathogenic meningococcus. Re-acquisition of meningococci after chemoprophylaxis does occur, albeit slowly, and may explain some failures of chemoprophylaxis.

It is important to appreciate that parenteral antibiotic treatment of systemic meningococcal disease is unreliable in eliminating meningococci from the nasopharynx; patients recovering from meningococcal disease may still be carriers[29] and are therefore a potential source of infection to their family contacts when they return home from hospital. Meningococcal disease patients should receive chemoprophylaxis before hospital discharge.

Co-primary cases, which occur within 24 hours of the index case, may not be amenable to prevention by chemoprophylaxis. Both the index case and the co-primary case are assumed to have been infected at the same time, probably from the same source. For this reason active surveillance of close contacts should be maintained for at least 24 hours after the index case.

2. To treat newly acquired infection in contacts who are non-immune and may be incubating the disease. The doses of rifampicin used for chemoprophylaxis are inadequate to treat incubating meningococcal infection reliably. An alternative strategy to achieve this aim is to give a course of protective chemotherapy. This approach was adopted in Norway, where a 7 day course of penicillin V was recommended for household contacts under 15 years of age[30]. A 5 day course of oral chloramphenicol or a single intramuscular injection of a long acting preparation of chloramphenicol are possible alternatives. No attempt is made to eliminate nasopharyngeal carriage. There is some evidence that this approach may be successful in preventing infections during the period of treatment[30], but individuals become susceptible to reinfection soon after cessation of therapy. It is no longer recommended.

3. To prevent susceptible contacts from acquiring infection by directly inhibiting colonisation. This approach could only be effective for the 2 days of prophylaxis.

Choice of prophylactic antibiotic

Successful eradication of nasopharyngeal carriage of meningococci can be achieved with several antibiotics. Sulphonamides were first used during epidemics in World War II, and a 2 day course is very effective in eradicating carriage of susceptible strains. Unfortunately resistance to sulphonamides is now widespread. Thirty-six per cent of serogroup B and 42% of serogroup C strains in England and Wales in 1991 had a minimum inhibitory concentration of sulphonamide of 10 mg/l or greater[4]. Therefore sulphonamides should not be used for prophylaxis unless the sensitivity of the meningococcus has been established.

Minocycline is also effective, either on its own or in combination with rifampicin. However, it is associated with an unacceptable level of side effects, particularly vestibular problems. It is contraindicated in children and in pregnant and lactating women.

Rifampicin is the most widely used chemoprophylactic agent at present. A 2 day course eradicates carriage in 70–95% of contacts[31]. Side effects include discoloration of soft contact lenses, interference with the oral contraceptive pill and orange-red colouring of urine, saliva, tears and other body secretions. Because of these side effects, compliance with the chemoprophylactic regimen may be sub-optimal. It is contraindicated in pregnancy[32], alcoholism and severe liver disease. Resistance to rifampicin is rare, and occurs mainly when it is used for mass prophylaxis. This was documented during an outbreak in Switzerland where rifampicin was administered to an entire school[33]. The other situation where resistance is encountered is when contacts become recolonised; between 10% and 25% of these recolonising strains may be resistant to rifampicin[34]. Rifampicin has a limited role in developing countries, where it is relatively expensive and where its use has been reserved for the treatment of tuberculosis.

Ceftriaxone is a third-generation cephalosporin which has recently become available in the UK. A study in Saudi Arabia during an outbreak of serogroup A disease showed that a single intramuscular injection of 250 mg for adults and 125 mg for children under 15 years old was 97% effective in eradicating meningococcal carriage in family contacts after one to two weeks[35]. The main advantages of ceftriaxone are the facility to use it in pregnancy and in young children and the documented high compliance achieved with a single dose parenteral preparation.

Ciprofloxacin as a single oral dose of 500 mg has recently been evaluated in a number of studies in adult contacts[36-39]. These have established an efficacy of 93–97% in eliminating carriage. It is an attractive option but its safety in children has yet to be established. The use of fluoroquinolones in children is discouraged because of animal studies which have raised concerns over bone development. However, it is unlikely that a single dose would affect bone growth adversely, and it has been used safely in children with severe infections and cystic fibrosis. No major side effects were recorded in a large study of ciprofloxacin in which 61% of the participants were children[40].

Swabbing

If the effectiveness of chemoprophylaxis is to be checked by culturing nasopharyngeal swabs from close contacts, it should be done 4–7 days after the course of antibiotics has been completed[16]. Swabbing to check for clearance is of limited value, as a single negative swab does not guarantee freedom from nasopharyngeal carriage. If the swab is positive, chemo-prophylaxis should be repeated.

Identifying meningococcal carriers among contacts in order to determine who should receive chemoprophylaxis is inappropriate for three reasons. It would delay the administration of chemoprophylaxis during the highest risk period; negative contacts may subsequently become carriers (or cases) and lastly, swabbing has a failure rate of at least 10% in identifying carriers[16].

However, because of the increasing use of parenteral penicillin in suspected cases of meningococcal disease prior to their admission to hospital, nasopharyngeal swabbing of contacts should be considered as a means of assisting in making the diagnosis. Close family contacts are more likely to be nasopharyngeal meningococcal carriers when the index case is aged under 3 years than when the index case is a teenager or adult. Isolation of a meningococcus from a close family contact may help to confirm the diagnosis in a culture-negative index case and may provide an isolate for determination of serogroup and serotype. Meningococci are part of the normal pharyngeal commensal flora, and 20–30% of young adults may carry meningococci at any one time (see Chapter 5). However, 90% of meningococcal strains from family contacts living at the same address as the index case are indistinguishable from the associated index case strain. If swabs are taken from close family contacts for diagnostic reasons, administration of chemoprophylaxis must not be delayed while results are awaited. Careful counselling is needed to ensure that parents or siblings whose nasopharyngeal swabs yield meningococci do not feel 'contaminated' or responsible for spreading infection.

In a community or institutional outbreak where widespread chemo-prophylaxis and/or vaccination are being contemplated, it may be useful to undertake more extensive swabbing in order to determine carriage rates of the outbreak strain and thereby define the population at risk to whom control measures should be applied.

VACCINATION

The development, safety, immunogenicity and efficacy of meningococcal vaccines have been described in detail in Chapter 10. Vaccines are currently available against four serogroups of meningococci: A, C, W-135 and Y. These vaccines are available as monovalent (A or C), bivalent (A + C) and quadrivalent (A + C + W-135 + Y) preparations. No effective serogroup B vaccine is presently available.

Vaccine efficacy and duration of protection

The efficacy of serogroup A and serogroup C polysaccharide vaccines in preventing meningococcal disease has been assessed in large-scale field trials among various populations, including army recruits in Finland[41] and the USA[42], young children in Finland[43], Egypt[44,45] and Burkina Faso[46]. The clinical efficacy of serogroup W-135 and serogroup Y vaccines has not been assessed (because the rate of disease due to these two serogroups is very low), but their immunogenicity has been established in adults and children aged over 2[47–49].

These studies have shown that the efficacy of a single dose of serogroup A and serogroup C vaccine is 90% or greater in adults and children over the age of 2. Serogroup C vaccines are not effective in children under the age of 2 and in this age group they appear to induce immunological tolerance, i.e. a reduced ability to respond to a second dose of vaccine some months later. Serogroup A vaccines are effective from 3 months of age provided a second dose is given 3 months later; further boosters at 18 months and 5 years may provide longer protection.

The duration of immunity from meningococcal vaccines is related to age. In children vaccinated at 4 years or older, the efficacy of serogroup A vaccine persists for at least 3 years[46], whereas in those vaccinated when younger than four years efficacy declines rapidly to approximately 50% after 2 years and less than 10% after 3 years[46]. The longterm effectiveness of serogroup C vaccines is not known. However, kinetic studies indicate that antibody levels decline more rapidly following serogroup C than serogroup A vaccine[50–52].

Use of vaccines for outbreak control

Despite these limitations, both serogroup A and serogroup C vaccines have been used successfully for outbreak control in military recruits[53], in the 'meningitis belt' of sub-Saharan Africa[46,54–59], in Nepal[60] and in New Zealand[61]. The most cost-effective strategy is one of selective vaccination, where only the age groups affected are included in the campaign. Family contacts of cases are at particular risk and should be given priority for vaccination during epidemics, particularly if resources and vaccine supplies are limited. A study in Nigeria showed that vaccination of these contacts can prevent secondary household cases[62].

After a few weeks family contacts may be at risk of disease despite adequate chemoprophylaxis[15]. This is the basis for the UK recommendation to vaccinate close contacts of sporadic and epidemic cases of serogroup A and serogroup C disease[63]. The protective antibody response to meningococcal vaccines takes 7–10 days to develop; therefore early secondary cases will not be prevented by this strategy and vaccination of close contacts should always be preceded by chemoprophylaxis.

Although vaccination protects individuals during an epidemic, there is evidence that it does not interrupt transmission. During epidemics in Rwanda[56] and The Gambia[64], carriage rates of serogroup A meningococci were not reduced by vaccination. In an outbreak in Nigeria, the incidence of meningococcal disease among non-vaccinated members of vaccinated villages was similar to that in control villages[54]. The implication for outbreak management is that the use of vaccine is only likely to reduce the incidence of disease in vaccinated individuals, strengthening the case for selective, rather than mass vaccination.

The point at which the incidence of serogroup A or serogroup C disease is sufficiently high to warrant vaccination beyond family contacts is not clear. When two or more cases occur within a well defined, closed or semi-closed population such as an army training camp or a residential school, the use of vaccine is justified on the basis that rapid spread may occur in the absence of vaccine, and that meningococcal vaccines are effective in school-age children and adults. The situation is more difficult to assess in community outbreaks. In sub-Saharan Africa, a threshold of 15 cases/100 000/week averaged over 2 weeks was 72–93% sensitive and 92–100% specific in detecting epidemics exceeding 100 cases/100 000/year[65]. In developed countries, this threshold is seldom reached. Attack rates during epidemics in developing countries are greatest in children aged 5 to 14 years, whereas in developed countries they tend to be greatest in children under 2 who do not respond optimally to vaccination. An epidemic of serogroup C disease occurred recently in Canada[66]; the maximum reported incidence rate did not exceed 10/100 000/year overall (22/100 000 in children under 2 years). Mass vaccination was nevertheless implemented in various age groups ranging from 6 months to 29 years[67]. The outbreak has since subsided but it is not clear to what extent vaccination played a part, since the incidence of disease was declining by the time the campaign began. The cost of the campaign in one of the metropolitan areas affected was estimated at US$ 4.2 million.

Prospects for new vaccines

Conjugate serogroup A and C vaccines have now been developed and are undergoing clinical trials[68]. If these provide long-lasting protection in young infants, they are likely to have a role in outbreak management as well as in routine infant immunisation programmes. Serogroup B vaccines are also under development. Studies in Brazil, Cuba and Norway have given efficacy estimates ranging from 57 to 83% against local serogroup B epidemic strains in older children and young adults[69–71], but little or no protection in young children.

RECOMMENDATIONS FOR OUTBREAK MANAGEMENT

The recommendations in this chapter are based on UK guidelines which have been produced by the Public Health Laboratory Service (PHLS) Meningococcal Infections Working Group[16,72]. They are generally consistent with guidelines that have been developed in Canada[73] and the USA[74]. The main principles are summarised in Table 11.2.

Management of single cases including uncertain diagnoses

The case

Patients with suspected meningococcal disease should be given parenteral penicillin before admission to hospital[75]. Cases should be nursed in respiratory isolation for 24 hours after the start of antibiotic treatment[74]. Thorough investigation and diagnosis of suspected cases is important not

Table 11.2 Summary of control measures for meningococcal disease

Action	Target group	Timescale
Notification to public health physician	Confirmed and suspected cases	Immediate
Emergency treatment (parenteral penicillin)	Confirmed and suspected cases	Immediate
Laboratory investigations	Confirmed and suspected cases	On admission to hospital (CSF and blood cultures) Other investigations within 24 hours
Chemoprophylaxis	Confirmed and suspected cases	Before discharge from hospital
	Household and mouth kissing contacts of cases	Within 24 hours (but beneficial up to 10 days)
	Nursery, crèche or playgroup contacts of cases	Within 24 hours (up to 10 days)
Clinical surveillance	Contacts of cases (as listed above)	For 24 hours after starting chemoprophylaxis
Vaccination	Contacts (as listed above) of cases due to vaccine-preventable strains (A, C, Y W-135)	When group of strain is known
Nasopharyngeal swabbing	Close contacts of younger sporadic cases	Before starting chemoprophylaxis
Information dissemination	Parents, teachers and the media	When there is public concern

only for their clinical management but also to determine epidemiological links between cases during outbreaks. Investigations should include clinical evaluation, CSF film and culture, blood culture, nasopharyngeal swab culture and paired sera for subsequent examination for meningococcal and viral antibodies[16]. Blood and CSF cultures should be taken as soon as possible, particularly if parenteral penicillin has been given before hospital admission. All meningococcal isolates should be sent to a reference laboratory for serogrouping, serotyping and determination of sulphonamide sensitivity.

Sending case isolates to a reference laboratory also provides an invaluable source of epidemiological data on the incidence of the disease and on the relative importance of different meningococcal strains. As new meningococcal strains are evolving constantly, these data are critical for vaccine development and control of secondary disease. In the UK, the national reference units are based in the Manchester Public Health Laboratory and at Ruchill Hospital in Glasgow.

Suspected cases of meningitis and septicaemia should be promptly notified to the relevant public health physician. In the UK, this is the consultant in Communicable Disease Control (CCDC). The trigger for notification is clinical suspicion; notification must not be delayed while results of laboratory investigations are awaited.

The contacts

Definition of a close contact. In sporadic cases of meningococcal disease, only those who have been in close contact with the patient in the 10 days before the onset of symptoms require public health intervention. Close contacts are defined as:

1. People sleeping in the same household as the case.
2. Anyone who has had mouth kissing contact with the case.
3. Anyone who has performed mouth to mouth resuscitation on the case.

If the case occurs in a pre-school nursery, crèche or playgroup, where the extent and nature of contact may resemble that within a household, then attenders of the group should also be considered close contacts[72]. Where the case occurs in a school, other children in the same school are not generally considered to be close contacts (unless they have shared sleeping quarters or had mouth kissing contact with the case).

These recommendations are general guidelines. Circumstances will vary from case to case. The CCDC should make a careful assessment and define the close contacts, based on the duration, frequency and intensity of exposure to the case.

Surveillance of contacts. Close contacts should be alerted to the increased risk of subsequent disease which is greatest within the first few days but which may persist for several months, especially if chemoprophylaxis is given. Contacts should be advised to seek urgent medical advice if fever or headache develops, even if chemoprophylaxis is given; they should be kept under active surveillance for 24 hours after chemoprophylaxis has started.

Chemoprophylaxis. Chemoprophylaxis should be given to close contacts. The recommended schedule is rifampicin 600 mg every 12 hours for 2 days in adults, 10 mg/kg/dose for children over one year of age, and 5 mg/kg/dose for children aged less than one year. Chemoprophylaxis is not normally recommended for children under 3 months of age. Pregnancy, severe liver disease and alcoholism are contraindications. Ideally, rifampicin should be administered simultaneously to all the close contacts and within 24 hours of the diagnosis being made in the index case. If administration of chemoprophylaxis is delayed, it may still be beneficial up to 10 days after the most recent exposure; some authorities recommend extending this period to 30 days for household contacts[73]. Contacts should be informed of the side effects of rifampicin and a fact sheet detailing these should be prepared for patients and GPs. Women taking the oral contraceptive pill should be given the advice published in the British National Formulary as for a 'missed pill'[76].

Ciprofloxacin as a single oral dose of 500 mg is a suitable alternative for adults, but cannot yet be recommended for children or for pregnant women. A single intramuscular dose of ceftriaxone 250 mg is suitable for chemoprophylaxis of pregnant contacts or where compliance with rifampicin may be poor. The dose for children under 12 years of age is 125 mg. It is contraindicated in patients with a history of hypersensitivity to cephalosporins and in children aged under 6 weeks.

Swabbing. Nasopharyngeal swabs should be taken from close contacts of younger sporadic cases, but only for diagnostic purposes. If, on repeat swabbing, a contact is still carrying the organism, repeated chemoprophylaxis is recommended.

Vaccination. Close contacts of sporadic cases caused by serogroup A or C strains should receive a single dose of the appropriate monovalent (A or C), bivalent (A + C) or quadrivalent (A + C + W-135 + Y) polysaccharide vaccine. Vaccination is not generally recommended for contacts of serogroup C disease who are aged less than 18 months. Serogroup A vaccine is recommended for contacts aged from 2 months; children aged between 2 and 18 months should receive two doses 3 months apart, whereas older children and adults only require a single dose.

As the principal aim of vaccinating close contacts is to prevent late, and not early, secondary cases, vaccination can be deferred until the serogroup of the organism from the case is identified. The decision on whether to vaccinate close contacts of cases where the serogroup is not known should be based on the local epidemiology of the disease. In England and Wales, the proportion of cases caused by vaccine-prevention strains is currently decreasing and was only 25% in 1993[77].

Management of clusters

Where two or more cases of meningococcal disease occur in a family, nursery, playgroup, crèche, school, military establishment or other setting where close contact may have taken place, the possibility of an outbreak should be considered. Responsibility for the public health aspects of managing the outbreak should be clearly laid out and the necessary resources made available.

Good communications must be maintained between hospital clinicians, the microbiologist and the public health physician to ensure that suspected cases are reported early and investigated promptly. During major incidents, an outbreak control team should be established which should meet frequently to review control measures and issue press statements. All communications with the press should be through a single, agreed channel. (In the current UK health service structure, a representative of a Trust hospital and a representative of the Health Authority should agree joint statements, making them together.) The advice of the appropriate reference laboratory or the national communicable disease epidemiology unit should be sought.

Household and kissing contacts should be given chemoprophylaxis, and vaccine if the infection is caused by a vaccine-preventable strain. The decision to extend chemoprophylaxis and/or vaccination beyond these immediate contacts should only be taken after a careful assessment of the risk of further cases. An extension of control measures is likely to cause public alarm and pressure for additional, unwarranted measures.

In certain situations, there is a clear indication for extending prophylaxis to a wider contact network. In closed populations such as military training establishments, the spread of meningococcal infection may be rapid and early action is indicated[78]. Chemoprophylaxis should be offered to the whole population, unless the cases are concentrated within one sector of the population that has minimal or no contact with other sectors, e.g. a single platoon. If the strain is of serogroup A or C, then vaccination of the contacts should also be undertaken. It is now the policy of the UK armed forces to vaccinate new military recruits. In the course of a vaccine-preventable outbreak in a military population, it would only be appropriate to offer vaccine to unvaccinated contacts or to those vaccinated more than 3 years previously.

Other closed populations where early widespread measures would be indicated include residential homes and boarding schools (during term-time).

The decision to extend control measures beyond immediate contacts is more difficult for outbreaks in semi-closed or open populations. A single case in a nursery, playgroup or crèche is justification for extending prophylaxis[72]. There are, however, two situations that are particularly difficult to assess.

Two or more cases of the same serogroup and serotype in a school

If the cases occur during the same term, it is possible they are linked through school contact. Chemoprophylaxis (and vaccine if the strain is vaccine-preventable) should be offered to the classroom contacts if both cases are in the same class. If the cases are in different classes, it may be worth swabbing a sample of school attenders (and possibly, a control group at an adjacent comparable school without cases) to identify subpopulations with increased carriage rates at whom prophylaxis could be directed. If a swabbing exercise is to be done, it must be carried out swiftly. The possibility that transmission is occurring predominantly through social networks outside the school, rather than in the school, must be considered. If this is the case, the prophylaxis of school contacts would be inappropriate. Both the local and reference laboratories should be consulted before undertaking any extensive swabbing. Where the cases are caused by a vaccine-preventable strain, the threshold for prophylaxis is lower, as serogroup C strains have a greater capacity for rapid spread than serogroup B strains. The occurrence of two cases of the same vaccine-preventable strain in the same term in a school, even in children attending different classes, might therefore justify more widespread vaccination.

If the cases occur in different terms, it is more likely that transmission has occurred outside the school, and extension of prophylaxis to school contacts is not indicated unless further cases occur in the school.

Cases occurring in school holidays are less likely to be linked through school contact, unless the date of onset is within 10 days of the end of term. Therefore it would not be appropriate to extend prophylaxis to school contacts in this situation. A single case (or two cases caused by different strains) in the same school does not warrant extension of prophylaxis beyond immediate household and kissing contacts.

Two or more cases of the same serogroup and serotype in a local neighbourhood

In developed countries widespread prophylaxis is rarely administered in community outbreaks, which are usually caused by serogroup B strains. Extensive antibiotic chemoprophylaxis in this situation has no proven value, is likely to induce a false sense of security, and would encourage the selection and emergence of resistant strains. Where the outbreak strain is of serogroup A or serogroup C, consideration should be given to the use of vaccine. In sub-Saharan Africa, widespread selective vaccination has been used with success for control of community outbreaks. In developed countries, however, the strategy is unproven and remains controversial. Vaccination appears to have been successful in halting an outbreak of serogroup A disease in Auckland[61]. However, most outbreaks in developing countries are caused by serogroup C strains, with the highest attack rates in young children among whom serogroup C vaccines are ineffective.

The threshold at which a small cluster of cases will develop into an epidemic cannot readily be predicted, although certain strains of serogroup C organisms (notably C2a[66]) are prone to cause epidemic disease. Mass vaccination poses logistic problems including vaccine supply, definition of a target population and poor compliance. Factors which should influence the decision to initiate vaccination include the attack rate, case fatality ratio, age distribution and risk of further spread. An outbreak affecting older children and adults is more likely to be controlled by vaccination than one affecting pre-school children. Carriage studies may be helpful in defining populations at greatest risk of subsequent disease. If widespread vaccination is implemented, priority should be given to the immediate contacts of cases.

The most important aspect of a community outbreak is information dissemination; this is considered below.

Information dissemination

During an outbreak, or whenever there is public concern, public health physicians should brief the local press officer, distribute information leaflets and be prepared to talk to the media, concerned parents groups or others. Public alarm may quickly develop into widespread panic, especially if fuelled by media sensationalism[62,79]. The death of one or more cases provokes a quite disproportionate level of alarm and may best be handled proactively. The media have a useful role to play when clusters of cases occur, or the incidence of the disease in the community is high. Local newspapers and radio can provide easily accessible information for the general public on symptoms and signs of early infection. In briefing the media, it is worth concentrating on the significance of a haemorrhagic rash, rather than on the symptoms of meningitis[79,80]; a haemorrhagic rash is a marker of more severe disease, and these are the patients most likely to benefit from early recognition and intervention with parenteral antibiotics[75]. Mortality and morbidity are very low in patients who do not have a haemorrhagic rash. There is some anecdotal evidence that such publicity achieves its objective of increasing parental awareness[81] (Brandtzaeg P, personal communication).

The occurrence of a single case in a nursery or school should prompt the distribution of information to parents. In the UK, the National Meningitis Trust has prepared a series of leaflets for parents and professionals which are suitable for distribution when a case or an outbreak of meningococcal disease occurs.

Ongoing education should also be provided to general practitioners and to casualty officers so they learn to recognise the symptoms of meningococcal disease quickly, give penicillin before admission and notify suspected cases. The advice should be stressed when outbreaks of influenza occur, as there is evidence that influenza A increases both the incidence and severity of meningococcal disease[82,83].

In conclusion, the management of outbreaks of meningococcal disease is complex and requires effective collaboration between health professionals, the media and parents. Control measures should be based on rational decision making, and not in response to public pressure.

REFERENCES

1. Centers for Disease Control. Case definitions for public health surveillance. MMWR 1990; *39* (RR-13): 23–4.
2. The Advisory Committee on Epidemiology and the Bureau of Communicable Disease Epidemiology. Canadian Communicable Disease Surveillance System. Disease-specific case definitions and surveillance methods. Ottawa: Laboratory Centre for Disease Control, 1991; 24.
3. Last JM ed. *A Dictionary of Epidemiology.* 2nd edition. Oxford: Oxford University Press, 1988.
4. Jones DM, Kaczarmarski EB. Meningococcal infections in England and Wales: 1991. Communicable Disease Report 1992; *2*: R61–5.
5. Cartwright K, Reilly S, White D, Stuart J. Early treatment with parenteral penicillin in meningococcal disease. Br Med J 1992; *305*: 143–7.
6. Ni H, Knight AI, Cartwright K, Palmer WH, McFadden J. Polymerase chain reaction for diagnosis of meningococcal meningitis. Lancet 1992; *340*: 1432–4.
7. Munford RS, Taunay AE, de Morais JS, Fraser DW, Feldman RA. Spread of meningococcal infection within households. Lancet 1974; *i*: 1275–8.
8. Cartwright KAV, Stuart JM, Robinson PM. Meningococcal carriage in close contacts of cases. Epidemiol Infect 1991; *106*: 133–41.
9. Cartwright KAV, Stuart JM, Noah ND. An outbreak of meningococcal disease in Gloucestershire. Lancet 1986; *ii*: 558–61.
10. Dawson JA, Wilkinson PJ, Rickard J. Meningococcal disease in the South-West

of England. Lancet 1986; *ii*: 806–7.

11. Jones DM, Eldridge J, Sutcliffe EM. Emergence of group B type 15 strains as a cause of meningococcal infection in England and Wales. In: *International Symposium: Meningococcal Disease in North West Europe*. Antonie van Leeuwenhoek 1986; *52*: 206–7.

12. Peltola H, Kataja JM, Mäkelä PH. Shift in the age distribution of meningococcal disease as predictor of an epidemic? Lancet 1982; *ii*: 595–7.

13. De Wals P, Hertoghe L, Borlée-Grimée I, De Maeyer-Cleempoel S, Reginster-Haneuse G, A *et al*. Meningococcal disease in Belgium. Secondary attack rate among household, day-care nursery and pre-elementary school contacts. J Infect 1981; *3* (Supl 1): S53–61.

14. Meningococcal Disease Surveillance Group. Meningococcal disease. Secondary attack rate and chemoprophylaxis in the United States, 1974. JAMA 1976; *235*: 261–5.

15. Stuart JM, Cartwright KAV, Robinson PM, Noah ND. Does eradication of meningococcal carriage in household contacts prevent secondary cases of meningococcal disease? Br Med J 1989; *298*: 569–70.

16. PHLS Meningococcal Infections Working Party. The epidemiology and control of meningococcal disease. Communicable Disease Report 1989; (8): 3–6. Internal publication of the Public Health Laboratory Service, London.

17. Cooke RPD, Riordan T, Jones DM, Painter MJ. Secondary cases of meningococcal infection among household contacts in England and Wales, 1984–7. Br Med J 1989; *298*: 555–8.

18. Kaiser AB, Hennekens CH, Saslaw MS, Hayes PS, Bennett JV. Seroepidemiology and chemoprophylaxis of disease due to sulfonamide-resistant *Neisseria meningitidis* in a civilian population. J Infect Dis 1974; *130*: 217–24.

19. Jacobson JA, Filice GA, Holloway JT. Meningococcal disease in day-care centres. Pediatrics 1977; *59*: 299–300.

20. Marks MI, Frasch CE, Shapera RM. Meningococcal colonization and infection in children and their household contacts. Am J Epidemiol 1979; *109*: 563–71.

21. Jacobson JA, Camargos PAM, Ferreira JT, McCormick JB. The risk of meningitis among classroom contacts during an epidemic of meningococcal disease. Am J Epidemiol 1976; *104*: 552–5.

22. Wall R, Wilson J, MacArdle B, Vellani Z. Meningococcal infection: evidence for school transmission. J Infect 1991; *23*: 155–9.

23. Hudson PJ, Voght RL, Heun EM, Brondum J, Coffin RR, Plikaytis BD *et al*. Evidence for school transmission of *Neisseria meningitidis* during a Vermont outbreak. Pediatr Infect Dis 1986; *5*: 213–17.

24. Feigin RD, Baker CJ, Herwaldt LA, Lampe RM, Mason EO, Whitney SE. Epidemic meningococcal disease in an elementary-school classroom. N Engl J Med 1982; *307*: 1255–7.

25. Morrow HW, Slaten DD, Riengold AL, Werner SB, Fenstersheib MD. Risk factors associated with a school-related outbreak of serogroup C meningococcal disease. Pediatr Infect Dis J 1990; *9*: 394–8.

26. Erikson NHR, Espersen F, Laursen L, Skinhoj P, Høiby N, Lind I. Nosocomial outbreak of group C meningococcal disease. Br Med J 1989; *298*: 568–9.

27. Shapiro ED. Prophylaxis for bacterial meningitis. Med Clin N Am 1985; *69*: 269–80.

28. Wilson HD. Prophylaxis in bacterial meningitis. Arch Dis Child 1981; 56:817–19.

29. Abramson JS, Spika JS. Persistence of *Neisseria meningitidis* in the upper respiratory tract after intravenous therapy for systemic meningococcal

disease. J Infect Dis 1985; *151*: 370–1.

30. Høiby EA, Moe PJ, Lystad A, Frøholm LO, Bøvre K. Phenoxymethyl-penicillin treatment of household contacts of meningococcal disease patients. Antonie van Leeuwenhoek 1986; *52*: 255–7.

31. Munford RS, de Vasconcelos ZJS, Phillips CJ, Gelli DS, Gorman GW, Risi JB *et al*. Eradication of *Neisseria meningitidis* in families: a study in Brazil. J Infect Dis 1974; *129*: 644–9.

32. Steen JSM, Stainton-Ellis DM. Rifampicin in pregnancy. Lancet 1977; *ii*: 1239–42.

33. Schübiger G, Munzinger J, Dudli C, Wipfli U. Meningokokken-epidemic in einer Internatsschule. Secundarerkrankung mit rifampicin-resistantem Erreger unter Chemoprophylaxe. Schweiz Med Wschr 1986; *116*: 1172–5.

34. Blakeborough IS, Gilles HM. The effect of rifampicin on meningococcal carriage in family contacts in Northern Nigeria. J Infect 1980; *2*: 137–43.

35. Schwartz B, Al-Tobaiqi A, Al-Ruwais A, Fontaine RE, A'Ashi J, Hightower AW *et al*. Comparative efficacy of ceftriaxone and rifampicin in eradicating pharyngeal carriage of group A *Neisseria meningitidis*. Lancet 1988; *i*: 1239–42.

36. Gaunt PN, Lambert BE. Single dose ciprofloxacin for the eradication of pharyngeal carriage of *Neisseria meningitidis*. J Antimicrob Chemother 1988; *21*: 489–96.

37. Pugsley MP, Dworzack DL, Horowitz EA, Cuevas TA, Sanders WE, Sanders CC. Efficacy of ciprofloxacin in the treatment of nasopharyngeal carriers of *Neisseria meningitidis*. J Infect Dis 1987; *156*: 211–13.

38. Renkonen OV, Sivonen A, Visakorpi R. Effect of ciprofloxacin on carrier rate of *Neisseria meningitidis* in army recruits in Finland. Antimicrob Agents Chemother 1987; *31*: 962–3.

39. Dworzack L, Sanders CC, Horowitz EA, Allais JM, Sookpranee M *et al*. Evaluation of single-dose ciprofloxacin in the eradication of *Neisseria meningitidis* from nasopharyngeal carriers. Antimicrob Agents Chemother 1988; *32*: 1740–1.

40. Cuevas LE, Hart CA. Chemoprophylaxis of bacterial meningitis. J Antimicrob Chemother 1993; *31* (suppl B): 79–91.

41. Mäkelä PH, Käyhty H, Weckstrom P, Sivonen A, Renkonen O-V. Effect of group A meningococcal vaccine in army recruits in Finland. Lancet 1975; *ii*: 883–6.

42. Artenstein MS, Gold R, Zimmerly JG, Wyle FA, Schnieder H, Harkins C. Prevention of meningococcal disease by group C polysaccharide vaccine. N Eng J Med 1970; *282*: 417–20.

43. Peltola H, Mäkelä PH, Käyhty H, Jousimies H, Herva E, Hallstrom K *et al*. Clinical efficacy of meningococcus group A capsular polysaccharide vaccine in children three months to five years of age. N Engl J Med 1977; *ii*: 686–91.

44. Wahdan MH, Rizk F, El-Akkad AM, El Ghoroury A, Hablas R, Girgis NI *et al*. A controlled field trial of a serogroup A meningococcal polysaccharide vaccine. Bull WHO 1973; *48*: 667–73.

45. Wahdan MH, Sallam SA, Hassan MN, Gawad AA, Rakha AS, Sippel JE *et al*. A second controlled field trial of a serogroup A meningococcal polysaccharide vaccine in Alexandria. Bull WHO 1977; *55*: 645–51.

46. Reingold AL, Broome CV, Hightower AW, Ajello GW, Bolan GA, Adamson C. Age-specific differences in duration of clinical protection after vaccination with meningococcal polysaccharide A vaccine. Lancet 1985; *ii*: 114–18.

47. Griffiss JM, Brandt BL, Altieri PL, Pier GB, Berman SL. Safety and immunogenicity of group Y and group W-135 meningococcal polysaccharide vaccine in adults. Infect Immun 1981; *34*: 725–32.

48. Armand J, Arminjon F, Mynard MC, Lafaix C. Tetravalent meningococcal

polysaccharide vaccine groups A, C, Y, W-135: clinical and serological evaluation. J Biol Stand 1982; *10*: 335–9.

49. Ambrosch F, Wiedermann G, Crooy P, George AM. Immunogenicity and side-effects of a new tetravalent meningococcal polysaccharide vaccine. Bull WHO 1983; *61*: 317–23.

50. Gold R, Lepow ML, Goldschneider I, Draper TF, Gotschlich EC. Kinetics of antibody production to group A and group C meningococcal polysaccharide vaccines administered during the first six years of life: prospects for routine immunization of infants and children. J Infect Dis 1979; *140*: 690–7.

51. Lepow ML, Goldschneider I, Gold R, Randolph M, Gotschlich EC. Persistence of antibody following immunization of children with groups A and C meningococcal polysaccharide vaccines. Pediatrics 1977; *60*: 673–80.

52. Käyhty H, Karanko V, Peltola H, Sarna S, Mäkelä PH. Serum antibodies to capsular polysaccharide vaccine of group A *Neisseria meningitidis* followed for three years in infants and children. J Infect Dis 1980; *142*: 861–8.

53. Stroffolini T. Vaccination campaign against meningococcal disease in army recruits in Italy. Epidemiol Infect 1990; *105*: 579–83.

54. Greenwood BM, Wali SS. Control of meningococcal disease in the African meningitis belt by selective vaccination. Lancet 1980; *i*: 729–32.

55. World Health Organization. Control of a cerebrospinal meningitis epidemic. Weekly Epidemiol Rec 1998; *68*: 237–8.

56. Bosmans E, Vimont-Vicary P, Andre FE, Crooy PJ, Roelnts P, Vandepitte J. Protective efficacy of a bivalent (A + C) meningococcal vaccine during a cerebrospinal epidemic in Rwanda. Ann Soc Belge Med Trop 1980; *60*: 297–306.

57. Mohommed I, Zaruba K. Control of epidemic meningococcal meningitis by mass vaccination. Lancet 1981; *ii*: 80–3.

58. Binkin N, Band J. Epidemic of meningococcal meningitis in Bamako, Mali: epidemiological features and analysis of vaccine efficacy. Lancet 1982; *ii*: 315–18.

59. Erwa HH, Haseeb MA, Idris AA, Lapeyssonnie L, Sanborn WR, Sippel JE. A serogroup A meningococcal polysaccharide vaccine. Studies in the Sudan to combat cerebrospinal meningitis caused by *Neisseria meningitidis* group A. Bull WHO 1973; *49*: 301–5.

60. Cochi SL, Markowitz LE, Joshi DD, Owens R, Stenhouse DH, Regmi DN *et al.* Control of epidemic group A meningococcal meningitis in Nepal. Int J Epidemiol 1987; *16*: 91–7.

61. Lennon D, Gellin B, Hood D, Voss L, Heffernan H, Thakur S. Successful intervention in a group A meningococcal outbreak in Auckland, New Zealand. Pediatr Infect Dis J 1992; *11*: 617–23.

29. Greenwood BM, Hassan-King M, Whittle HC. Prevention of secondary cases of meningococcal disease in household contacts by vaccination. Br Med J 1978; *i*: 1317–19.

63. UK Health Departments. *Immunisation against Infectious Disease.* 1992 edition. London, HMSO: 1992.

64. Hassan-King MKA, Wall RA, Greenwood BM. Meningococcal carriage, meningococcal disease and vaccination. J Infect 1988; *16*: 55–9.

65. Moore PS, Plikaytis BD, Bolan GA, Oxtoby MJ, Yada A, Zoubga A *et al.* Detection of meningitis epidemics in Africa: a population-based analysis. Int J Epidemiol 1992; *21*: 155–62.

66. Ashton FE, Ryan JA, Borczyk A, Caugant DA, Mancino L, Huang D. Emergence of a virulent clone of *Neisseria meningitidis* serotype 2a that is associated with meningococcal group C disease in Canada. J Clin Microbiol

1991; *29*: 2489–93.
67. Hume SE. Mass voluntary immunization campaigns for meningococcal disease in Canada: media hysteria. JAMA 1992; *267*: 1833–8.
68. Costantino P, Viti S, Podda A, Velmonte MA, Nencioni L, Rappuoli R. Development and phase 1 clinical testing of a conjugate vaccine against meningococcus A and C. Vaccine 1992; *10*: 691–8.
69. Bjune G, Høiby EA, Grønnesby JK, Arnesen Ø, Fredriksen JH, Halstensen A *et al.* Effect of outer membrane vesicle vaccine against group B meningococcal disease in Norway. Lancet 1991; *338*: 1093–6.
70. Sierra GVG, Campa HC, Varcacel NBP, Garcia IL, Izquierdo PL, Sotolongo PF *et al.* Vaccine against group B *Neisseria meningitidis*: protection trial and mass vaccination results in Cuba. NIPH Ann 1991; *14*: 195–204.
71. Costa W, Saachi CT, Ramos S, Milagnes L, Prigenzi LS. Meningococcal disease in São Paulo, Brazil. NIPH Ann 1991; *14*: 215–16.
72. PHLS Meningococcal Infections Working Group. Sporadic cases of meningococcal disease in schools. Comm Dis Rep Weekly 1992; *2*: 209.
73. Advisory Committee on Epidemiology. Guidelines for control of meningococcal disease. Can Dis Weekly Rep 1991; *17*: 245–9.
74. Benenson AS ed. *Control of Communicable Diseases in Man.* 15th edition. Washington, American Public Health Association: 1990.
75. Cartwright K, Reilly S, White D, Stuart J, Begg N, Constantine C. Management of early meningococcal disease. Lancet 1993; *342*: 985–6.
76. British Medical Association and the Royal Pharmaceutical Society of Great Britain. Contraceptives. In: *British National Formulary, No. 26.* London: the Pharmaceutical Press, 1993; 292–9.
77. Jones DM, Kaczmarski EB. Meningococcal infections in England and Wales: 1993. Comm Dis Rep Rev; 1994; *4*: R97–100.
78. Evans CW, Lambert BE, Gaunt PN. A description of the outbreak of meningitis in HMS Raleigh in February 1987. J Roy Nav Med Serv 1988; *74*: 187–94.
79. Thomson APJ, Hayhurst GK. Press publicity in meningococcal disease. Arch Dis Child 1993; *69*: 166–9.
80. Peltola H. Early meningococcal disease: advising the public and the profession. Lancet 1993; *342*: 509–10.
81. Riordan FAI, Thompson APJ. Early presentation of meningococcal disease after media publicity. Arch Dis Child 1993; *69*: 711.
82. Cartwright KAV, Jones DM, Smith AJ, Stuart JM, Kaczmarski EB, Palmer SR. Influenza A and meningococcal disease. Lancet 1991; *338*: 554–7.
83. Hubert B, Watier L, Garnerin P, Richardson S. Meningococcal disease and influenza-like syndrome: a new approach to an old question. J Infect Dis 1992; *166*: 542–5.

Index

Index compiled by Campbell Purton